*TO OUR SPOUSES AND CHILDREN*

*Rob, Ryan and Tyler Smith,*
*Jan, Megan, Bridget, Erin, Courtney,*
*Chelsea and Dana Fish*

*who are always there for us.*

# INTRODUCTION

*Pure Practice for ECGs* has been designed to provide extensive practice in interpreting a variety of ECG rhythm strips, including cardiac dysrhythmias, conduction defects, and pacemaker rhythms. The authors, Louise Fish Smith, MS, RN and Frank H. Fish, MD, have selected actual patient rhythm strips for interpretation followed by a detailed analysis.

## THE FOUR PART WORKBOOK INCLUDES:

### Part I: Basic Dysrhythmias

Commonly encountered ECG rhythm strips including simple cardiac dysrhythmias and conduction defects

**Prerequisite:** A sound knowledge of the basic principles of electrophysiology and electrocardiography and a beginning level course in cardiac dysrhythmias

### Part II: Complex Dysrhythmias

Less commonly encountered ECG rhythm strips including complex cardiac dysrhythmias and conduction defects

**Prerequisite:** Mastery in basic dysrhythmia interpretation is recommended before attempting this section

### Part III: Pacemaker Rhythm Strips

ECG rhythm strips from patients with mechanical pacemakers, including normally functioning pacemakers and pacemaker malfunction

**Prerequisite:** In addition to advanced cardiac rhythm interpretive skills, a thorough understanding of the basic types and modes of operation of commonly used pacemakers is essential for interpreting the rhythm strips in this section. The *Pacemaker ECG Rhythm Strip Analysis Guide* in Part III provides content to assist you in acquiring the appropriate knowledge.

### Part IV: Continuing Education

Seven comprehensive dysrhythmia strips are offered for analysis. Questions related to the rhythm analysis and interpretation are in a multiple choice format. Instructions for completing and meeting contact hour approval requirements precede this section.

**Prerequisite:** Completion of Parts I, II, and III

## OBJECTIVES

### After completing this workbook, you will be able to:

1. Use a systematic format for cardiac and pacemaker rhythm strip analysis

2. Identify simple and complex cardiac rhythm disturbances faster and more accurately
3. Delineate the type of pacemaker and mode of operation on an ECG rhythm strip
4. Assess pacemaker function and recognize any abnormalities present

## PRODUCT ADAPTABILITY

**Individuals:** The *Pure Practice for ECGs* workbook is for all health care professionals, including physicians, nurses, and ECG technicians, who are required to interpret ECG rhythms.

**Instructors:** The *Pure Practice for ECGs Instructor's Kit,* consists of the workbook and **294** rhythm strip slides. The slides are identical to the rhythm strips contained in the workbook and provide the visual support to complete the learning experience.

## WORKBOOK FORMAT AND USE

Each rhythm strip is presented in a worksheet format. The worksheet provides a systematic approach to rhythm strip analysis to enhance and simplify learning and facilitate a comprehensive and accurate interpretation. After completing the worksheet, compare your analysis to the data analysis located on the backside of the corresponding worksheet. All rhythm strips have been reviewed by a cardiologist to provide accurate feedback and reinforcement of the interpretation. For a complete and successful analysis, carefully follow each of the steps listed below:

1. **Rhythm**
   Determine the regularity of the atrial and ventricular rhythms

2. **Rate**
   Calculate the atrial and ventricular rates

3. **P Wave**
   Examine the P wave for presence, appearance, consistency, and relation to QRS complex

   **Remember:**
   - Identification of "atrial abnormalities" from rhythm strips is difficult as monitor leads often distort P wave morphology. A 12 lead ECG is usually necessary to accurately diagnose left or right atrial abnormalities.

# PURE PRACTICE FOR ECGs

## A Practice Workbook

**Louise Fish Smith,** MS, RN, CCRN

Professor of Nursing
New Hampshire Technical Institute
Concord, New Hampshire

**Frank Henry Fish,** MD, FACC

Chief of Cardiology
Memorial Hospital of Burlington County
Mt. Holly, New Jersey

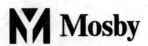

St. Louis  Baltimore  Boston  Carlsbad  Chicago  Naples  New York  Philadelphia  Portland
London  Madrid  Mexico City  Singapore  Sydney  Tokyo  Toronto  Wiesbaden

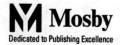
**Mosby**
Dedicated to Publishing Excellence

**A Times Mirror**
**Company**

Jay Katz, Senior Vice-President, Division of Continuing Education and Training

Jacqueline Katz, Vice-President, Division of Continuing Education and Training

Barbara Watts, Executive Secretary

Project Manager: Peg Fagen

Production Editor: Donna Walls

Manufacturing Supervisor: Pat Stinecipher

Cover Art: GW Graphics, Inc.

Printed in the United States of America
Composition by Nucomp, Inc.
Printing/binding by Plus Communications

Mosby-Year Book, Inc.
11830 Westline Industrial Drive
St. Louis, Missouri 63146

ISBN 0-8151-7923-5

95 96 97 98 99 / 9 8 7 6 5 4 3 2

## 4. P-R Interval
Calculate the P-R interval

## 5. QRS Complex
Examine QRS complex for presence, appearance, consistency, and duration

## 6. Data Analysis

### Remember:

- Monitor leads may distort QRS morphology. The presence of a "notched" QRS alone does not mean an intraventricular conduction problem exists. A 12 lead ECG may be necessary to accurately diagnose specific bundle branch disorders.

**Note** : Empirically, if the QRS complex measures 0.12 seconds or more, it is classified intraventricular conduction "delay." If the QRS complex measures 0.11 seconds or 0.10 seconds with an "abnormal" QRS configuration it is classified intraventricular conduction "defect."

## Data Analysis

### Analyze the data collected:

a. Determine which values are normal or abnormal
b. Summarize these findings

## 7. Interpretation
Interpret the rhythm strip - Your interpretation explains the data analysis and classifies the rhythm and any abnormalities present.

*After completing the worksheet, compare your findings with the appropriate corresponding analysis.*

**A special note regarding Part III:** For Pacemaker Rhythm Strips, steps 1 through 5 of the pacemaker analysis worksheet follows the same format used in Parts I and II, but applies only to the intrinsic (non-mechanical pacemaker–induced) rhythm. Steps 6 through 12 are specifically designed for analyzing mechanical pacemaker activity. The introduction to Part III discusses the interpretation process in detail.

# ECG ANALYSIS GUIDE

## 1. Determine the regularity of the atrial and ventricular rhythms.

**Atrial:** Locate the P waves and measure the interval between consecutive P waves (P-P interval). When the P-P interval remains constant, the atrial rhythm is regular.

**Ventricular:** Locate the R waves and measure the interval between consecutive R waves (R-R interval). When the R-R interval remains constant, the ventricular rhythm is regular.

### Remember:

- Normal sinus rhythm is typically **not** a perfectly regular rhythm, but is "essentially regular," meaning that the rhythm may vary slightly.
- If the rhythm is not regular, see if there is some pattern to the irregularity or whether the rhythm is irregularly irregular.

## 2. Calculate the atrial and ventricular rates.

**Atrial:** One commonly used method to calculate the atrial rate is counting the number of P waves in a six second interval and then multiplying this number by ten.

**Ventricular:** Count the number of QRS complexes in a six second strip and multiply this number by ten.

### Remember:

- You can use these and other rapid methods of estimating rates (e.g., ECG rulers) most reliably only when the atrial and ventricular rhythms are regular.

## 3. Examine the P waves.

**Presence:** Whether P waves are easily identified.

**Appearance:** Whether configuration is normal.

**Consistency:** Whether appearance varies or remains constant.

**Relation to QRS:** The number of P waves that precede each QRS and where they are located relative to the QRS complex.

## 4. Calculate the duration of the P-R interval.

**Duration:** Measure from the beginning of the P wave to the beginning of the QRS complex.

**Consistency:** Measure a number of P-R intervals to determine whether they remain the same or vary.

## 5. Examine the QRS complex.

**Presence:** Whether QRS complexes are easily identified.

**Appearance:** Whether the configuration is normal.

**Consistency:** Whether appearance varies or remains constant.

**Duration:** Measure from the beginning of the Q wave (or R wave if there is no Q wave) to the end of the S wave.

# TABLE OF NORMAL ECG VALUES

**Rhythm:**

    **Atrial** - essentially regular (constant P-P intervals)

    **Ventricular** - essentially regular (constant R-R intervals)

**Rates:**

    **Atrial** - 60 to 100 per minute

    **Ventricular** - 60 to 100 per minute

**P Waves:**

    Readily identifiable

    Smooth, rounded contour with same appearance for all P waves

    1:1 relation to QRS complexes

**P-R interval:**

    0.12 to 0.20 seconds

    Remains constant

**QRS complex:**

    Readily identifiable

    Configurations may vary with lead monitored; Q wave may not be observable

    Appearance remains constant

    0.05 to 0.10 seconds duration

# CONTENTS

# • Part I •

## Basic Dysrhythmias

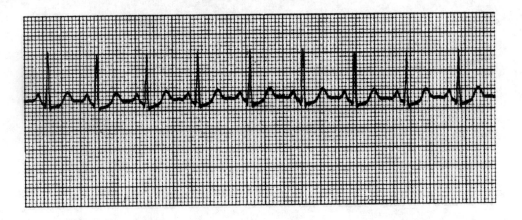

Figure 1-1A

# ECG RHYTHM STRIP #1

## 1. RHYTHM

Atrial:

Ventricular:

## 2. RATE

Atrial:

Ventricular:

## 3. P WAVE

Presence:

Appearance:

Consistency:

Relation to QRS:

## 4. P-R INTERVAL

Duration:

Consistency:

## 5. QRS COMPLEX

Presence:

Appearance:

Consistency:

Duration:

## 6. DATA ANALYSIS

## 7. INTERPRETATION

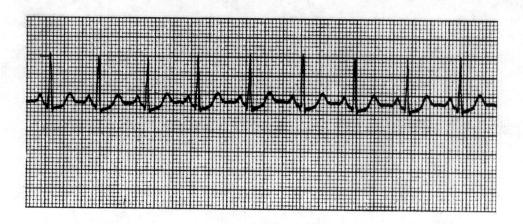

Figure 1-1B

## ECG RHYTHM STRIP #1

### 1. RHYTHM

Atrial: Regular

Ventricular: Regular

### 2. RATE

Atrial: 107

Ventricular: 107

### 3. P WAVE

Presence: Yes

Appearance: Normal

Consistency: Consistent

Relation to QRS: 1:1

### 4. P-R INTERVAL

Duration: 0.14 seconds

Consistency: Consistent

### 5. QRS COMPLEX

Presence: Yes

Appearance: Normal

Consistency: Consistent

Duration: 0.07 seconds

### 6. DATA ANALYSIS

All values are normal, except that the rates are 107 per minute in both the atria and ventricles.

### 7. INTERPRETATION

Sinus tachycardia

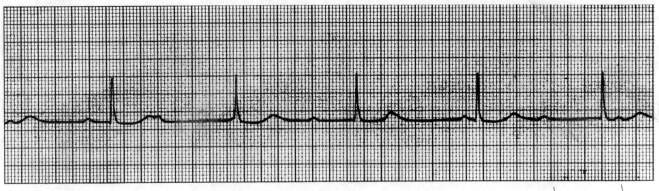

Figure 1-2A

# ECG RHYTHM STRIP #2

## 1. RHYTHM

Atrial:

Ventricular:

## 2. RATE

Atrial:

Ventricular:

## 3. P WAVE

Presence:

Appearance:

Consistency:

Relation to QRS:

## 4. P-R INTERVAL

Duration:

Consistency:

## 5. QRS COMPLEX

Presence:

Appearance:

Consistency:

Duration:

## 6. DATA ANALYSIS

## 7. INTERPRETATION

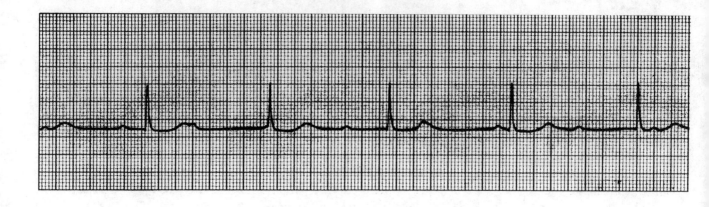

Figure 1-2B

# ECG RHYTHM STRIP #2

## I. RHYTHM

Atrial: Regular

Ventricular: Regular

## 2. RATE

Atrial: 70

Ventricular: 40

## 3. P WAVE

Presence: Yes

Appearance: Normal

Consistency: Consistent

Relation to QRS: Variable

## 4. P-R INTERVAL

Duration: Variable

Consistency: Inconsistent

## 5. QRS COMPLEX

Presence: Yes

Appearance: Normal

Consistency: Consistent

Duration: 0.08 seconds

## 6. DATA ANALYSIS

Regular P-P and R-R intervals with variable P-R intervals indicate that the atria and ventricles are functioning independently of each other —i.e., that AV dissociation exists. A sinus rhythm is driving the atria. The "narrow QRS" (a QRS of normal duration) indicates that the ventricles are controlled by a supraventricular pacemaking site.

## 7. INTERPRETATION

Sinus rhythm with 3rd degree (complete) AV block and a junctional escape rhythm

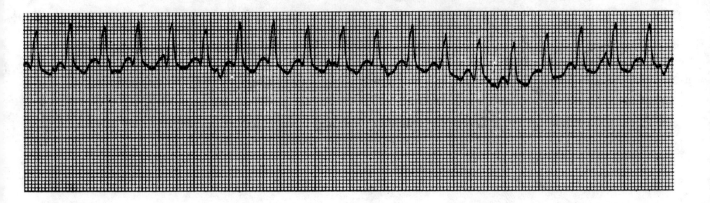

Figure 1-3A

# ECG RHYTHM STRIP #3

## I. RHYTHM

Atrial:

Ventricular:

## 2. RATE

Atrial:

Ventricular:

## 3. P WAVE

Presence:

Appearance:

Consistency:

Relation to QRS:

## 4. P-R INTERVAL

Duration:

Consistency:

## 5. QRS COMPLEX

Presence:

Appearance:

Consistency:

Duration:

## 6. DATA ANALYSIS

## 7. INTERPRETATION

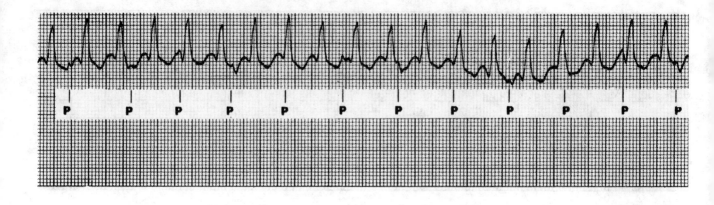

Figure 1-3B

# ECG RHYTHM STRIP #3

## I. RHYTHM

Atrial: Regular

Ventricular: Regular

## 2. RATE

Atrial: 95

Ventricular: 155

## 3. P WAVE

Presence: Yes, some hidden in QRS complexes

Appearance: Normal when observable

Consistency: Consistent, some distortion due to locations in QRS and ST segments

Relation to QRS: Variable

## 4. P-R INTERVAL

Duration: Variable

Consistency: Inconsistent

## 5. QRS COMPLEX

Presence: Yes

Appearance: Abnormal (widened, bizarre)

Consistency: Consistent

Duration: 0.14 seconds

## 6. DATA ANALYSIS

P waves are difficult to identify because of their varying location before, within, and following the QRS complexes. Where P waves are not seen (e.g, 8th and 9th complexes), their presence is accountable within the QRS complex. The variable P-R intervals with constant P-P and R-R intervals suggest independence of the atrial and ventricular rhythms (AV dissociation). The ventricular rhythm is rapid with wide, bizarre QRS complexes.

## 7. INTERPRETATION

Ventricular tachycardia

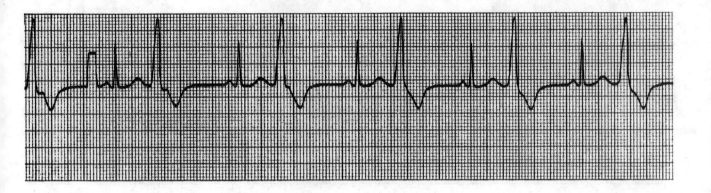

Figure 1-4A

# ECG RHYTHM STRIP #4

## 1. RHYTHM

Atrial:

Ventricular:

## 2. RATE

Atrial:

Ventricular:

## 3. P WAVE

Presence:

Appearance:

Consistency:

Relation to QRS:

## 4. P-R INTERVAL

Duration:

Consistency:

## 5. QRS COMPLEX

Presence:

Appearance:

Consistency:

Duration:

## 6. DATA ANALYSIS

## 7. INTERPRETATION

9

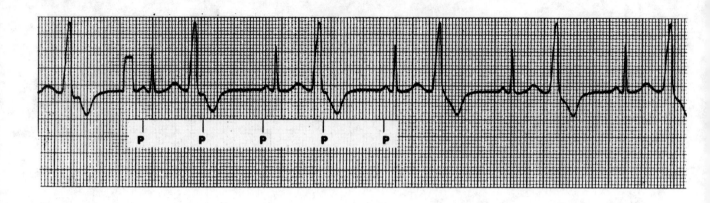

Figure 1-4B

# ECG RHYTHM STRIP #4

## 1. RHYTHM

Atrial: Regular

Ventricular: Regularly irregular

## 2. RATE

Atrial: 80

Ventricular: 80

## 3. P WAVE

Presence: Yes

Appearance: Normal

Consistency: Consistent

Relation to QRS: P waves preceding QRS complex alternate with P waves that immediately follow QRS complex

## 4. P-R INTERVAL

Duration: 0.16 seconds on P waves preceding QRS

Consistency: Consistent in conducted beats where P precedes QRS

## 5. QRS COMPLEX

Presence: Yes

Appearance: Normal alternate with abnormal (wide, bizarre) complexes

Consistency: No, though alternating pattern remains consistent

Duration: 0.06 seconds with normal complexes; 0.15 seconds with abnormal complexes

## 6. DATA ANALYSIS

The atrial rate, rhythm, and P waves are normal, indicating a sinus rhythm in the atria. Every other QRS complex is wide, abnormal, and unrelated to the P wave that follows it. The ventricular rhythm is irregular due to premature QRS complexes. There is a regularity (bigeminy) in the ventricular rhythm.

## 7. INTERPRETATION

Sinus rhythm with ventricular bigeminy

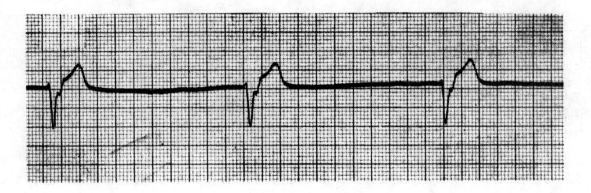

Figure 1-5A

# ECG RHYTHM STRIP #5

## I. RHYTHM

Atrial:

Ventricular:

## 2. RATE

Atrial:

Ventricular:

## 3. P WAVE

Presence:

Appearance:

Consistency:

Relation to QRS:

## 4. P-R INTERVAL

Duration:

Consistency:

## 5. QRS COMPLEX

Presence:

Appearance:

Consistency:

Duration:

## 6. DATA ANALYSIS

## 7. INTERPRETATION

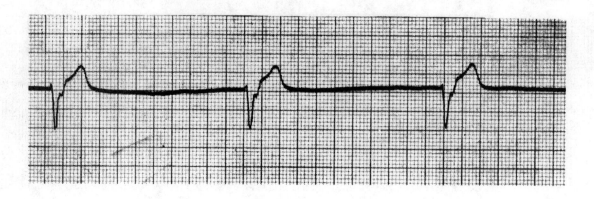

Figure 1-5B

# ECG RHYTHM STRIP #5

## I. RHYTHM

Atrial: Unable to determine

Ventricular: Regular

## 2. RATE

Atrial: —

Ventricular: 27

## 3. P WAVE

Presence: No

Appearance: —

Consistency: —

Relation to QRS: —

## 4. P-R INTERVAL

Duration: —

Consistency: —

## 5. QRS COMPLEX

Presence: Yes

Appearance: Abnormal

Consistency: Yes

Duration: 0.16 seconds

## 6. DATA ANALYSIS

There is no identifiable atrial activity. QRS complexes are wide and bizarre in appearance. The ventricular rate is slow and the rhythm is regular.

## 7. INTERPRETATION

Idioventricular rhythm

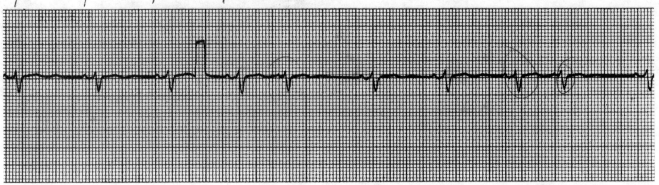

Figure 1-6A

# ECG RHYTHM STRIP #6

**1. RHYTHM**

    Atrial:

    Ventricular:

**2. RATE**

    Atrial:

    Ventricular:

**3. P WAVE**

    Presence:

    Appearance:

    Consistency:

    Relation to QRS:

**4. P-R INTERVAL**

    Duration:

    Consistency:

**5. QRS COMPLEX**

    Presence:

    Appearance:

    Consistency:

    Duration:

**6. DATA ANALYSIS**

**7. INTERPRETATION**

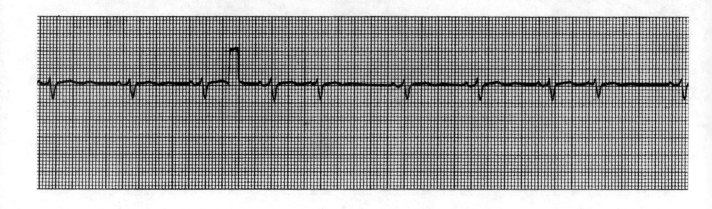

Figure 1-6B

# ECG RHYTHM STRIP #6

## I. RHYTHM

Atrial: Irregular

Ventricular: Irregular

## 2. RATE

Atrial: 70

Ventricular: 70 (ECG standard marking between beats 3 and 4

## 3. P WAVE

Presence: Yes

Appearance: Normal

Consistency: Consistent except for 5th and 9th beats

Relation to QRS: 1:1

## 4. P-R INTERVAL

Duration: 0.12 seconds

Consistency: Consistent except in 5th and 9th cycles where it shortens

## 5. QRS COMPLEX

Presence: Yes

Appearance: Normal

Consistency: Consistent

Duration: 0.09 seconds

## 6. DATA ANALYSIS

The underlying rhythm varies in a cyclic pattern in both atria and ventricles. There are two premature beats that have slightly different configurations compared to the patient's sinus P waves; the QRS complexes in premature beats are identical to those in the sinus beats. P-R intervals in the two premature beats are shorter than those in sinus beats; QRS duration is the same in both cases.

## 7. INTERPRETATION

Sinus arrhythmia with 2 PACs (5th, 9th beats)

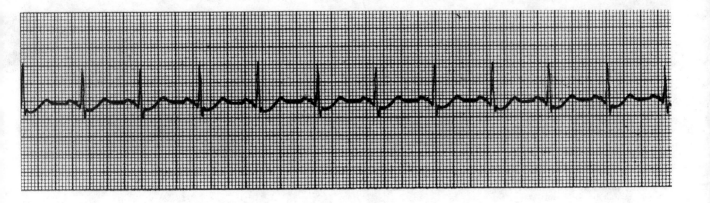

Figure 1-7A

# ECG RHYTHM STRIP #7

## 1. RHYTHM

Atrial:

Ventricular:

## 2. RATE

Atrial:

Ventricular:

## 3. P WAVE

Presence:

Appearance:

Consistency:

Relation to QRS:

## 4. P-R INTERVAL

Duration:

Consistency:

## 5. QRS COMPLEX

Presence:

Appearance:

Consistency:

Duration:

## 6. DATA ANALYSIS

## 7. INTERPRETATION

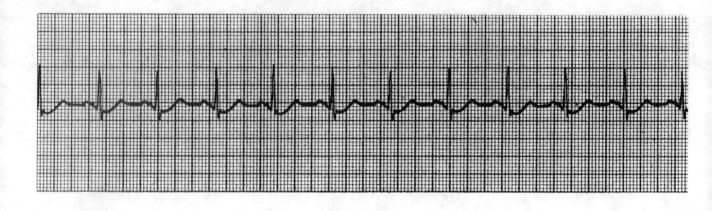

Figure 1-7B

## ECG RHYTHM STRIP #7

**I. RHYTHM**

Atrial: Regular

Ventricular: Regular

**2. RATE**

Atrial: 90

Ventricular: 90

**3. P WAVE**

Presence: Yes

Appearance: Normal

Consistency: Consistent

Relation to QRS: 1:1

**4. P-R INTERVAL**

Duration: 0.16 seconds

Consistency: Consistent

**5. QRS COMPLEX**

Presence: Yes

Appearance: Normal

Consistency: Consistent

Duration: 0.08 seconds

**6. DATA ANALYSIS**

All values are within normal limits

**7. INTERPRETATION**

(Normal) Sinus rhythm

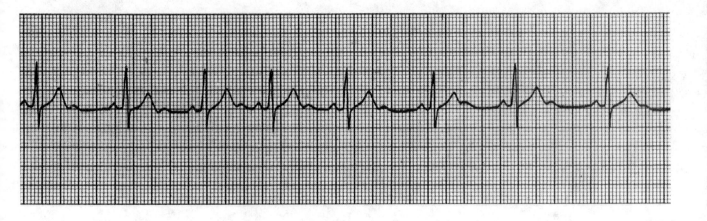

Figure 1-8A

# ECG RHYTHM STRIP #8

## 1. RHYTHM

Atrial:

Ventricular:

## 2. RATE

Atrial:

Ventricular:

## 3. P WAVE

Presence:

Appearance:

Consistency:

Relation to QRS:

## 4. P-R INTERVAL

Duration:

Consistency:

## 5. QRS COMPLEX

Presence:

Appearance:

Consistency:

Duration:

## 6. DATA ANALYSIS

## 7. INTERPRETATION

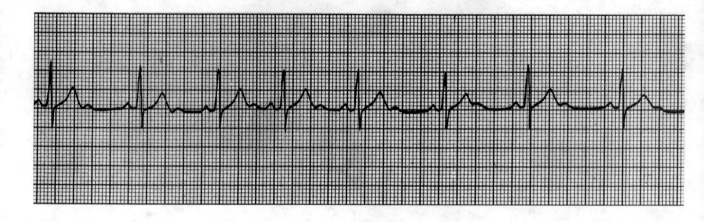

Figure 1-8B

## ECG RHYTHM STRIP #8

### 1. RHYTHM

Atrial: Irregular

Ventricular: Irregular; pattern of slow-fast-slow
for both

### 2. RATE

Atrial: 70

Ventricular: 70

### 3. P WAVE

Presence: Yes

Appearance: Normal

Consistency: Consistent

Relation to QRS: 1:1

### 4. P-R INTERVAL

Duration: 0.16 seconds

Consistency: Consistent

### 5. QRS COMPLEX

Presence: Yes

Appearance: Normal

Consistency: Consistent

Duration: 0.08 seconds

### 6. DATA ANALYSIS

All values are normal, except for the cyclical pattern of slow-fast-slow rhythm. P waves are normal and similar in appearance, suggesting that the variation in rhythm is due to the respiratory cycle's effect on the sinus node.

### 7. INTERPRETATION

Sinus arrhythmia

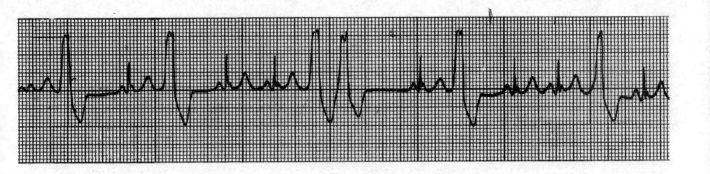

Figure 1-9A

## ECG RHYTHM STRIP #9

**1. RHYTHM**

    Atrial:

    Ventricular:

**2. RATE**

    Atrial:

    Ventricular:

**3. P WAVE**

    Presence:

    Appearance:

    Consistency:

    Relation to QRS:

**4. P-R INTERVAL**

    Duration:

    Consistency:

**5. QRS COMPLEX**

    Presence:

    Appearance:

    Consistency:

    Duration:

**6. DATA ANALYSIS**

**7. INTERPRETATION**

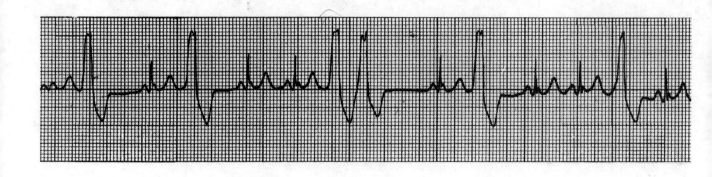

Figure 1-9B

# ECG RHYTHM STRIP #9

## I. RHYTHM

Atrial: Essentially regular

Ventricular: Irregular

## 2. RATE

Atrial: 110

Ventricular: 110

## 3. P WAVE

Presence: Yes — some hidden by QRS complex

Appearance: Normal

Consistency: Consistent

Relation to QRS: 1:1 except with premature QRS complexes

## 4. P-R INTERVAL

Duration: 0.12 seconds

Consistency: Consistent in all conducted beats

## 5. QRS COMPLEX

Presence: Yes

Appearance: Some normal; premature QRS complexes are abnormally wide and bizarre

Consistency: Inconsistent (2 forms)

Duration: 0.08 seconds in normal QRS; 0.16 seconds in abnormal QRS

## 6. DATA ANALYSIS

The underlying atrial and ventricular rates are fast, but otherwise normal. There are six premature QRS complexes, which are wide and bizarre but uniform in their appearance; two of these premature QRS complexes occur as consecutive beats. The atrial rhythm (P-P interval) is not disrupted by the premature QRS complexes.

## 7. INTERPRETATION

Sinus tachycardia with frequent uniform (unifocal) PVCs, including one pair of consecutive PVCs.

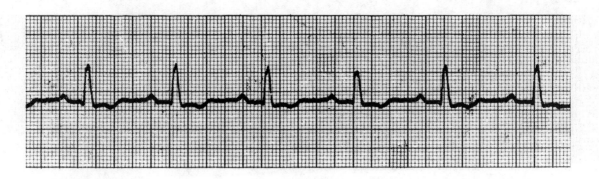

Figure 1-10A

# ECG RHYTHM STRIP #10

## 1. RHYTHM

Atrial:

Ventricular:

## 2. RATE

Atrial:

Ventricular:

## 3. P WAVE

Presence:

Appearance:

Consistency:

Relation to QRS:

## 4. P-R INTERVAL

Duration:

Consistency:

## 5. QRS COMPLEX

Presence:

Appearance:

Consistency:

Duration:

## 6. DATA ANALYSIS

## 7. INTERPRETATION

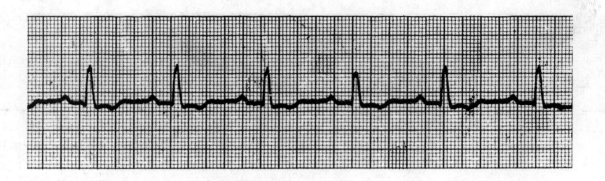

Figure 1-10B

## ECG RHYTHM STRIP #10

### 1. RHYTHM

Atrial: Regular

Ventricular: Regular

### 2. RATE

Atrial: 60

Ventricular: 60

### 3. P WAVE

Presence: Yes

Appearance: Normal

Consistency: Consistent

Relation to QRS: 1:1

### 4. P-R INTERVAL

Duration: 0.26 seconds

Consistency: Consistent

### 5. QRS COMPLEX

Presence: Yes

Appearance: Widened

Consistency: Consistent

Duration: 0.12 seconds

### 6. DATA ANALYSIS

Values are normal, except that the P-R interval and the QRS duration are prolonged. These prolongations remain consistent throughout.

### 7. INTERPRETATION

Sinus rhythm with first degree AV block and an intraventricular conduction delay

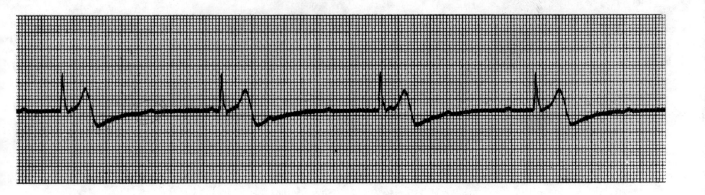

Figure 1-11A

## ECG RHYTHM STRIP #11

**1. RHYTHM**

　　Atrial:

　　Ventricular:

**2. RATE**

　　Atrial:

　　Ventricular:

**3. P WAVE**

　　Presence:

　　Appearance:

　　Consistency:

　　Relation to QRS:

**4. P-R INTERVAL**

　　Duration:

　　Consistency:

**5. QRS COMPLEX**

　　Presence:

　　Appearance:

　　Consistency:

　　Duration:

**6. DATA ANALYSIS**

**7. INTERPRETATION**

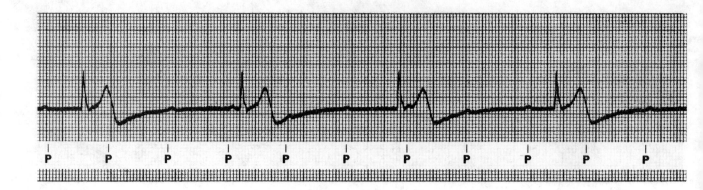

Figure 1-11B

# ECG RHYTHM STRIP #11

## 1. RHYTHM

Atrial: Regular

Ventricular: Regular

## 2. RATE

Atrial: 85

Ventricular: 30

## 3. P WAVE

Presence: Yes

Appearance: Normal

Consistency: Consistent

Relation to QRS: Variable

## 4. P-R INTERVAL

Duration: Variable

Consistency: Inconsistent

## 5. QRS COMPLEX

Presence: Yes

Appearance: Normal

Consistency: Consistent

Duration: 0.09 seconds

## 6. DATA ANALYSIS

The atrial and ventricular rates are different; atrial rate is significantly faster than the ventricular rate. The P-P intervals remain constant as do the R-R intervals, but there is no relation between P waves and QRS complexes as evidenced by the widely varying P-R intervals (AV dissociation). The QRS complexes are of normal duration, suggesting a supraventricular origin.

## 7. INTERPRETATION

Sinus rhythm with third degree (complete) AV block and a junctional escape rhythm

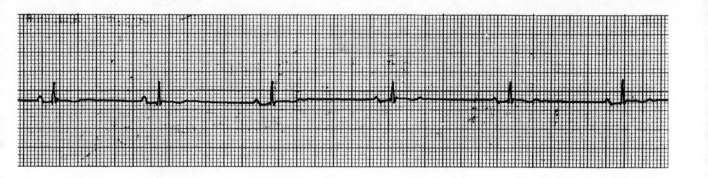

Figure 1-12A

# ECG RHYTHM STRIP #12

## 1. RHYTHM

Atrial:

Ventricular:

## 2. RATE

Atrial:

Ventricular:

## 3. P WAVE

Presence:

Appearance:

Consistency:

Relation to QRS:

## 4. P-R INTERVAL

Duration:

Consistency:

## 5. QRS COMPLEX

Presence:

Appearance:

Consistency:

Duration:

## 6. DATA ANALYSIS

## 7. INTERPRETATION

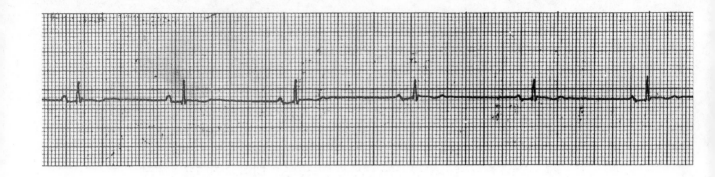

Figure 1-12B

# ECG RHYTHM STRIP #12

## I. RHYTHM

Atrial: Essentially regular

Ventricular: Essentially regular

## 2. RATE

Atrial: 50

Ventricular: 50

## 3. P WAVE

Presence: Yes

Appearance: Grossly normal

Consistency: Varies somewhat

Relation to QRS: 1:1

## 4. P-R INTERVAL

Duration: 0.16 seconds

Consistency: Gets slightly longer when rate slows

## 5. QRS COMPLEX

Presence: Yes

Appearance: Normal

Consistency: Consistent

Duration: 0.06 seconds

## 6. DATA ANALYSIS

The atrial and ventricular rates are slow. P wave configuration changes after the initial two beats following an increase in the P-P interval. The P-R interval lengthens as the rate slows.

## 7. INTERPRETATION

Wandering atrial pacemaker at a slow (bradycardic) rate

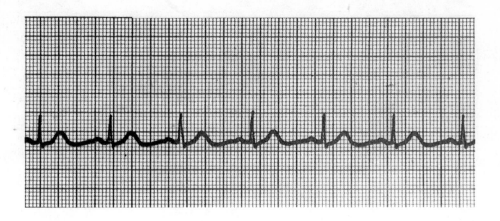

Figure 1-13A

# ECG RHYTHM STRIP #13

## 1. RHYTHM

Atrial:

Ventricular:

## 2. RATE

Atrial:

Ventricular:

## 3. P WAVE

Presence:

Appearance:

Consistency:

Relation to QRS:

## 4. P-R INTERVAL

Duration:

Consistency:

## 5. QRS COMPLEX

Presence:

Appearance:

Consistency:

Duration:

## 6. DATA ANALYSIS

## 7. INTERPRETATION

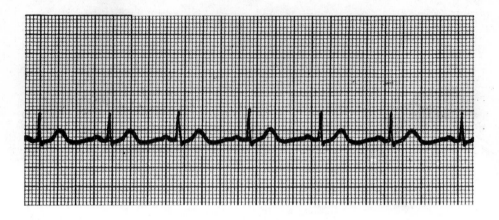

Figure 1-13B

# ECG RHYTHM STRIP #13

## 1. RHYTHM

Atrial: Regular

Ventricular: Regular

## 2. RATE

Atrial: 80

Ventricular: 80

## 3. P WAVE

Presence: Yes

Appearance: Normal

Consistency: Consistent

Relation to QRS: 1:1

## 4. P-R INTERVAL

Duration: 0.16 seconds

Consistency: Consistent

## 5. QRS COMPLEX

Presence: Yes

Appearance: Normal

Consistency: Consistent

Duration: 0.06 seconds

## 6. DATA ANALYSIS

All values are within normal limits.

## 7. INTERPRETATION

(Normal) Sinus rhythm

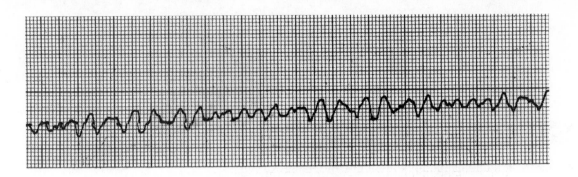

Figure 1-14A

# ECG RHYTHM STRIP #14

**1. RHYTHM**

    Atrial:

    Ventricular:

**2. RATE**

    Atrial:

    Ventricular:

**3. P WAVE**

    Presence:

    Appearance:

    Consistency:

    Relation to QRS:

**4. P-R INTERVAL**

    Duration:

    Consistency:

**5. QRS COMPLEX**

    Presence:

    Appearance:

    Consistency:

    Duration:

**6. DATA ANALYSIS**

**7. INTERPRETATION**

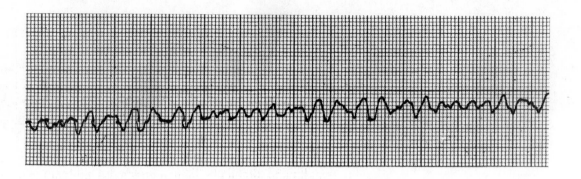

Figure 1-14B

# ECG RHYTHM STRIP #14

## I. RHYTHM

Atrial:  Unable to determine

Ventricular:  Unable to determine

## 2. RATE

Atrial:  —

Ventricular:  —

## 3. P WAVE

Presence:  No

Appearance:  —

Consistency:  —

Relation to QRS:  —

## 4. P-R INTERVAL

Duration:  Unable to determine

Consistency:  —

## 5. QRS COMPLEX

Presence:  Not distinctly identifiable

Appearance:  Coarse fibrillatory waveforms

Consistency:  Waves vary in size, shape, and configuration

Duration:  Unable to determine

## 6. DATA ANALYSIS

There is no identifiable evidence of atrial activity. Ventricular activity is evidenced as coarse, fibrillatory undulations of the baseline.

## 7. INTERPRETATION

(Coarse) Ventricular fibrillation

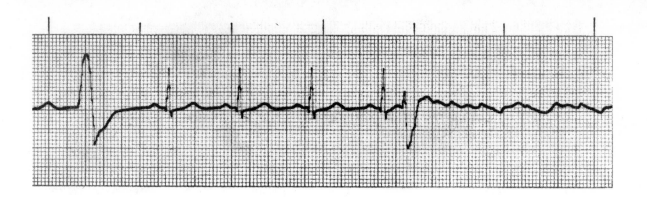

Figure 1-15A

# ECG RHYTHM STRIP #15

## I. RHYTHM

Atrial:

Ventricular:

## 2. RATE

Atrial:

Ventricular:

## 3. P WAVE

Presence:

Appearance:

Consistency:

Relation to QRS:

## 4. P-R INTERVAL

Duration:

Consistency:

## 5. QRS COMPLEX

Presence:

Appearance:

Consistency:

Duration:

## 6. DATA ANALYSIS

## 7. INTERPRETATION

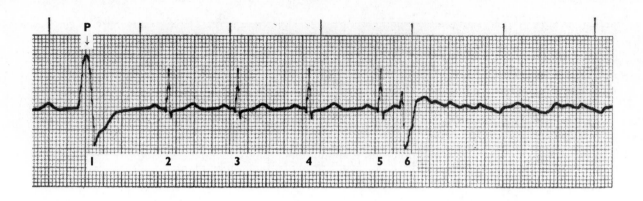

Figure 1-15B

# ECG RHYTHM STRIP #15

## 1. RHYTHM

Atrial: Initially Regular

Ventricular: Irregular

## 2. RATE

Atrial: 75 then indeterminable

Ventricular: Same as atrial

## 3. P WAVE

Presence: Yes

Appearance: Normal

Consistency: Consistent

Relation to QRS: 1:1 with conducted beats

## 4. P-R INTERVAL

Duration: 0.16 seconds

Consistency: Consistent

## 5. QRS COMPLEX

Presence: Yes; No distinguishable complex after
the 6th QRS

Appearance: Some normal; premature QRS
complexes are wide and bizarre

Consistency: Inconsistent

Duration: 0.06 seconds in normal QRS; 0.16
to 0.20 seconds in abnormal QRS
complexes

## 6. DATA ANALYSIS

The 2nd through 5th beats are normal and
indicate a basic sinus rhythm at 75 per minute.
The first P wave is obscured by the early QRS
complex.

The 1st and 6th QRS complexes are premature,
wide, bizarre, and multiform in configuration.
Beat #6 (second premature QRS) falls on the T
wave of the preceding sinus beat. It is followed
by fibrillatory undulations of the baseline with
no evidence of atrial activity.

## 7. INTERPRETATION

Sinus rhythm with multiform PVCs; R on T
phenomenon going into ventricular fibrillation

32

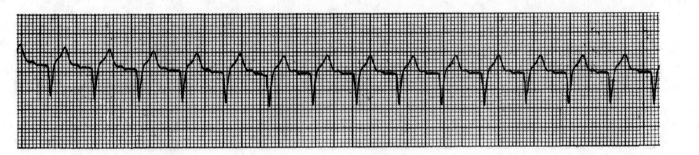

Figure 1-16A

# ECG RHYTHM STRIP #16

## I. RHYTHM

Atrial:

Ventricular:

## 2. RATE

Atrial:

Ventricular:

## 3. P WAVE

Presence:

Appearance:

Consistency:

Relation to QRS:

## 4. P-R INTERVAL

Duration:

Consistency:

## 5. QRS COMPLEX

Presence:

Appearance:

Consistency:

Duration:

## 6. DATA ANALYSIS

## 7. INTERPRETATION

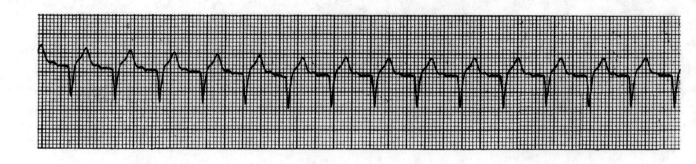

Figure 1-16B

## ECG RHYTHM STRIP #16

### 1. RHYTHM

Atrial: Regular

Ventricular: Regular

### 2. RATE

Atrial: 130

Ventricular: 130

### 3. P WAVE

Presence: Yes

Appearance: Normal

Consistency: Consistent

Relation to QRS: 1:1

### 4. P-R INTERVAL

Duration: 0.20 seconds

Consistency: Consistent

### 5. QRS COMPLEX

Presence: Yes

Appearance: Normal

Consistency: Consistent

Duration: 0.08 seconds

### 6. DATA ANALYSIS

All values are normal, except the atrial and ventricular rates, which are rapid.

### 7. INTERPRETATION

Sinus tachycardia

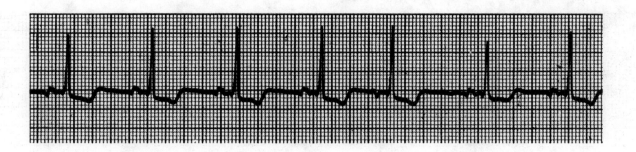

Figure 1-17A

# ECG RHYTHM STRIP #17

**1. RHYTHM**

    Atrial:

    Ventricular:

**2. RATE**

    Atrial:

    Ventricular:

**3. P WAVE**

    Presence:

    Appearance:

    Consistency:

    Relation to QRS:

**4. P-R INTERVAL**

    Duration:

    Consistency:

**5. QRS COMPLEX**

    Presence:

    Appearance:

    Consistency:

    Duration:

**6. DATA ANALYSIS**

**7. INTERPRETATION**

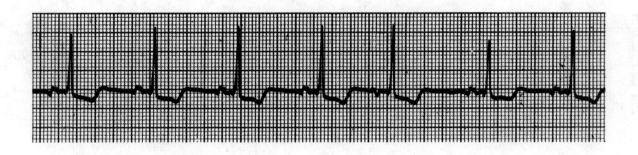

Figure 1-17B

# ECG RHYTHM STRIP #17

## I. RHYTHM

Atrial: Regular except for one premature cycle

Ventricular: Regular except for one premature cycle

## 2. RATE

Atrial: 70

Ventricular: 70

## 3. P WAVE

Presence: Yes

Appearance: Normal (variant)

Consistency: Consistent except for 5th beat

Relation to QRS: 1:1

## 4. P-R INTERVAL

Duration: 0.18 seconds

Consistency: Consistent

## 5. QRS COMPLEX

Presence: Yes

Appearance: Normal

Consistency: Consistent—amplitude of 6th beat is less

Duration: 0.09 seconds

## 6. DATA ANALYSIS

All values are normal, except for one complete P-QRS-T cycle that is premature and preceded by a P wave different from the sinus P waves. The QRS complex associated with the premature P wave is identical to the QRS of the sinus beats.

## 7. INTERPRETATION

Sinus rhythm with 1 PAC

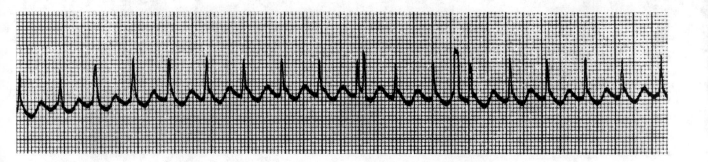

Figure 1-18A

# ECG RHYTHM STRIP #18

## 1. RHYTHM

Atrial:

Ventricular:

## 2. RATE

Atrial:

Ventricular:

## 3. P WAVE

Presence:

Appearance:

Consistency:

Relation to QRS:

## 4. P-R INTERVAL

Duration:

Consistency:

## 5. QRS COMPLEX

Presence:

Appearance:

Consistency:

Duration:

## 6. DATA ANALYSIS

## 7. INTERPRETATION

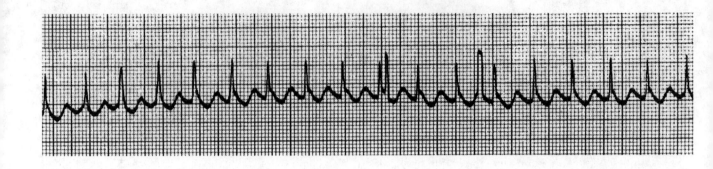

Figure 1-18B

# ECG RHYTHM STRIP #18

## 1. RHYTHM

Atrial: Regular

Ventricular: Regular

## 2. RATE

Atrial: 300

Ventricular: 150

## 3. P WAVE

Presence: Evidence of atrial activity present

Appearance: Flutter waves (sawtooth) rather than discrete P waves

Consistency: Consistent

Relation to QRS: 2:1

## 4. P-R INTERVAL

Duration: Unable to determine

Consistency: —

## 5. QRS COMPLEX

Presence: Yes

Appearance: Normal—distorted somewhat by flutter waves

Consistency: Consistent

Duration: 0.04 seconds

## 6. DATA ANALYSIS

Discrete P waves have been replaced by sawtooth flutter waves at a rate of 300 per minute. Flutter waves partially distort the QRS complex at regular intervals. The ventricular rate is exactly half of the atrial rate.

## 7. INTERPRETATION

Atrial flutter with 2:1 conduction ratio

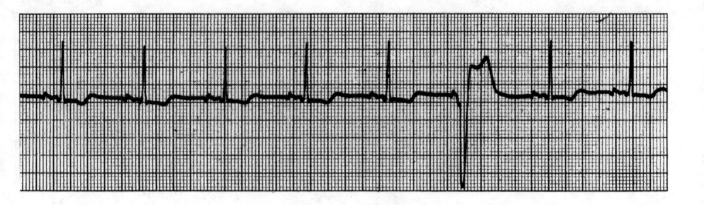

Figure 1-19A

# ECG RHYTHM STRIP #19

## 1. RHYTHM

Atrial:

Ventricular:

## 2. RATE

Atrial:

Ventricular:

## 3. P WAVE

Presence:

Appearance:

Consistency:

Relation to QRS:

## 4. P-R INTERVAL

Duration:

Consistency:

## 5. QRS COMPLEX

Presence:

Appearance:

Consistency:

Duration:

## 6. DATA ANALYSIS

## 7. INTERPRETATION

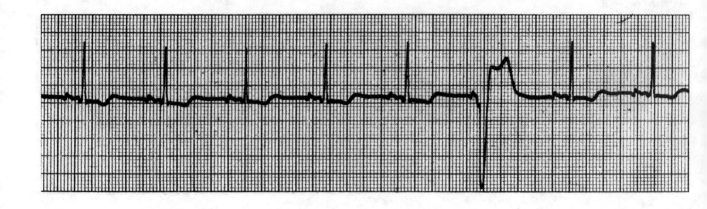

Figure 1-19B

# ECG RHYTHM STRIP #19

## 1. RHYTHM

Atrial: Regular

Ventricular: Regular except for 6th beat

## 2. RATE

Atrial: 62

Ventricular: 62

## 3. P WAVE

Presence: Yes

Appearance: Normal (variant)

Consistency: Consistent

Relation to QRS: 1:1

## 4. P-R INTERVAL

Duration: 0.18 seconds

Consistency: Consistent

## 5. QRS COMPLEX

Presence: Yes

Appearance: Normal except in 6th beat

Consistency: Consistent except in 6th beat

Duration: 0.09 seconds in all but 6th beat
(0.12 seconds)

## 6. DATA ANALYSIS

Values are normal except for the 6th cycle where the P wave occurs on time, but the wide and distorted QRS complex is premature. Sinus rhythm appears to continue without disruption by the premature ventricular beat.

## 7. INTERPRETATION

Sinus rhythm with one PVC (late diastolic PVC)

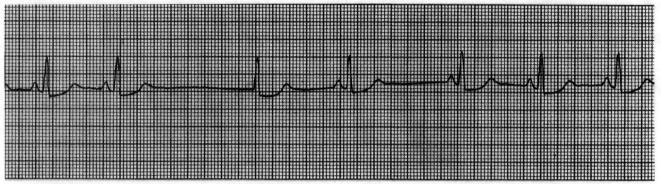

Figure 1-20A

# ECG RHYTHM STRIP #20

## 1. RHYTHM

Atrial:

Ventricular:

## 2. RATE

Atrial:

Ventricular:

## 3. P WAVE

Presence:

Appearance:

Consistency:

Relation to QRS:

## 4. P-R INTERVAL

Duration:

Consistency:

## 5. QRS COMPLEX

Presence:

Appearance:

Consistency:

Duration:

## 6. DATA ANALYSIS

## 7. INTERPRETATION

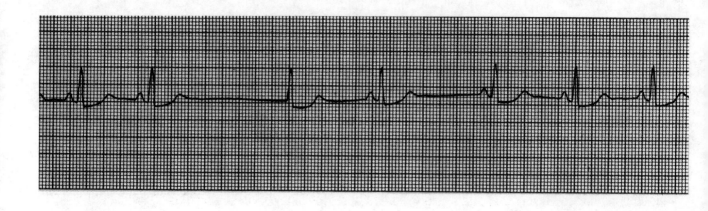

Figure 1-20B

# ECG RHYTHM STRIP #20

## I. RHYTHM

Atrial: Irregular

Ventricular: Irregular (slow-fast cycle)

## 2. RATE

Atrial: 40

Ventricular: 50

## 3. P WAVE

Presence: Yes—except in 3rd beat

Appearance: Normal

Consistency: Consistent

Relation to QRS: 1:1

## 4. P-R INTERVAL

Duration: 0.14 seconds

Consistency: Consistent

## 5. QRS COMPLEX

Presence: Yes

Appearance: Normal

Consistency: Consistent

Duration: 0.08 seconds

## 6. DATA ANALYSIS

The atrial rate is less than the ventricular rate, owing to the lack of an identifiable P wave in the 3rd cycle. Both atrial and ventricular rhythms are irregular. The initial pause in the rhythm occurs when the sinus node fails to produce a beat. The pause is ended by a late (escape) beat with a narrow QRS and no P wave. The rhythm following the initial pause remains irregular.

## 7. INTERPRETATION

Sinus arrhythmia with one episode of sinus pause followed by a junctional escape beat

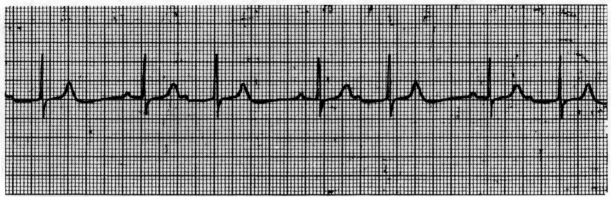

Figure 1-21A

# ECG RHYTHM STRIP #21

## I. RHYTHM

Atrial:

Ventricular:

## 2. RATE

Atrial:

Ventricular:

## 3. P WAVE

Presence:

Appearance:

Consistency:

Relation to QRS:

## 4. P-R INTERVAL

Duration:

Consistency:

## 5. QRS COMPLEX

Presence:

Appearance:

Consistency:

Duration:

## 6. DATA ANALYSIS

## 7. INTERPRETATION

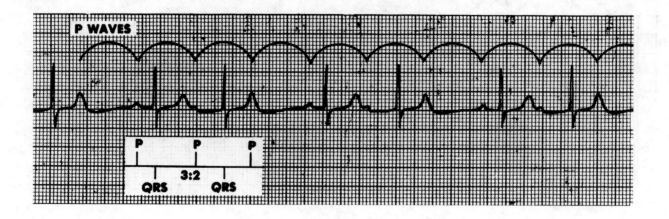

Figure 1-21B

# ECG RHYTHM STRIP #21

## 1. RHYTHM

Atrial: Regular

Ventricular: Irregular with pattern of grouped beats

## 2. RATE

Atrial: 95

Ventricular: 70

## 3. P WAVE

Presence: Yes—some are hidden in QRS or T waves

Appearance: Normal

Consistency: Consistent

Relation to QRS: 3:2

## 4. P-R INTERVAL

Duration: 0.20 and 0.36 seconds

Consistency: Progressively increases until QRS dropped

## 5. QRS COMPLEX

Presence: Yes

Appearance: Normal

Consistency: Consistent

Duration: 0.06 seconds

## 6. DATA ANALYSIS

Atrial rate exceeds ventricular rate, suggesting the presence of AV block. P waves are normal and rhythmic. P-R interval progressively increases until a QRS complex is dropped. There are three P waves for every two QRS complexes.

## 7. INTERPRETATION

Sinus rhythm with 2nd degree AV block, Mobitz I (Wenckeback) and 3:2 conduction

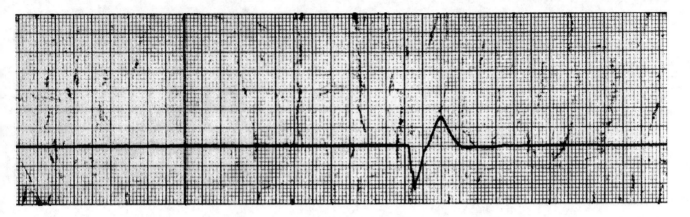

Figure 1-22A

# ECG RHYTHM STRIP #22

## 1. RHYTHM

Atrial:

Ventricular:

## 2. RATE

Atrial:

Ventricular:

## 3. P WAVE

Presence:

Appearance:

Consistency:

Relation to QRS:

## 4. P-R INTERVAL

Duration:

Consistency:

## 5. QRS COMPLEX

Presence:

Appearance:

Consistency:

Duration:

## 6. DATA ANALYSIS

## 7. INTERPRETATION

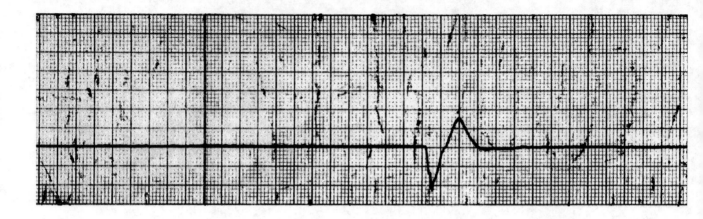

Figure 1-22B

# ECG RHYTHM STRIP #22

## 1. RHYTHM

Atrial: —

Ventricular: Unable to determine

## 2. RATE

Atrial: —

Ventricular: 10 or less

## 3. P WAVE

Presence: No

Appearance: —

Consistency: —

Relation to QRS: —

## 4. P-R INTERVAL

Duration: —

Consistency: —

## 5. QRS COMPLEX

Presence: Single complex

Appearance: Wide, bizarre

Consistency: —

Duration: 0.20 seconds

## 6. DATA ANALYSIS

The only evidence of cardiac electrical activity is a single, wide, and bizarre QRS complex without a preceding P wave. Otherwise there is complete asystole.

## 7. INTERPRETATION

Asystole with one ventricular (escape) beat as seen in agonal rhythm/dying heart

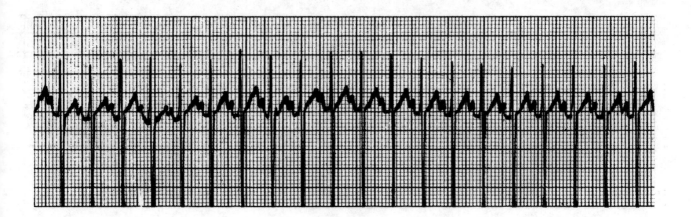

Figure 1-23A

# ECG RHYTHM STRIP #23

**1. RHYTHM**

Atrial:

Ventricular:

**2. RATE**

Atrial:

Ventricular:

**3. P WAVE**

Presence:

Appearance:

Consistency:

Relation to QRS:

**4. P-R INTERVAL**

Duration:

Consistency:

**5. QRS COMPLEX**

Presence:

Appearance:

Consistency:

Duration:

**6. DATA ANALYSIS**

**7. INTERPRETATION**

47

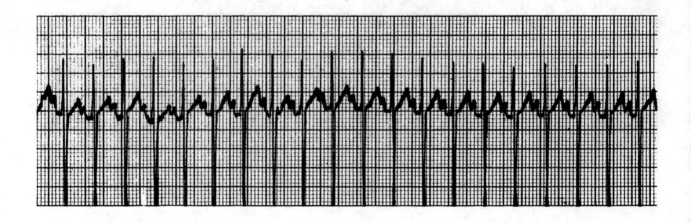

Figure 1-23B

# ECG RHYTHM STRIP #23

## I. RHYTHM

Atrial: Regular

Ventricular: Regular

## 2. RATE

Atrial: 187

Ventricular: 187

## 3. P WAVE

Presence: Yes

Appearance: Normal, assuming preceding waveform is a T wave

Consistency: Consistent

Relation to QRS: 1:1

## 4. P-R INTERVAL

Duration: 0.12 seconds

Consistency: Consistent

## 5. QRS COMPLEX

Presence: Yes

Appearance: Normal

Consistency: Consistent

Duration: 0.06 seconds

## 6. DATA ANALYSIS

Both atrial and ventricular rates are very rapid. The P-R interval is consistent with a tachycardia. It is difficult to differentiate whether the tachycardia is sinus, atrial, or junctional since P waves are assumed to follow a T wave; these waveforms could conceivably represent a biphasic or notched P wave or even an inverted P wave. Without a 12 lead ECG to assist in differentiating the origin, a narrow QRS tachycardia may be designated as supraventricular in origin.

## 7. INTERPRETATION

Supraventricular tachycardia (SVT)

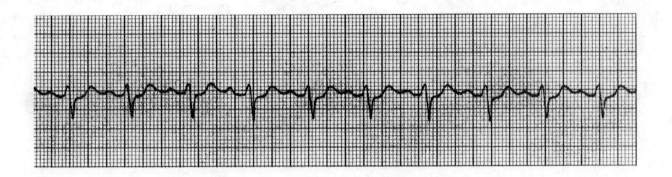

Figure 1-24A

# ECG RHYTHM STRIP #24

**1. RHYTHM**

    Atrial:

    Ventricular:

**2. RATE**

    Atrial:

    Ventricular:

**3. P WAVE**

    Presence:

    Appearance:

    Consistency:

    Relation to QRS:

**4. P-R INTERVAL**

    Duration:

    Consistency:

**5. QRS COMPLEX**

    Presence:

    Appearance:

    Consistency:

    Duration:

**6. DATA ANALYSIS**

**7. INTERPRETATION**

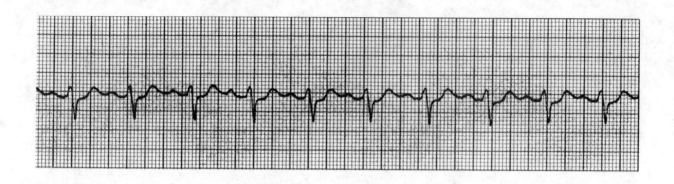

Figure 1-24B

# ECG RHYTHM STRIP #24

## 1. RHYTHM

Atrial: Regular

Ventricular: Regular

## 2. RATE

Atrial: 95

Ventricular: 95

## 3. P WAVE

Presence: Yes

Appearance: Normal

Consistency: Consistent

Relation to QRS: 1:1

## 4. P-R INTERVAL

Duration: 0.22 seconds

Consistency: Consistent

## 5. QRS COMPLEX

Presence: Yes

Appearance: Normal—wide

Consistency: Consistent

Duration: 0.12 seconds

## 6. DATA ANALYSIS

Rates and rhythm are normal for atria and ventricles. The P-R interval and QRS duration are both abnormally prolonged.

## 7. INTERPRETATION

Sinus rhythm with first degree AV block and intraventricular conduction delay

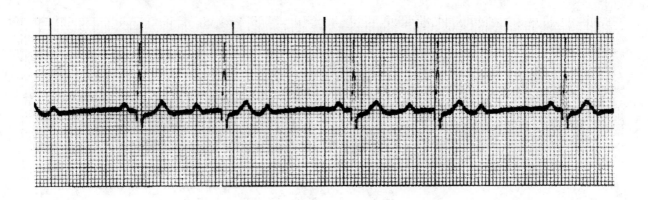

Figure 1-25A

# ECG RHYTHM STRIP #25

**1. RHYTHM**

Atrial:

Ventricular:

**2. RATE**

Atrial:

Ventricular:

**3. P WAVE**

Presence:

Appearance:

Consistency:

Relation to QRS:

**4. P-R INTERVAL**

Duration:

Consistency:

**5. QRS COMPLEX**

Presence:

Appearance:

Consistency:

Duration:

**6. DATA ANALYSIS**

**7. INTERPRETATION**

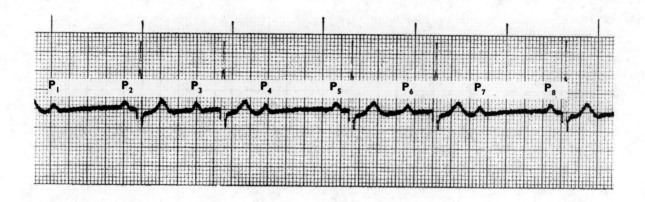

Figure 1-25B

# ECG RHYTHM STRIP #25

## I. RHYTHM

Atrial: Regular

Ventricular: Irregular

## 2. RATE

Atrial: 80

Ventricular: 50

## 3. P WAVE

Presence: Yes

Appearance: Normal

Consistency: Consistent

Relation to QRS: 3:2

## 4. P-R INTERVAL

Duration: Varies between 0.18 to 0.32 seconds

Consistency: Progressively lengthens

## 5. QRS COMPLEX

Presence: Yes

Appearance: Normal

Consistency: Consistent

Duration: 0.06 seconds

## 6. DATA ANALYSIS

The atrial rate, rhythm, and P waves are consistent with an underlying sinus rhythm. The 1st, 4th, and 7th P waves are not followed by a QRS complex, indicating that these P waves were not conducted. Prior to the 4th and 7th P waves, the P-R interval progressively increases. The ventricular rhythm is characterized by "group beating" caused by pauses in the rhythm created by the nonconducted P waves.

## 7. INTERPRETATION

Sinus rhythm with second degree AV block, Type 1 (Wenckebach) with 3:2 conduction ratio

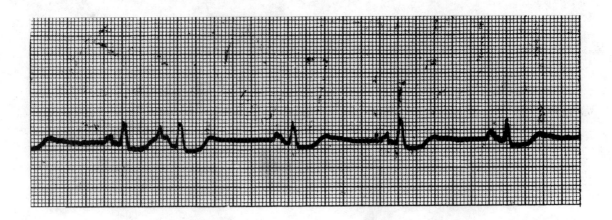

Figure 1-26A

## ECG RHYTHM STRIP #26

**1. RHYTHM**

    Atrial:

    Ventricular:

**2. RATE**

    Atrial:

    Ventricular:

**3. P WAVE**

    Presence:

    Appearance:

    Consistency:

    Relation to QRS:

**4. P-R INTERVAL**

    Duration:

    Consistency:

**5. QRS COMPLEX**

    Presence:

    Appearance:

    Consistency:

    Duration:

**6. DATA ANALYSIS**

**7. INTERPRETATION**

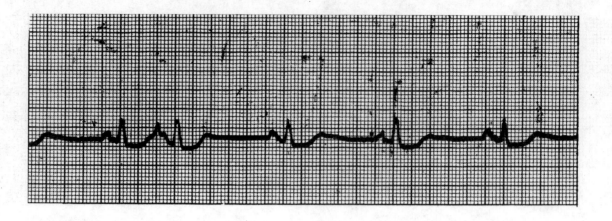

Figure 1-26B

# ECG RHYTHM STRIP #26

## 1. RHYTHM

Atrial: Irregular

Ventricular: Irregular

## 2. RATE

Atrial: 50

Ventricular: 50

## 3. P WAVE

Presence: Yes

Appearance: Some distortion

Consistency: Consistent, except for 2nd beat
(peaked P on T wave)

Relation to QRS: 1:1

## 4. P-R INTERVAL

Duration: 0.20 seconds

Consistency: Consistent

## 5. QRS COMPLEX

Presence: Yes

Appearance: Normal

Consistency: Consistent

Duration: 0.08 seconds

## 6. DATA ANALYSIS

Atrial and ventricular rates are both slow at 50 per minute. The rhythm irregularity is due to an early P-QRS cycle that is initiated by a P wave different from the other P waves; the QRS of the early beat is similar to the other QRS complexes. Following this premature cycle, the atrial and ventricular rhythms are restored.

## 7. INTERPRETATION

Sinus bradycardia with one PAC

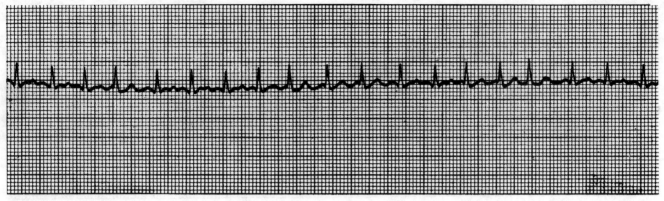

Figure 1-27A

# ECG RHYTHM STRIP #27

## I. RHYTHM

Atrial:

Ventricular:

## 2. RATE

Atrial:

Ventricular:

## 3. P WAVE

Presence:

Appearance:

Consistency:

Relation to QRS:

## 4. P-R INTERVAL

Duration:

Consistency:

## 5. QRS COMPLEX

Presence:

Appearance:

Consistency:

Duration:

## 6. DATA ANALYSIS

## 7. INTERPRETATION

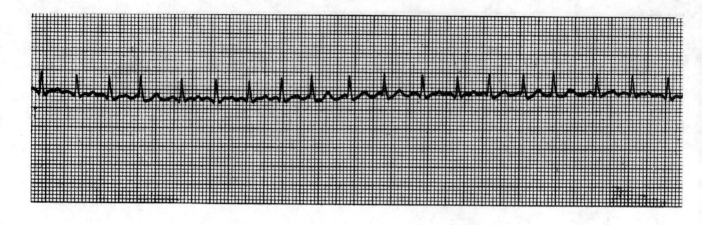

Figure 1-27B

# ECG RHYTHM STRIP #27

## I. RHYTHM

Atrial: Irregular

Ventricular: Irregularly irregular

## 2. RATE

Atrial: Unable to determine

Ventricular: 160

## 3. P WAVE

Presence: Discrete P waves are not identifiable

Appearance: Fibrillatory waves

Consistency: Inconsistent

Relation to QRS: Unable to determine without distinct P waves

## 4. P-R INTERVAL

Duration: Unable to determine

Consistency: —

## 5. QRS COMPLEX

Presence: Yes

Appearance: Normal

Consistency: Consistent

Duration: 0.06 seconds

## 6. DATA ANALYSIS

The ventricular rate is very rapid. The QRS is of normal duration, indicating that the rapid rate is of supraventricular origin. P waves are not distinctly identifiable but are relpaced by irregular undulations of the baseline. The ventricular rhythm is irregularly irregular.

## 7. INTERPRETATION

Atrial fibrillation with a rapid (uncontrolled) ventricular response

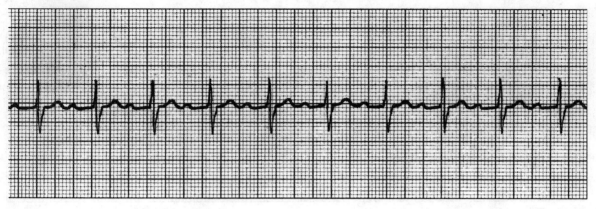

Figure 1-28A

# ECG RHYTHM STRIP #28

## 1. RHYTHM

Atrial:

Ventricular:

## 2. RATE

Atrial:

Ventricular:

## 3. P WAVE

Presence:

Appearance:

Consistency:

Relation to QRS:

## 4. P-R INTERVAL

Duration:

Consistency:

## 5. QRS COMPLEX

Presence:

Appearance:

Consistency:

Duration:

## 6. DATA ANALYSIS

## 7. INTERPRETATION

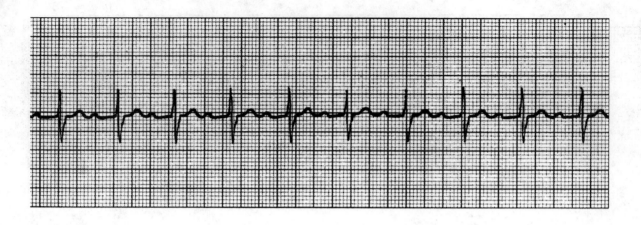

Figure 1-28B

## ECG RHYTHM STRIP #28

### I. RHYTHM

Atrial: Regular

Ventricular: Regular

### 2. RATE

Atrial: 95

Ventricular: 95

### 3. P WAVE

Presence: Yes

Appearance: Normal

Consistency: Consistent

Relation to QRS: 1:1

### 4. P-R INTERVAL

Duration: 0.26 seconds

Consistency: Consistent

### 5. QRS COMPLEX

Presence: Yes

Appearance: Normal

Consistency: Consistent

Duration: 0.08 seconds

### 6. DATA ANALYSIS

All values are normal except that the P-R interval is prolonged. This indicates delayed conduction through the AV junction.

### 7. INTERPRETATION

Sinus rhythm with first degree AV block

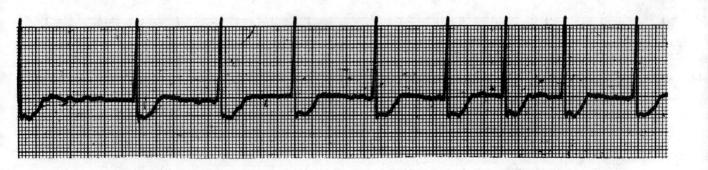

Figure 1-29A

# ECG RHYTHM STRIP #29

**I. RHYTHM**

    Atrial:

    Ventricular:

**2. RATE**

    Atrial:

    Ventricular:

**3. P WAVE**

    Presence:

    Appearance:

    Consistency:

    Relation to QRS:

**4. P-R INTERVAL**

    Duration:

    Consistency:

**5. QRS COMPLEX**

    Presence:

    Appearance:

    Consistency:

    Duration:

**6. DATA ANALYSIS**

**7. INTERPRETATION**

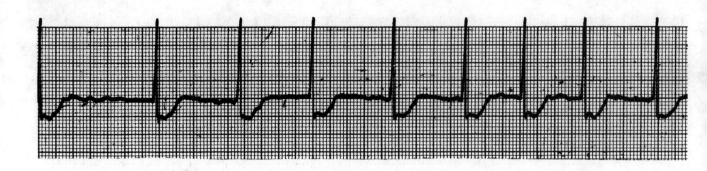

Figure 1-29B

# ECG RHYTHM STRIP #29

## I. RHYTHM

Atrial: Unable to determine

Ventricular: Irregularly irregular

## 2. RATE

Atrial: Unable to determine

Ventricular: 70

## 3. P WAVE

Presence: No—unable to identify discrete P waves

Appearance: Fine fibrillatory waves

Consistency: Inconsistent

Relation to QRS: Unable to determine without discrete P waves

## 4. P-R INTERVAL

Duration: Unable to calculate

Consistency: —

## 5. QRS COMPLEX

Presence: Yes

Appearance: Normal

Consistency: Consistent

Duration: 0.08 seconds

## 6. DATA ANALYSIS

The presence of an irregularly irregular ventricular rhythm where QRS complexes are preceded by fine undulations of the baseline rather than identifiable P waves suggests a fibrillatory mechanism in the atria as the origin of the rhythm. QRS complexes are of normal duration.

## 7. INTERPRETATION

Atrial fibrillation with a controlled ventricular reponse

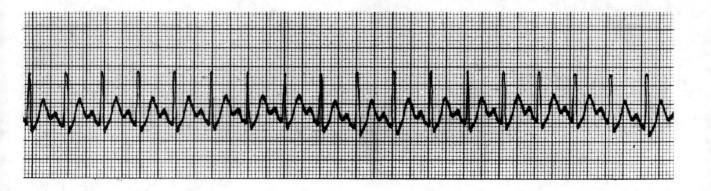

Figure 1-30A

# ECG RHYTHM STRIP #30

## 1. RHYTHM

Atrial:

Ventricular:

## 2. RATE

Atrial:

Ventricular:

## 3. P WAVE

Presence:

Appearance:

Consistency:

Relation to QRS:

## 4. P-R INTERVAL

Duration:

Consistency:

## 5. QRS COMPLEX

Presence:

Appearance:

Consistency:

Duration:

## 6. DATA ANALYSIS

## 7. INTERPRETATION

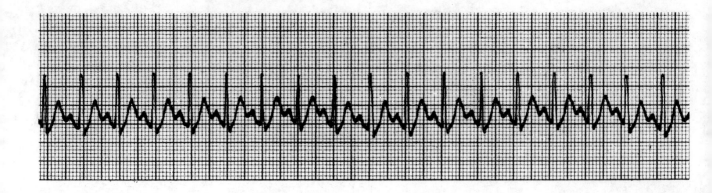

Figure 1-30B

# ECG RHYTHM STRIP #30

## I. RHYTHM

Atrial: Regular

Ventricular: Regular

## 2. RATE

Atrial: 150

Ventricular: 150

## 3. P WAVE

Presence: Yes

Appearance: Normal

Consistency: Consistent

Relation to QRS: 1:1

## 4. P-R INTERVAL

Duration: 0.14 seconds

Consistency: Consistent

## 5. QRS COMPLEX

Presence: Yes

Appearance: Normal

Consistency: Consistent

Duration: 0.06 seconds

## 6. DATA ANALYSIS

All values are normal, except that both the atrial and ventricular rates are very rapid. P waves appear normal. A 12 lead ECG would be helpful to confirm the exact origin of this tachycardia. The rhythm originates above the ventricles since the QRS duration is normal.

## 7. INTERPRETATION

Supraventricular tachycardia (SVT)—probably a sinus tachycardia

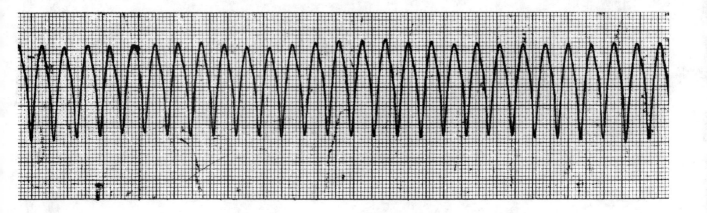

Figure 1-31A

# ECG RHYTHM STRIP #31

## 1. RHYTHM

Atrial:

Ventricular:

## 2. RATE

Atrial:

Ventricular:

## 3. P WAVE

Presence:

Appearance:

Consistency:

Relation to QRS:

## 4. P-R INTERVAL

Duration:

Consistency:

## 5. QRS COMPLEX

Presence:

Appearance:

Consistency:

Duration:

## 6. DATA ANALYSIS

## 7. INTERPRETATION

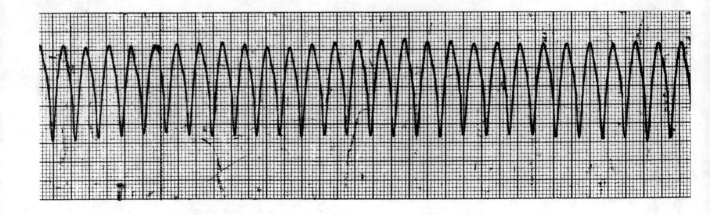

Figure 1-31B

# ECG RHYTHM STRIP #31

## 1. RHYTHM

Atrial: Unable to determine

Ventricular: Regular

## 2. RATE

Atrial: Unable to determine

Ventricular: 250

## 3. P WAVE

Presence: Not identifiable

Appearance: —

Consistency: —

Relation to QRS: —

## 4. P-R INTERVAL

Duration: Unable to determine

Consistency: —

## 5. QRS COMPLEX

Presence: Yes

Appearance: Unable to distinguish specific
waveforms; sine wave appearance

Consistency: Consistent

Duration: Unable to determine without discrete
waveforms

## 6. DATA ANALYSIS

There is no identifiable evidence of atrial activity. The ventricular rate is very rapid and regular. The QRS complex has no discrete waveforms which can be identified. The QRS has been replaced by a wide sine-like waveform.

## 7. INTERPRETATION

Ventricular tachycardia (flutter)

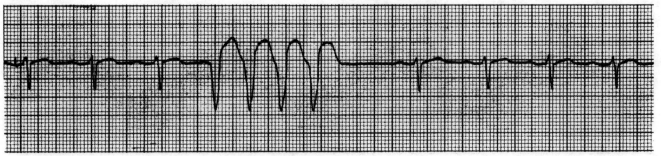

Figure 1-32A

# ECG RHYTHM STRIP #32

**1. RHYTHM**

    Atrial:

    Ventricular:

**2. RATE**

    Atrial:

    Ventricular:

**3. P WAVE**

    Presence:

    Appearance:

    Consistency:

    Relation to QRS:

**4. P-R INTERVAL**

    Duration:

    Consistency:

**5. QRS COMPLEX**

    Presence:

    Appearance:

    Consistency:

    Duration:

**6. DATA ANALYSIS**

**7. INTERPRETATION**

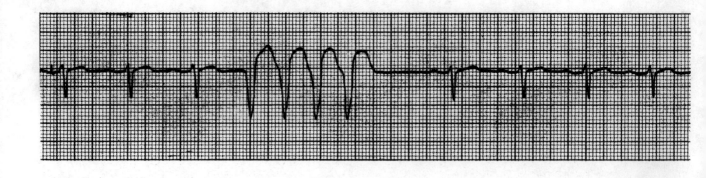

Figure 1-32B

## ECG RHYTHM STRIP #32

### I. RHYTHM

Atrial: Regular

Ventricular: Regular underlying rhythm; short run of rapid, regular rhythm

### 2. RATE

Atrial: 80

Ventricular: 80 with normal QRS; 150 with wide QRS

### 3. P WAVE

Presence: Yes

Appearance: Normal

Consistency: Consistent

Relation to QRS: 1:1 with normal QRS; P waves obscured by wide QRS complexes

### 4. P-R INTERVAL

Duration: 0.24 seconds

Consistency: Consistent

### 5. QRS COMPLEX

Presence: Yes

Appearance: Normal (first 3 and last 4); abnormal (4th to 7th beats)

Consistency: Inconsistent (two types)

Duration: 0.08 with normal QRS; 0.14 with abnormal QRS

### 6. DATA ANALYSIS

The underlying rhythm is normal except for the prolonged P-R interval. A short (4 beat) run of a rapid rhythm with wide QRS complexes interrupts the underlying sinus rhythm. The P-P interval remains constant even through the run of rapid rhythm where P waves are obscured by the QRS complexes.

### 7. INTERPRETATION

Sinus rhythm with first degree AV block and a 4-beat run of ventricular tachycardia

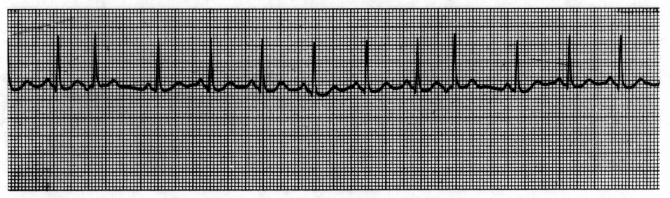

Figure 1-33A

# ECG RHYTHM STRIP #33

## 1. RHYTHM

Atrial:

Ventricular:

## 2. RATE

Atrial:

Ventricular:

## 3. P WAVE

Presence:

Appearance:

Consistency:

Relation to QRS:

## 4. P-R INTERVAL

Duration:

Consistency:

## 5. QRS COMPLEX

Presence:

Appearance:

Consistency:

Duration:

## 6. DATA ANALYSIS

## 7. INTERPRETATION

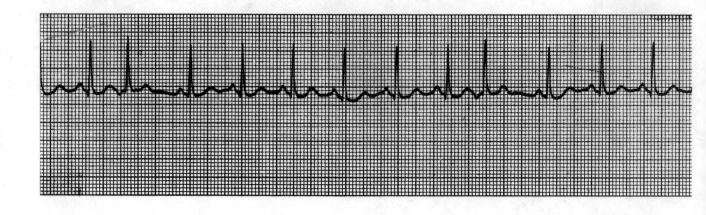

Figure 1-33B

## ECG RHYTHM STRIP #33

### I. RHYTHM

Atrial: Irregular

Ventricular: Irregular

### 2. RATE

Atrial: 100

Ventricular: 100

### 3. P WAVE

Presence: Yes

Appearance: Normal in all but 2nd and 9th beats (inverted/negative)

Consistency: Consistent except in all but 2nd and 9th beats

Relation to QRS: 1:1

### 4. P-R INTERVAL

Duration: 0.12 seconds except 0.08 seconds in 2nd and 9th beats

Consistency: Consistent except shorter when P waves are negative

### 5. QRS COMPLEX

Presence: Yes

Appearance: Normal

Consistency: Consistent

Duration: 0.06 seconds

### 6. DATA ANALYSIS

The normal underlying rhythm is interrupted by two premature cycles in which the P wave becomes a negative deflection in a lead where it is normally a positive deflection. P wave inversion suggests retrograde atrial conduction. The shortened P-R interval that occurs with the negative P waves is consistent with beats originating in the AV junction.

### 7. INTERPRETATION

Sinus rhythm with two premature junctional beats (PJCs)

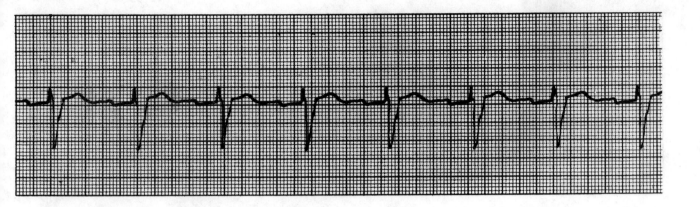

Figure 1-34A

# ECG RHYTHM STRIP #34

## I. RHYTHM

Atrial:

Ventricular:

## 2. RATE

Atrial:

Ventricular:

## 3. P WAVE

Presence:

Appearance:

Consistency:

Relation to QRS:

## 4. P-R INTERVAL

Duration:

Consistency:

## 5. QRS COMPLEX

Presence:

Appearance:

Consistency:

Duration:

## 6. DATA ANALYSIS

## 7. INTERPRETATION

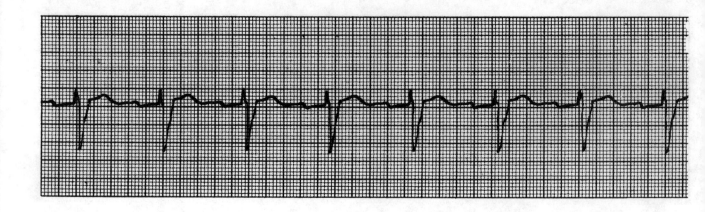

Figure 1-34B

## ECG RHYTHM STRIP #34

### 1. RHYTHM

Atrial: Regular

Ventricular: Regular

### 2. RATE

Atrial: 60

Ventricular: 60

### 3. P WAVE

Presence: Yes

Appearance: Normal

Consistency: Consistent

Relation to QRS: 1:1

### 4. P-R INTERVAL

Duration: 0.32 seconds

Consistency: Consistent

### 5. QRS COMPLEX

Presence: Yes

Appearance: Normal—wide

Consistency: Consistent

Duration: 0.16 seconds

### 6. DATA ANALYSIS

The rate is at the lower limit of normal. The P-R interval and QRS duration are both prolonged, indicating, respectively, delay of conduction through the AV junction and delay through the ventricles.

### 7. INTERPRETATION

Sinus rhythm with first degree AV block and an intraventricular conduction delay

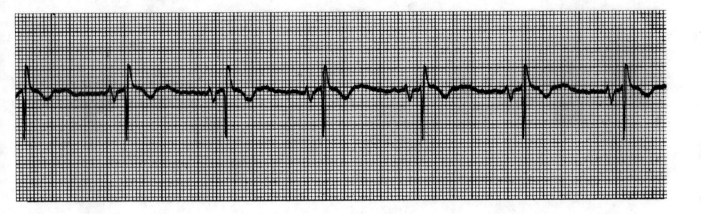

Figure 1-35A

# ECG RHYTHM STRIP #35

## 1. RHYTHM

Atrial:

Ventricular:

## 2. RATE

Atrial:

Ventricular:

## 3. P WAVE

Presence:

Appearance:

Consistency:

Relation to QRS:

## 4. P-R INTERVAL

Duration:

Consistency:

## 5. QRS COMPLEX

Presence:

Appearance:

Consistency:

Duration:

## 6. DATA ANALYSIS

## 7. INTERPRETATION

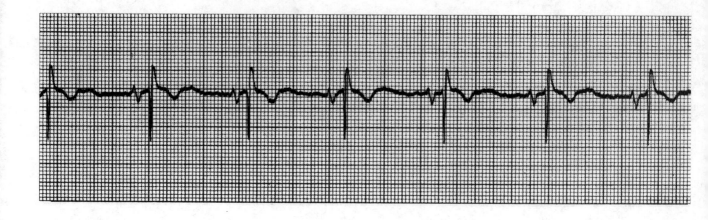

Figure 1-35B

## ECG RHYTHM STRIP #35

### 1. RHYTHM

Atrial: Regular

Ventricular: Regular

### 2. RATE

Atrial: 56

Ventricular: 56

### 3. P WAVE

Presence: Yes

Appearance: Normal (variant)

Consistency: Consistent

Relation to QRS: 1:1

### 4. P-R INTERVAL

Duration: 0.20 seconds

Consistency: Consistent

### 5. QRS COMPLEX

Presence: Yes

Appearance: Normal

Consistency: Consistent

Duration: 0.10 seconds

### 6. DATA ANALYSIS

Atrial and ventricular rates are uniformly slow. The P-R interval is consistent with a bradycardia.

### 7. INTERPRETATION

Sinus bradycardia

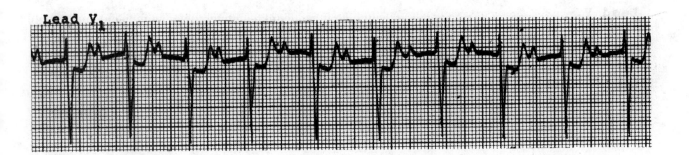

Lead V₁

Figure 1-36A

# ECG RHYTHM STRIP #36

## 1. RHYTHM

Atrial:

Ventricular:

## 2. RATE

Atrial:

Ventricular:

## 3. P WAVE

Presence:

Appearance:

Consistency:

Relation to QRS:

## 4. P-R INTERVAL

Duration:

Consistency:

## 5. QRS COMPLEX

Presence:

Appearance:

Consistency:

Duration:

## 6. DATA ANALYSIS

## 7. INTERPRETATION

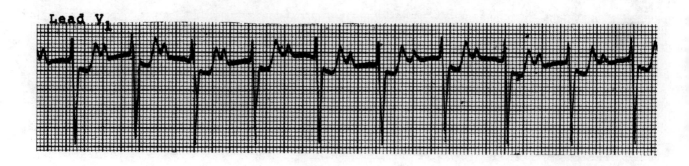

Figure 1-36B

# ECG RHYTHM STRIP #36

## I. RHYTHM

Atrial: Regular

Ventricular: Regular

## 2. RATE

Atrial: 90

Ventricular: 90

## 3. P WAVE

Presence: Yes

Appearance: Normal

Consistency: Consistent

Relation to QRS: 1:1

## 4. P-R INTERVAL

Duration: 0.32 seconds

Consistency: Consistent

## 5. QRS COMPLEX

Presence: Yes

Appearance: Normal

Consistency: Consistent

Duration: 0.10 seconds

## 6. DATA ANALYSIS

All values are normal except that the P-R interval is prolonged.

## 7. INTERPRETATION

Sinus rhythm with first degree AV block

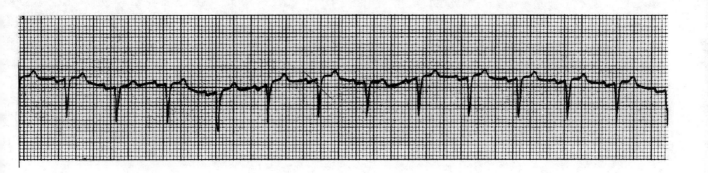

Figure 1-37A

# ECG RHYTHM STRIP #37

## I. RHYTHM

Atrial:

Ventricular:

## 2. RATE

Atrial:

Ventricular:

## 3. P WAVE

Presence:

Appearance:

Consistency:

Relation to QRS:

## 4. P-R INTERVAL

Duration:

Consistency:

## 5. QRS COMPLEX

Presence:

Appearance:

Consistency:

Duration:

## 6. DATA ANALYSIS

## 7. INTERPRETATION

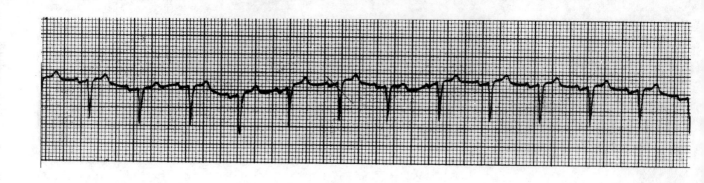

Figure 1-37B

# ECG RHYTHM STRIP #37

## I. RHYTHM

Atrial: Regular

Ventricular: Regular

## 2. RATE

Atrial: 104

Ventricular: 104

## 3. P WAVE

Presence: Yes

Appearance: Normal

Consistency: Consistent

Relation to QRS: 1:1

## 4. P-R INTERVAL

Duration: 0.14 seconds

Consistency: Consistent

## 5. QRS COMPLEX

Presence: Yes

Appearance: Normal

Consistency: Consistent

Duration: 0.08 seconds

## 6. DATA ANALYSIS

All values are normal except the rates are over 100 per minute.

## 7. INTERPRETATION

Sinus tachycardia

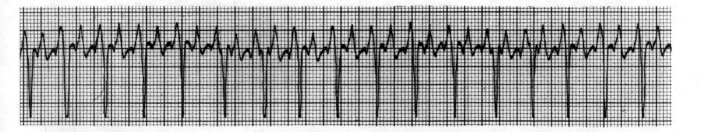

Figure 1-38A

# ECG RHYTHM STRIP #38

## 1. RHYTHM

Atrial:

Ventricular:

## 2. RATE

Atrial:

Ventricular:

## 3. P WAVE

Presence:

Appearance:

Consistency:

Relation to QRS:

## 4. P-R INTERVAL

Duration:

Consistency:

## 5. QRS COMPLEX

Presence:

Appearance:

Consistency:

Duration:

## 6. DATA ANALYSIS

## 7. INTERPRETATION

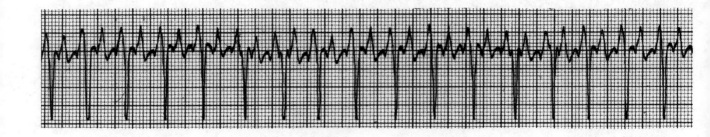

Figure 1-38B

# ECG RHYTHM STRIP #38

## I. RHYTHM

Atrial: Regular

Ventricular: Regular

## 2. RATE

Atrial: 280

Ventricular: 140

## 3. P WAVE

Presence: Yes

Appearance: Sharply pointed sawtooth

Consistency: Consistent

Relation to QRS: 2:1

## 4. P-R INTERVAL

Duration: Unable to determine

Consistency: —

## 5. QRS COMPLEX

Presence: Yes

Appearance: Normal

Consistency: Consistent

Duration: 0.06 seconds

## 6. DATA ANALYSIS

The atrial rate is extremely rapid and is twice the ventricular rate. P waves are replaced by a sawtooth pattern that partially merges with some of the QRS complexes. The atrial rhythm is precisely regular rather than "essentially" regular as it usually is in sinus rhythm. The AV conduction ratio remains constant at 2:1.

## 7. INTERPRETATION

Atrial flutter with a constant 2:1 AV conduction ratio

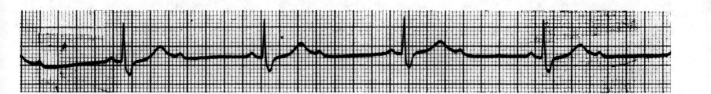

Figure 1-39A

# ECG RHYTHM STRIP #39

## 1. RHYTHM

Atrial:

Ventricular:

## 2. RATE

Atrial:

Ventricular:

## 3. P WAVE

Presence:

Appearance:

Consistency:

Relation to QRS:

## 4. P-R INTERVAL

Duration:

Consistency:

## 5. QRS COMPLEX

Presence:

Appearance:

Consistency:

Duration:

## 6. DATA ANALYSIS

## 7. INTERPRETATION

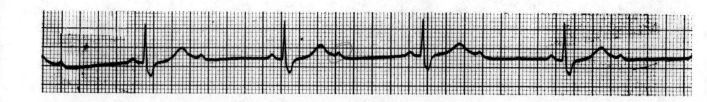

Figure 1-39B

# ECG RHYTHM STRIP #39

## I. RHYTHM

Atrial: Regular

Ventricular: Regular

## 2. RATE

Atrial: 80

Ventricular: 40

## 3. P WAVE

Presence: Yes

Appearance: Normal

Consistency: Consistent

Relation to QRS: 2:1

## 4. P-R INTERVAL

Duration: 0.16 seconds

Consistency: Consistent

## 5. QRS COMPLEX

Presence: Yes

Appearance: Normal—widened

Consistency: Consistent

Duration: 0.12 seconds

## 6. DATA ANALYSIS

The atrial rhythm and rate are normal. The ventricular rhythm is regular, but the rate is half that of the atria. Two P waves precede each QRS complex. The P-R interval of all conducted beats remains constant. The faster atrial rate suggests the presence of AV block. The constant P-R interval of the conducted beats negates the presence of a complete AV block. There are no instances of a complete AV block. There are no instances of 2 or more consecutively conducted beats, making a more definitive determination impossible.

## 7. INTERPRETATION

Sinus rhythm with second degree AV block and constant 2:1 conduction ratios. Since there are no examples of 2 or more consecutively conducted beats, cannot distinguish Mobitz 1 from Mobitz II. An intraventricular conduction delay is present.

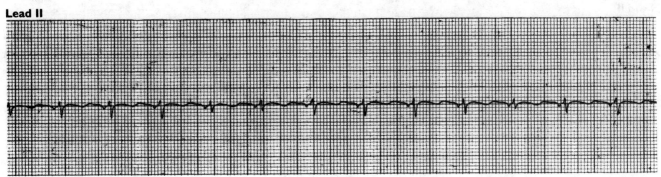

Figure 1-40A

## ECG RHYTHM STRIP #40

**1. RHYTHM**

  Atrial:

  Ventricular:

**2. RATE**

  Atrial:

  Ventricular:

**3. P WAVE**

  Presence:

  Appearance:

  Consistency:

  Relation to QRS:

**4. P-R INTERVAL**

  Duration:

  Consistency:

**5. QRS COMPLEX**

  Presence:

  Appearance:

  Consistency:

  Duration:

**6. DATA ANALYSIS**

**7. INTERPRETATION**

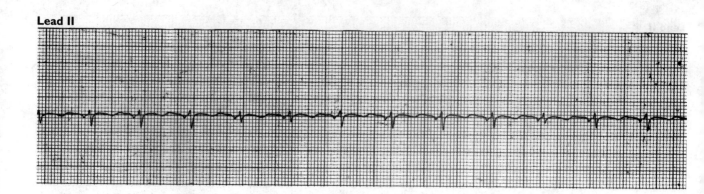

**Lead II**

Figure 1-40B

## ECG RHYTHM STRIP #40

### I. RHYTHM

Atrial: Regular

Ventricular: Regular

### 2. RATE

Atrial: 100

Ventricular: 100

### 3. P WAVE

Presence: Yes

Appearance: Negative deflection in Lead II

Consistency: Consistent

Relation to QRS: 1:1

### 4. P-R INTERVAL

Duration: 0.07 seconds

Consistency: Consistent

### 5. QRS COMPLEX

Presence: Yes

Appearance: Normal

Consistency: Consistent

Duration: 0.07 seconds

### 6. DATA ANALYSIS

All values are normal except that the P waves are negative deflections in a lead where they are normally positive. This suggests retrograde atrial depolarization, further supported by the shortened P-R interval. The QRS of normal duration indicates the rhythm has a supraventricular origin. Junctional rhythms normally have rates between 40 and 60 per minute.

### 7. INTERPRETATION

Junctional tachycardia (accelerated junctional rhythm)

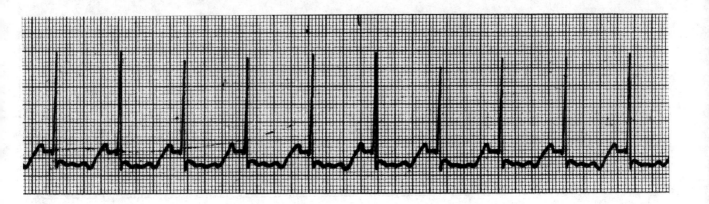

Figure 1-41A

# ECG RHYTHM STRIP #41

## 1. RHYTHM

Atrial:

Ventricular:

## 2. RATE

Atrial:

Ventricular:

## 3. P WAVE

Presence:

Appearance:

Consistency:

Relation to QRS:

## 4. P-R INTERVAL

Duration:

Consistency:

## 5. QRS COMPLEX

Presence:

Appearance:

Consistency:

Duration:

## 6. DATA ANALYSIS

## 7. INTERPRETATION

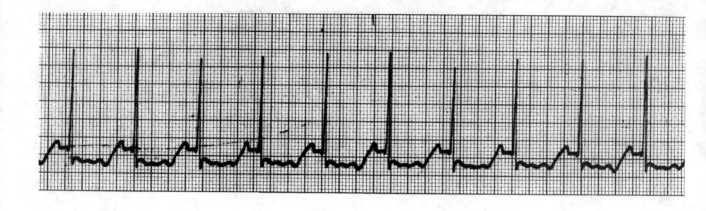

Figure 1-41B

# ECG RHYTHM STRIP #41

## I. RHYTHM

Atrial: Regular

Ventricular: Regular

## 2. RATE

Atrial: 84

Ventricular: 84

## 3. P WAVE

Presence: Yes

Appearance: Normal; onset hard to distinguish

Consistency: Consistent

Relation to QRS: 1:1

## 4. P-R INTERVAL

Duration: 0.16 seconds

Consistency: Consistent

## 5. QRS COMPLEX

Presence: Yes

Appearance: Normal

Consistency: Consistent

Duration: 0.08 seconds

## 6. DATA ANALYSIS

All values are within normal limits. The irregular baseline (S-T segment and T wave) preceding each P wave should not be confused with the distinct P wave located before each QRS complex.

## 7. INTERPRETATION

(Normal) Sinus rhythm

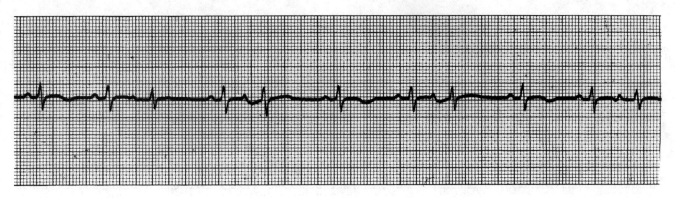

Figure 1-42A

# ECG RHYTHM STRIP #42

**1. RHYTHM**

    Atrial:

    Ventricular:

**2. RATE**

    Atrial:

    Ventricular:

**3. P WAVE**

    Presence:

    Appearance:

    Consistency:

    Relation to QRS:

**4. P-R INTERVAL**

    Duration:

    Consistency:

**5. QRS COMPLEX**

    Presence:

    Appearance:

    Consistency:

    Duration:

**6. DATA ANALYSIS**

**7. INTERPRETATION**

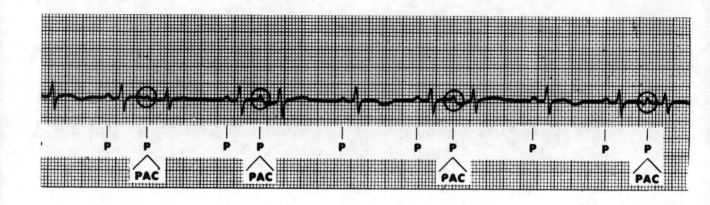

Figure 1-42B

# ECG RHYTHM STRIP #42

## I. RHYTHM

Atrial: Irregular

Ventricular: Irregular

## 2. RATE

Atrial: 80

Ventricular: 80

## 3. P WAVE

Presence: Yes

Appearance: Two types: normal with underlying rhythm and a variant with early beats

Consistency: Inconsistent

Relation to QRS: 1:1

## 4. P-R INTERVAL

Duration: 0.16 seconds in normal P waves: 0.24 seconds in premature P waves

Consistency: Inconsistent

## 5. QRS COMPLEX

Presence: Yes

Appearance: Normal

Consistency: Consistent

Duration: 0.08 seconds

## 6. DATA ANALYSIS

There is a basic underlying rhythm that is disrupted by premature P-QRS cycles where the P wave differs from the sinus P wave and the P-R interval lengthens. These early P waves suggest ectopic atrial activity. The premature atrial activity may occur so early that the impulse finds the AV junction not quite capable (refractory) of conducting as quickly as it normally would. This would prolong the P-R interval of the early P-QRS cycles.

## 7. INTERPRETATION

Sinus rhythm with PACs

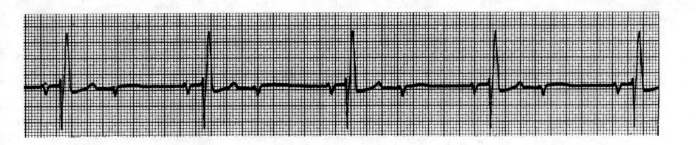

Figure 1-43A

# ECG RHYTHM STRIP #43

## I. RHYTHM

Atrial:

Ventricular:

## 2. RATE

Atrial:

Ventricular:

## 3. P WAVE

Presence:

Appearance:

Consistency:

Relation to QRS:

## 4. P-R INTERVAL

Duration:

Consistency:

## 5. QRS COMPLEX

Presence:

Appearance:

Consistency:

Duration:

## 6. DATA ANALYSIS

## 7. INTERPRETATION

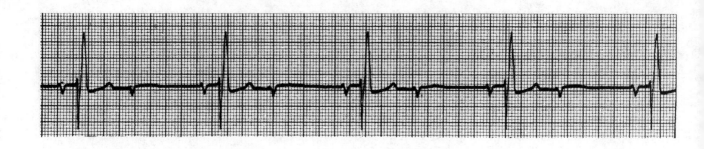

Figure 1-43B

# ECG RHYTHM STRIP #43

## I. RHYTHM

Atrial: Regular

Ventricular: Regular

## 2. RATE

Atrial: 64

Ventricular: 32

## 3. P WAVE

Presence: Yes

Appearance: Normal—variant

Consistency: Consistent

Relation to QRS: 2:1

## 4. P-R INTERVAL

Duration: 0.24 seconds

Consistency: Consistent

## 5. QRS COMPLEX

Presence: Yes

Appearance: Abnormal (rSR' pattern)

Consistency: Consistent

Duration: 0.16 seconds

## 6. DATA ANALYSIS

The ventricular rate is half the atrial rate and is very slow at 32 per minute. There are two P waves for each QRS. On the conducted beats, the P-R interval remains constant at a prolonged duration of 0.24 seconds. No instances of 2 consecutively conducted beats are present, limiting the ability to distinguish between the forms of 2nd degree AV block. The QRS duration is prolonged, suggesting block located below the level of the AV junction.

## 7. INTERPRETATION

Sinus rhythm with 1st degree and 2nd degree AV block with 2:1 AV conduction ratios and an intraventricular conduction delay.

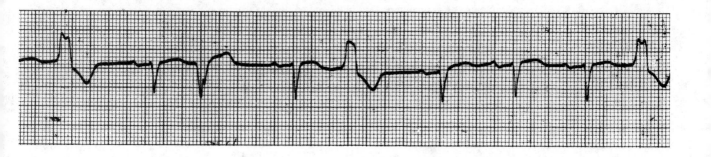

Figure 1-44A

# ECG RHYTHM STRIP #44

**I. RHYTHM**

Atrial:

Ventricular:

**2. RATE**

Atrial:

Ventricular:

**3. P WAVE**

Presence:

Appearance:

Consistency:

Relation to QRS:

**4. P-R INTERVAL**

Duration:

Consistency:

**5. QRS COMPLEX**

Presence:

Appearance:

Consistency:

Duration:

**6. DATA ANALYSIS**

**7. INTERPRETATION**

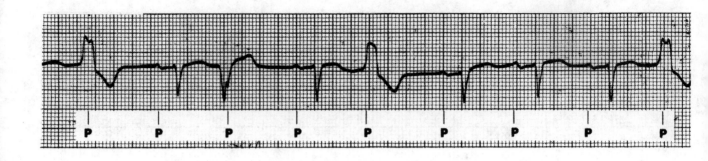

Figure 1-44B

## ECG RHYTHM STRIP #44

### I. RHYTHM

Atrial: Regular

Ventricular: Irregular

### 2. RATE

Atrial: 75

Ventricular: 75

### 3. P WAVE

Presence: Yes

Appearance: Normal

Consistency: Consistent

Relation to QRS: 1:1 except with premature QRS complexes

### 4. P-R INTERVAL

Duration: 0.22 seconds

Consistency: Consistent

### 5. QRS COMPLEX

Presence: Yes

Appearance: Normal and three types of abnormal

Consistency: Inconsistent

Duration: 0.10 seconds in sinus beats; 0.16 seconds in premature beats

### 6. DATA ANALYSIS

The atrial rate, rhythm, and P waves are normal, indicating an underlying sinus rhythm. Some P waves are obscured by the early QRS complexes, but the P-P does "march out." The 1st, 3rd, 5th, and 9th QRS complexes are premature, wide, bizarre, and not preceded by a P wave; these early QRS complexes differ from one another in their configuration. The QRS duration of the sinus beats is at the upper limit of normal.

### 7. INTERPRETATION

Sinus rhythm with first degree AV block and frequent multiform PVCs

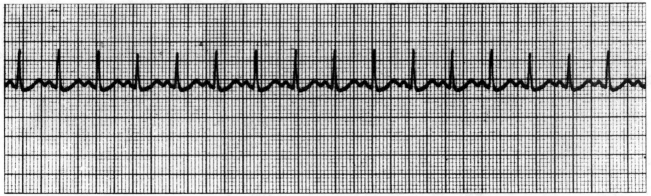

Figure 1-45A

# ECG RHYTHM STRIP #45

## 1. RHYTHM

Atrial:

Ventricular:

## 2. RATE

Atrial:

Ventricular:

## 3. P WAVE

Presence:

Appearance:

Consistency:

Relation to QRS:

## 4. P-R INTERVAL

Duration:

Consistency:

## 5. QRS COMPLEX

Presence:

Appearance:

Consistency:

Duration:

## 6. DATA ANALYSIS

## 7. INTERPRETATION

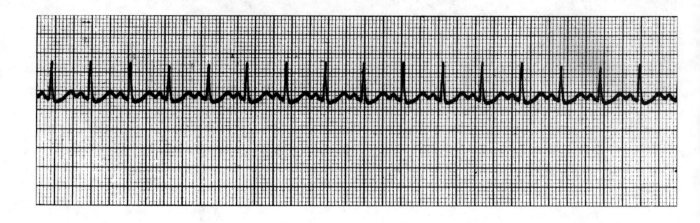

Figure 1-45B

## ECG RHYTHM STRIP #45

### I. RHYTHM

Atrial: Regular

Ventricular: Regular

### 2. RATE

Atrial: 140

Ventricular: 140

### 3. P WAVE

Presence: Yes

Appearance: Normal

Consistency: Consistent

Relation to QRS: 1:1

### 4. P-R INTERVAL

Duration: 0.12 seconds

Consistency: Consistent

### 5. QRS COMPLEX

Presence: Yes

Appearance: Normal

Consistency: Consistent

Duration: 0.06 seconds

### 6. DATA ANALYSIS

All values are normal, except that the rates are 140 per minute.

### 7. INTERPRETATION

Sinus tachycardia

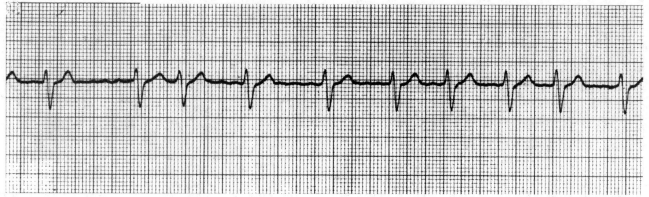

Figure 1-46A

# ECG RHYTHM STRIP #46

**1. RHYTHM**

    Atrial:

    Ventricular:

**2. RATE**

    Atrial:

    Ventricular:

**3. P WAVE**

    Presence:

    Appearance:

    Consistency:

    Relation to QRS:

**4. P-R INTERVAL**

    Duration:

    Consistency:

**5. QRS COMPLEX**

    Presence:

    Appearance:

    Consistency:

    Duration:

**6. DATA ANALYSIS**

**7. INTERPRETATION**

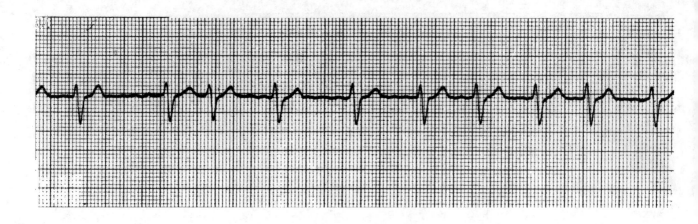

Figure 1-46B

# ECG RHYTHM STRIP #46

## 1. RHYTHM

Atrial: Irregular

Ventricular: Irregularly irregular

## 2. RATE

Atrial: Unable to determine

Ventricular: 90

## 3. P WAVE

Presence: Not as a discrete waveform

Appearance: Replaced by fine fibrillatory waves

Consistency: Inconsistent

Relation to QRS: Unable to determine

## 4. P-R INTERVAL

Duration: Unable to calculate

Consistency: —

## 5. QRS COMPLEX

Presence: Yes

Appearance: Normal—widened

Consistency: Consistent

Duration: 0.11 seconds

## 6. DATA ANALYSIS

P waves are not clearly identifiable, but atrial activity is manifested as wavelike undulations of the baseline that differ from one cycle to another. The QRS duration is prolonged. The ventricular rhythm is irregularly irregular.

## 7. INTERPRETATION

Atrial fibrillation with a controlled ventricular response and an intraventricular conduction defect

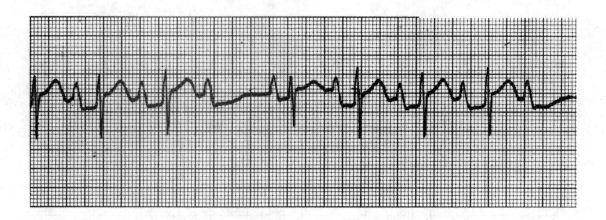

Figure 1-47A

## ECG RHYTHM STRIP #47

**1. RHYTHM**

    Atrial:

    Ventricular:

**2. RATE**

    Atrial:

    Ventricular:

**3. P WAVE**

    Presence:

    Appearance:

    Consistency:

    Relation to QRS:

**4. P-R INTERVAL**

    Duration:

    Consistency:

**5. QRS COMPLEX**

    Presence:

    Appearance:

    Consistency:

    Duration:

**6. DATA ANALYSIS**

**7. INTERPRETATION**

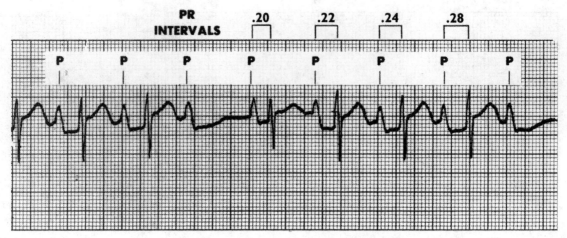

Figure 1-47B

# ECG RHYTHM STRIP #47

## I. RHYTHM

Atrial: Regular

Ventricular: Irregular—group beating

## 2. RATE

Atrial: 85

Ventricular: 70

## 3. P WAVE

Presence: Yes

Appearance: Normal, peaked

Consistency: Consistent

Relation to QRS: 5:4 in "group"

## 4. P-R INTERVAL

Duration: 0.20 to 0.28 seconds

Consistency: Progressively increases until QRS
is dropped

## 5. QRS COMPLEX

Presence: Yes

Appearance: Normal

Consistency: Consistent

Duration: 0.08 seconds

## 6. DATA ANALYSIS

The atrial rate exceeds the ventricular rate, suggesting some form of AV block. The 3rd and 8th P waves are not followed by a QRS complex, indicating these P waves were not conducted. Prior to the nonconducted P waves, the P-R interval progressively increases. The nonconducted P waves create pauses in the rhythm, leading to "group beating"

## 7. INTERPRETATION

Sinus rhythm with second degree AV block–Mobitz Type I (Wenckebach) with 5:4 conduction ratio

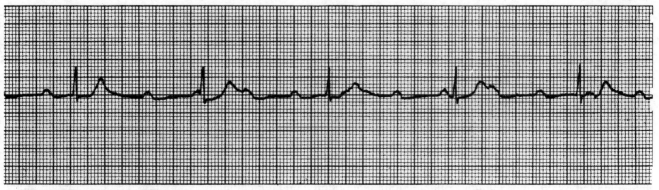

Figure 1-48A

# ECG RHYTHM STRIP #48

## I. RHYTHM

Atrial:

Ventricular:

## 2. RATE

Atrial:

Ventricular:

## 3. P WAVE

Presence:

Appearance:

Consistency:

Relation to QRS:

## 4. P-R INTERVAL

Duration:

Consistency:

## 5. QRS COMPLEX

Presence:

Appearance:

Consistency:

Duration:

## 6. DATA ANALYSIS

## 7. INTERPRETATION

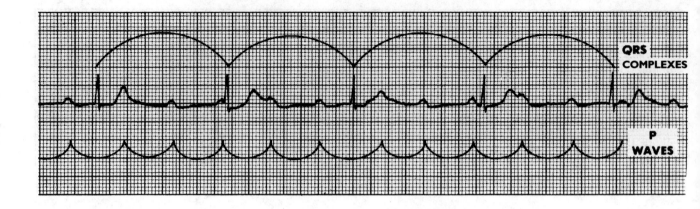

QRS
COMPLEXES

P
WAVES

Figure 1-48B

# ECG RHYTHM STRIP #48

## 1. RHYTHM

Atrial: Regular

Ventricular: Regular

## 2. RATE

Atrial: 110

Ventricular: 40

## 3. P WAVE

Presence: Yes

Appearance: Normal

Consistency: Consistent

Relation to QRS: Variable

## 4. P-R INTERVAL

Duration: Variable

Consistency: Totally inconsistent

## 5. QRS COMPLEX

Presence: Yes

Appearance: Normal

Consistency: Consistent

Duration: 0.06 seconds

## 6. DATA ANALYSIS

Both the atrial and ventricular rhythms are regular but are unrelated to each other. The ventricular rate is less than half of the rapid atrial rate. The variable P-R intervals support that AV dissociation is present, while the slower ventricular rate suggests that the dissociation is attributable to AV block. The QRS of normal duration indicates that the pacemaking site for the ventricles is located in the AV junction.

## 7. INTERPRETATION

Sinus tachycardia with third degree (complete) AV block and a junctional escape rhythm

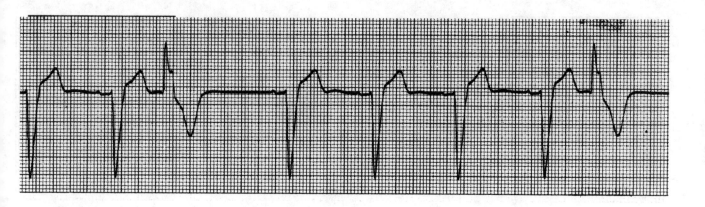
Figure 1-49A

# ECG RHYTHM STRIP #49

**I. RHYTHM**

    Atrial:

    Ventricular:

**2. RATE**

    Atrial:

    Ventricular:

**3. P WAVE**

    Presence:

    Appearance:

    Consistency:

    Relation to QRS:

**4. P-R INTERVAL**

    Duration:

    Consistency:

**5. QRS COMPLEX**

    Presence:

    Appearance:

    Consistency:

    Duration:

**6. DATA ANALYSIS**

**7. INTERPRETATION**

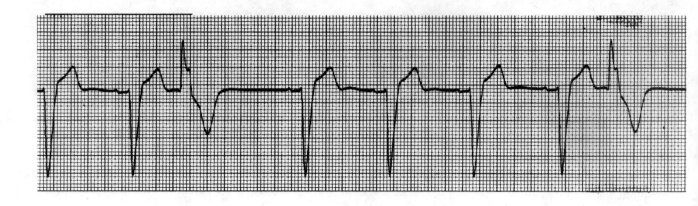

Figure 1-49B

## ECG RHYTHM STRIP #49

### 1. RHYTHM

Atrial: Regular

Ventricular: Irregular

### 2. RATE

Atrial: 60

Ventricular: 60 basic rhythm; 70 with ectopic beats

### 3. P WAVE

Presence: Yes

Appearance: Normal

Consistency: Consistent

Relation to QRS: 1:1 except for early QRS cycles

### 4. P-R INTERVAL

Duration: 0.16 seconds

Consistency: Consistent

### 5. QRS COMPLEX

Presence: Yes

Appearance: Normal and abnormal

Consistency: Inconsistent

Duration: 0.16 seconds

### 6. DATA ANALYSIS

The atrial rate and normal P waves are consistent with a sinus rhythm. The QRS complexes of the sinus beats are prolonged in duration, indicating an intraventricular conduction delay. The underlying rhythm is disrupted by 2 premature QRS complexes that are wide and bizarre in appearance as compared to the sinus beats. Both premature QRS complexes are similar in their configuration.

### 7. INTERPRETATION

Sinus rhythm with an intraventricular conduction delay and 2 uniform (unifocal) PVCs

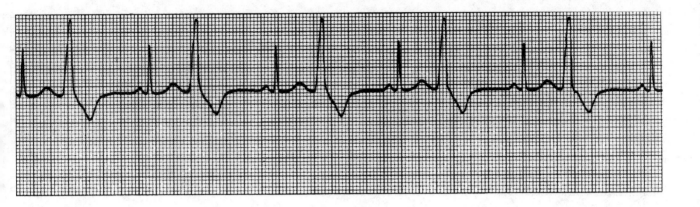

Figure 1-50A

# ECG RHYTHM STRIP #50

## I. RHYTHM

Atrial:

Ventricular:

## 2. RATE

Atrial:

Ventricular:

## 3. P WAVE

Presence:

Appearance:

Consistency:

Relation to QRS:

## 4. P-R INTERVAL

Duration:

Consistency:

## 5. QRS COMPLEX

Presence:

Appearance:

Consistency:

Duration:

## 6. DATA ANALYSIS

## 7. INTERPRETATION

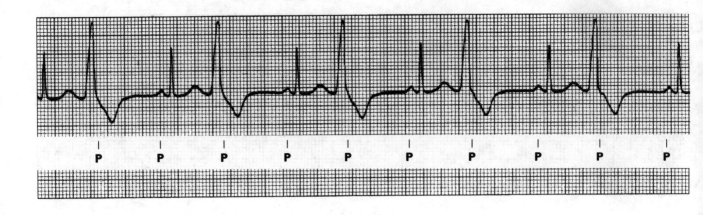

Figure 1-50B

# ECG RHYTHM STRIP #50

## I. RHYTHM

Atrial: Regular

Ventricular: Regularly irregular (pairs)

## 2. RATE

Atrial: 85

Ventricular: 85

## 3. P WAVE

Presence: Yes

Appearance: Normal—every other is hidden in the QRS

Consistency: Consistent

Relation to QRS: 1:1 in sinus beats

## 4. P-R INTERVAL

Duration: 0.14 seconds

Consistency: Consistent

## 5. QRS COMPLEX

Presence: Yes

Appearance: Normal alternates with abnormal

Consistency: Inconsistent

Duration: 0.06 seconds in sinus beats; 0.12 seconds in premature QRS complexes

## 6. DATA ANALYSIS

The atrial rate, rhythm, and P waves are normal, indicating that the underlying rhythm is sinus. Every other QRS complex is widened, abnormal, and premature relative to the sinus rhythm. A pause follows every early QRS complex, resulting in a consistent pattern of paired beats (bigeminy).

## 7. INTERPRETATION

Sinus rhythm with ventricular bigeminy

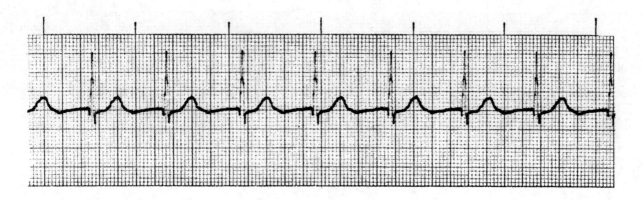

Figure 1-51A

## ECG RHYTHM STRIP #51

**1. RHYTHM**

    Atrial:

    Ventricular:

**2. RATE**

    Atrial:

    Ventricular:

**3. P WAVE**

    Presence:

    Appearance:

    Consistency:

    Relation to QRS:

**4. P-R INTERVAL**

    Duration:

    Consistency:

**5. QRS COMPLEX**

    Presence:

    Appearance:

    Consistency:

    Duration:

**6. DATA ANALYSIS**

**7. INTERPRETATION**

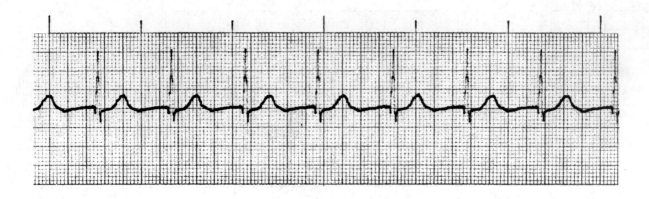

Figure 1-51B

## ECG RHYTHM STRIP #51

### I. RHYTHM

Atrial: Indeterminable

Ventricular: Regular

### 2. RATE

Atrial: Indeterminable

Ventricular: 75

### 3. P WAVE

Presence: None visible—may be hidden in QRS

Appearance: —

Consistency: —

Relation to QRS: —

### 4. P-R INTERVAL

Duration: Indeterminable

Consistency: —

### 5. QRS COMPLEX

Presence: Yes

Appearance: Normal

Consistency: Consistent

Duration: 0.07 seconds

### 6. DATA ANALYSIS

The origin of the rhythm is supraventricular, since the QRS complex is normal. Although we are unable to examine the morphology of the P wave, this must be junctional in origin since the rhythm is regular. The P waves are most likely hidden in the QRS complexes with retrograde atrial depolarization occurring simultaneously with antegrade ventricular depolarization. The rate is faster than the normal junctional rate of 40 to 60.

### 7. INTERPRETATION

Junctional tachycardia (accelerated junctional rhythm)

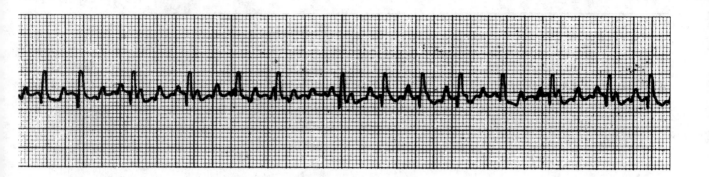

Figure 1-52A

# ECG RHYTHM STRIP #52

**1. RHYTHM**

    Atrial:

    Ventricular:

**2. RATE**

    Atrial:

    Ventricular:

**3. P WAVE**

    Presence:

    Appearance:

    Consistency:

    Relation to QRS:

**4. P-R INTERVAL**

    Duration:

    Consistency:

**5. QRS COMPLEX**

    Presence:

    Appearance:

    Consistency:

    Duration:

**6. DATA ANALYSIS**

**7. INTERPRETATION**

105

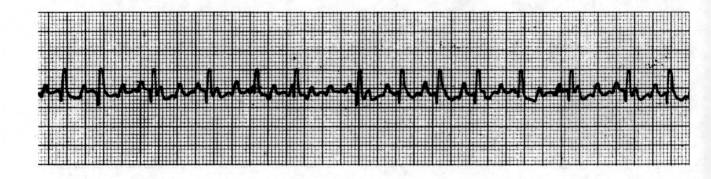

Figure 1-52B

# ECG RHYTHM STRIP #52

## I. RHYTHM

Atrial: Regular

Ventricular: Irregular

## 2. RATE

Atrial: 280

Ventricular: 120

## 3. P WAVE

Presence: Not as a single discrete P wave

Appearance: Sawtooth waves

Consistency: Consistent

Relation to QRS: Varies between 2:1 and 3:1

## 4. P-R INTERVAL

Duration: Unable to calculate

Consistency: —

## 5. QRS COMPLEX

Presence: Yes

Appearance: Normal-sawtooth distorts QRS complex at times

Consistency: Consistent when not distorted by sawtooth waves

Duration: 0.08 seconds

## 6. DATA ANALYSIS

The atrial rate is very rapid and much faster than the ventricular rate, suggesting AV block. The rapidity of the atrial rate, however, supports that the AV block is likely physiological rather than pathological. Atrial activity is manifested by the sawtooth pattern seen in flutter; the atrial rate is also consistent with atrial flutter. The AV junction physiologically blocks every 2nd or 3rd atrial impulse, resulting in AV conduction ratios of 2:1 and 3:1.

## 7. INTERPRETATION

Atrial flutter with variable (2:1 and 3:1) AV conduction ratios

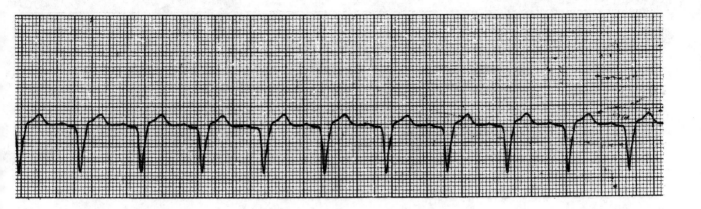

Figure 1-53A

# ECG RHYTHM STRIP #53

## 1. RHYTHM

Atrial:

Ventricular:

## 2. RATE

Atrial:

Ventricular:

## 3. P WAVE

Presence:

Appearance:

Consistency:

Relation to QRS:

## 4. P-R INTERVAL

Duration:

Consistency:

## 5. QRS COMPLEX

Presence:

Appearance:

Consistency:

Duration:

## 6. DATA ANALYSIS

## 7. INTERPRETATION

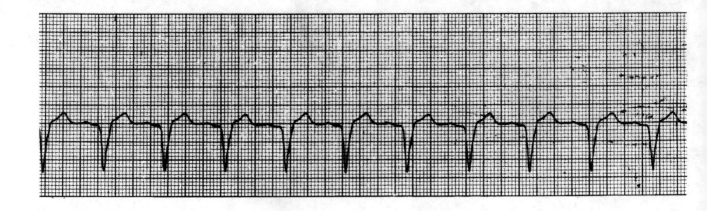

Figure 1-53B

## ECG RHYTHM STRIP #53

### I. RHYTHM

Atrial:  Regular

Ventricular:  Regular

### 2. RATE

Atrial:  90

Ventricular:  90

### 3. P WAVE

Presence:  Yes

Appearance:  Normal

Consistency:  Consistent

Relation to QRS:  1:1

### 4. P-R INTERVAL

Duration:  0.18 seconds

Consistency:  Consistent

### 5. QRS COMPLEX

Presence:  Yes

Appearance:  Normal—wide

Consistency:  Consistent

Duration:  0.14 seconds

### 6. DATA ANALYSIS

All values are within normal limits except for the prolonged QRS duration.

### 7. INTERPRETATION

Sinus rhythm with an intraventricular conduction delay

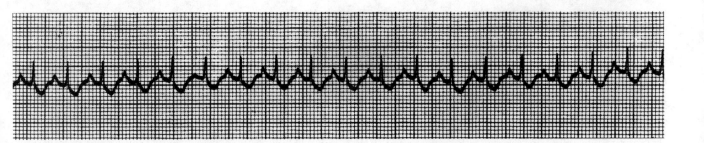

Figure 1-54A

# ECG RHYTHM STRIP #54

## 1. RHYTHM

Atrial:

Ventricular:

## 2. RATE

Atrial:

Ventricular:

## 3. P WAVE

Presence:

Appearance:

Consistency:

Relation to QRS:

## 4. P-R INTERVAL

Duration:

Consistency:

## 5. QRS COMPLEX

Presence:

Appearance:

Consistency:

Duration:

## 6. DATA ANALYSIS

## 7. INTERPRETATION

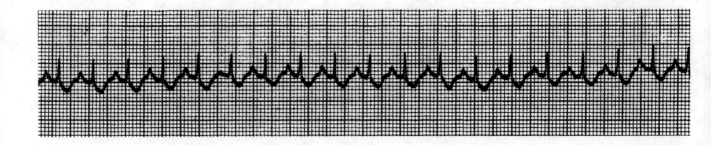

Figure 1-54B

# ECG RHYTHM STRIP #54

## 1. RHYTHM

Atrial: Regular

Ventricular: Regular

## 2. RATE

Atrial: 150

Ventricular: 150

## 3. P WAVE

Presence: Yes

Appearance: Normal

Consistency: Consistent

Relation to QRS: 1:1

## 4. P-R INTERVAL

Duration: 0.14 seconds

Consistency: Consistent

## 5. QRS COMPLEX

Presence: Yes

Appearance: Normal

Consistency: Consistent

Duration: 0.04 seconds

## 6. DATA ANALYSIS

Values are all within normal limits, except that the rates are over 100 per minute. This appears to be a sinus tachycardia since normal P waves precede each QRS complex. Since this is a rhythm strip, however, the exact origin of this supraventricular rhythm should be confirmed by a 12 lead ECG. The QRS of normal duration indicates that this tachycardia originates above the ventricles.

## 7. INTERPRETATION

Supraventricular tachycardia

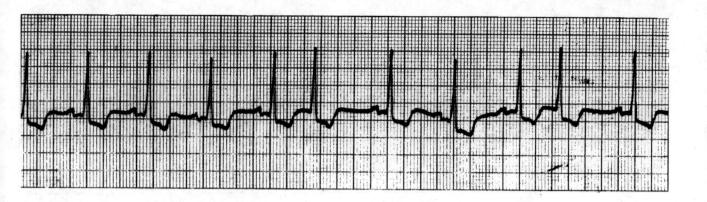

Figure 1-55A

# ECG RHYTHM STRIP #55

**1. RHYTHM**

    Atrial:

    Ventricular:

**2. RATE**

    Atrial:

    Ventricular:

**3. P WAVE**

    Presence:

    Appearance:

    Consistency:

    Relation to QRS:

**4. P-R INTERVAL**

    Duration:

    Consistency:

**5. QRS COMPLEX**

    Presence:

    Appearance:

    Consistency:

    Duration:

**6. DATA ANALYSIS**

**7. INTERPRETATION**

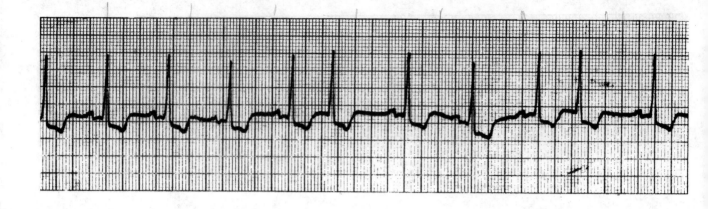

Figure 1-55B

# ECG RHYTHM STRIP #55

## I. RHYTHM

Atrial: Irregular

Ventricular: Irregular

## 2. RATE

Atrial: 80

Ventricular: 90

## 3. P WAVE

Presence: Yes

Appearance: Normal

Consistency: Some variation likely due to tracing artifact

Relation to QRS: 1:1 except in premature beats

## 4. P-R INTERVAL

Duration: 0.18 seconds

Consistency: Consistent

## 5. QRS COMPLEX

Presence: Yes

Appearance: Normal

Consistency: Consistent

Duration: 0.08 seconds

## 6. DATA ANALYSIS

The underlying rhythm is sinus as evidenced by normal rate and P waves. Two premature QRS complexes (cycles 6 and 10) interrupt the basic rhythm. These premature QRS complexes are similar to the sinus complexes in appearance and duration; they are not preceded by any evidence of atrial activity, suggesting a probable junctional origin.

## 7. INTERPRETATION

Sinus rhythm with 2 premature junctional beats (PJCs)

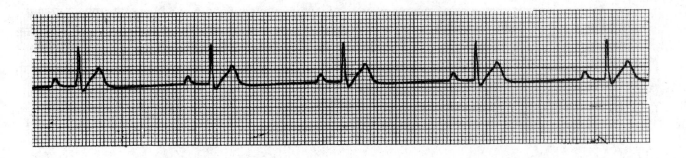

Figure 1-56A

# ECG RHYTHM STRIP #56

**I. RHYTHM**

Atrial:

Ventricular:

**2. RATE**

Atrial:

Ventricular:

**3. P WAVE**

Presence:

Appearance:

Consistency:

Relation to QRS:

**4. P-R INTERVAL**

Duration:

Consistency:

**5. QRS COMPLEX**

Presence:

Appearance:

Consistency:

Duration:

**6. DATA ANALYSIS**

**7. INTERPRETATION**

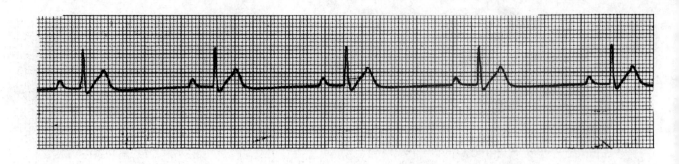

Figure 1-56B

# ECG RHYTHM STRIP #56

## I. RHYTHM

Atrial: Regular

Ventricular: Regular

## 2. RATE

Atrial: 40

Ventricular: 40

## 3. P WAVE

Presence: Yes

Appearance: Normal

Consistency: Consistent

Relation to QRS: 1:1

## 4. P-R INTERVAL

Duration: 0.26 seconds

Consistency: Consistent

## 5. QRS COMPLEX

Presence: Yes

Appearance: Normal

Consistency: Consistent

Duration: 0.09 seconds

## 6. DATA ANALYSIS

Both the atrial and ventricular rates are very slow. The P-R interval is prolonged. The peculiar peaking of the T waves raises the possibility of a superimposed second and premature P wave which is not conducted to the ventricles (nonconducted PAC). A 12 lead ECG would be helpful to clarify this.

## 7. INTERPRETATION

Sinus bradycardia with first degree AV block. Rule out atrial bigeminy with nonconducted PACs.

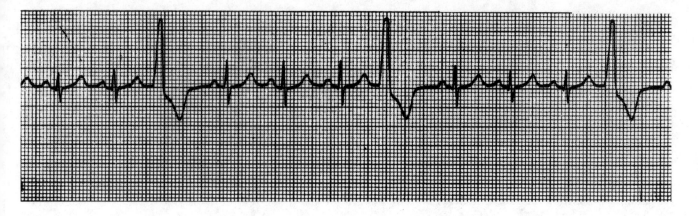

Figure 1-57A

## ECG RHYTHM STRIP #57

**1. RHYTHM**

    Atrial:

    Ventricular:

**2. RATE**

    Atrial:

    Ventricular:

**3. P WAVE**

    Presence:

    Appearance:

    Consistency:

    Relation to QRS:

**4. P-R INTERVAL**

    Duration:

    Consistency:

**5. QRS COMPLEX**

    Presence:

    Appearance:

    Consistency:

    Duration:

**6. DATA ANALYSIS**

**7. INTERPRETATION**

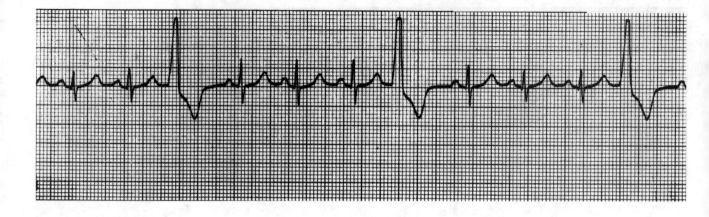

Figure 1-57B

# ECG RHYTHM STRIP #57

## 1. RHYTHM

Atrial: Regular

Ventricular: Irregular

## 2. RATE

Atrial: 100

Ventricular: 100

## 3. P WAVE

Presence: Yes

Appearance: Normal

Consistency: Consistent

Relation to QRS: 1:1 except with premature beats

## 4. P-R INTERVAL

Duration: 0.16 seconds

Consistency: Consistent

## 5. QRS COMPLEX

Presence: Yes

Appearance: Normal and abnormal

Consistency: Inconsistent

Duration: 0.08 seconds with normal; 0.12 seconds with abnormal

## 6. DATA ANALYSIS

Atrial rhythm and P waves are normal, indicating an underlying sinus rhythm. This rhythm is interrupted on three occassions by premature QRS complexes that are prolonged and bizarre with S-T segments and T waves oriented opposite to the major QRS complex waveform; the appearance of these premature beats is consistent with a ventricular origin. The ventricular ectopic beats are similar in appearance and duration.

## 7. INTERPRETATION

Sinus rhythm with frequent uniform (unifocal) PVCs

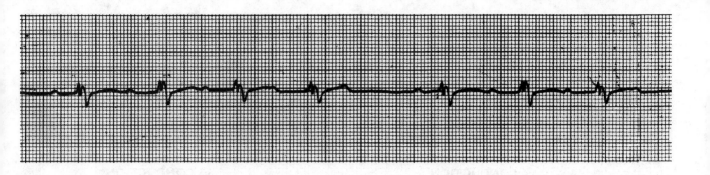

Figure 1-58A

# ECG RHYTHM STRIP #58

## 1. RHYTHM

Atrial:

Ventricular:

## 2. RATE

Atrial:

Ventricular:

## 3. P WAVE

Presence:

Appearance:

Consistency:

Relation to QRS:

## 4. P-R INTERVAL

Duration:

Consistency:

## 5. QRS COMPLEX

Presence:

Appearance:

Consistency:

Duration:

## 6. DATA ANALYSIS

## 7. INTERPRETATION

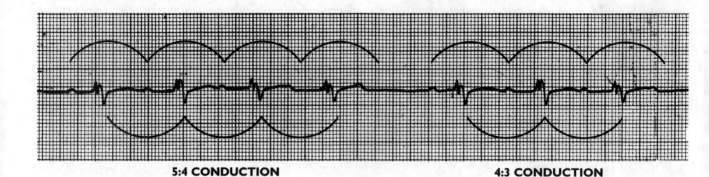

| 5:4 CONDUCTION | 4:3 CONDUCTION |

Figure 1-58B

# ECG RHYTHM STRIP #58

## I. RHYTHM

Atrial: Regular

Ventricular: Irregular (group beating)

## 2. RATE

Atrial: 70

Ventricular: 60

## 3. P WAVE

Presence: Yes

Appearance: Normal

Consistency: Slight variation

Relation to QRS: 5:4 and 4:3

## 4. P-R INTERVAL

Duration: Varies 0.28 to 0.44 seconds

Consistency: Inconsistent—progressively
lengthens

## 5. QRS COMPLEX

Presence: Yes

Appearance: Abnormal

Consistency: Consistent

Duration: 0.15 seconds

## 6. DATA ANALYSIS

The atrial rate, rhythm, and P waves are consistent with an underlying sinus rhythm. The shortest P-R interval is 0.28 seconds. The P-R progressively lengthens over 3 or 4 cycles until a QRS complex is dropped. This is consistent with progressive delay in conduction through the AV junction.

## 7. INTERPRETATION

Sinus rhythm with first degree AV block, second degree AV block, Type I (Wenckebach), and an intraventricular conduction delay

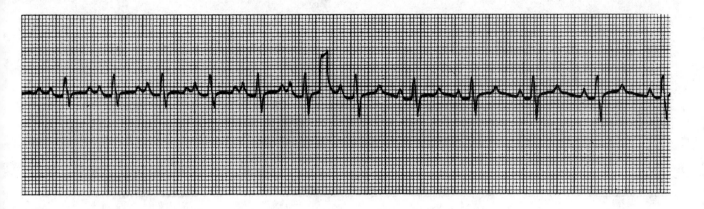

Figure 1-59A

# ECG RHYTHM STRIP #59

## 1. RHYTHM

Atrial:

Ventricular:

## 2. RATE

Atrial:

Ventricular:

## 3. P WAVE

Presence:

Appearance:

Consistency:

Relation to QRS:

## 4. P-R INTERVAL

Duration:

Consistency:

## 5. QRS COMPLEX

Presence:

Appearance:

Consistency:

Duration:

## 6. DATA ANALYSIS

## 7. INTERPRETATION

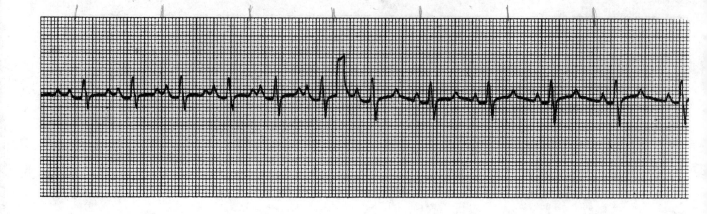

Figure 1-59B

# ECG RHYTHM STRIP #59

## I. RHYTHM

Atrial: Irregular

Ventricular: Irregular (both fast and slow)

## 2. RATE

Atrial: 100

Ventricular: 100 (ECG standard marking between beats 6 and 7)

## 3. P WAVE

Presence: Yes

Appearance: Normal

Consistency: Consistent

Relation to QRS: 1:1

## 4. P-R INTERVAL

Duration: 0.16 seconds

Consistency: Consistent

## 5. QRS COMPLEX

Presence: Yes

Appearance: Normal

Consistency: Consistent

Duration: 0.10 seconds

## 6. DATA ANALYSIS

All values are within normal limits except that the rhythm varies as the rate changes from faster to slower.

## 7. INTERPRETATION

Sinus arrhythmia

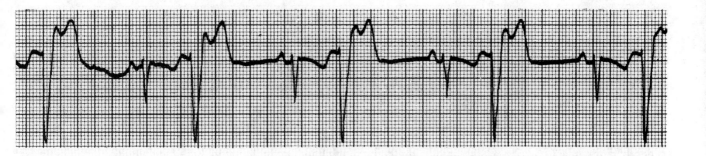

Figure 1-60A

# ECG RHYTHM STRIP #60

**1. RHYTHM**

Atrial:

Ventricular:

**2. RATE**

Atrial:

Ventricular:

**3. P WAVE**

Presence:

Appearance:

Consistency:

Relation to QRS:

**4. P-R INTERVAL**

Duration:

Consistency:

**5. QRS COMPLEX**

Presence:

Appearance:

Consistency:

Duration:

**6. DATA ANALYSIS**

**7. INTERPRETATION**

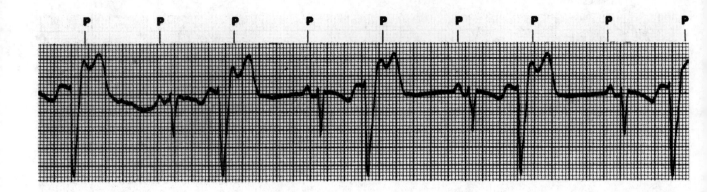

Figure 1-60B

## ECG RHYTHM STRIP #60

### I. RHYTHM

Atrial: Regular

Ventricular: Regularly irregular

### 2. RATE

Atrial: 70

Ventricular: 70

### 3. P WAVE

Presence: Yes—every other follows early QRS

Appearance: Normal

Consistency: Consistent

Relation to QRS: 1:1 except with premature beats

### 4. P-R INTERVAL

Duration: 0.14 seconds

Consistency: Consistent

### 5. QRS COMPLEX

Presence: Yes

Appearance: Normal alternates with abnormal

Consistency: Alternating pattern is consistent

Duration: 0.10 seconds with normal QRS; 0.14 seconds with abnormal QRS

### 6. DATA ANALYSIS

An alternating pattern of sinus beat and premature ectopic beat exists. The second P wave can be seen immediately following the premature QRS complex. The early ectopic beats are wide and bizarre in comparison with the normal QRS complex.

### 7. INTERPRETATION

Sinus rhythm with ventricular bigeminy

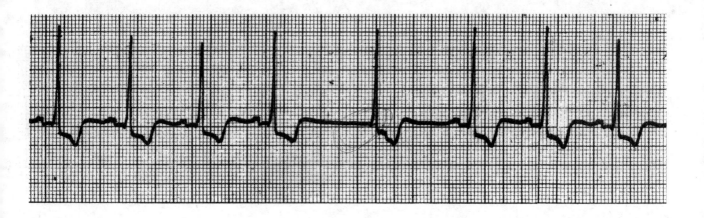

Figure 1-61A

# ECG RHYTHM STRIP #61

## 1. RHYTHM

Atrial:

Ventricular:

## 2. RATE

Atrial:

Ventricular:

## 3. P WAVE

Presence:

Appearance:

Consistency:

Relation to QRS:

## 4. P-R INTERVAL

Duration:

Consistency:

## 5. QRS COMPLEX

Presence:

Appearance:

Consistency:

Duration:

## 6. DATA ANALYSIS

## 7. INTERPRETATION

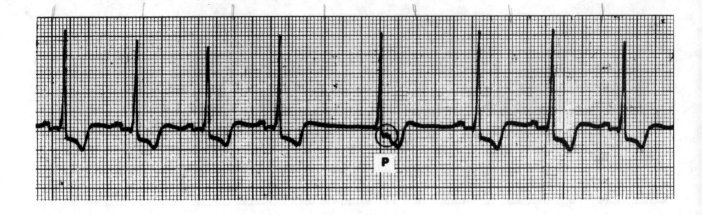

Figure 1-61B

# ECG RHYTHM STRIP #61

## I. RHYTHM

Atrial: Irregular

Ventricular: Irregular

## 2. RATE

Atrial: 70

Ventricular: 70

## 3. P WAVE

Presence: Yes

Appearance: Normal

Consistency: Consistent

Relation to QRS: 1:1, though P wave follows 5th QRS complex

## 4. P-R INTERVAL

Duration: 0.20 seconds

Consistency: Consistent

## 5. QRS COMPLEX

Presence: Yes

Appearance: Normal

Consistency: Consistent

Duration: 0.08 seconds

## 6. DATA ANALYSIS

A sinus rhythm at 75 per minute is interrupted by a pause during which the sinus node fails to fire and a narrow QRS followed by a retrograde P wave appears as an escape beat. The escape beat QRS is identical to that of the sinus QRS complexes. Following this escape beat, sinus rhythm is restored.

## 7. INTERPRETATION

Sinus rhythm with an episode of sinus pause and a junctional escape beat.

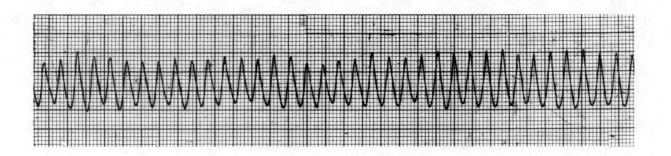

Figure 1-62A

# ECG RHYTHM STRIP #62

## 1. RHYTHM

Atrial:

Ventricular:

## 2. RATE

Atrial:

Ventricular:

## 3. P WAVE

Presence:

Appearance:

Consistency:

Relation to QRS:

## 4. P-R INTERVAL

Duration:

Consistency:

## 5. QRS COMPLEX

Presence:

Appearance:

Consistency:

Duration:

## 6. DATA ANALYSIS

## 7. INTERPRETATION

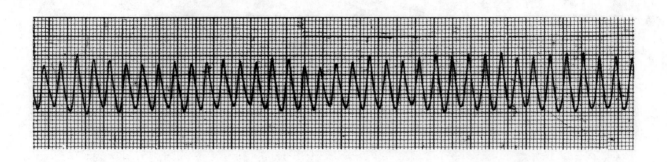

Figure 1-62B

## ECG RHYTHM STRIP #62

### I. RHYTHM

Atrial: Unable to determine

Ventricular: Regular

### 2. RATE

Atrial: Unable to determine

Ventricular: Over 300

### 3. P WAVE

Presence: No

Appearance: —

Consistency: —

Relation to QRS: —

### 4. P-R INTERVAL

Duration: Unable to determine

Consistency: —

### 5. QRS COMPLEX

Presence: Yes

Appearance: Waveforms not identifiable

Consistency: Consistent

Duration: Unable to determine (no identifiable waveforms)

### 6. DATA ANALYSIS

There is no evidence of atrial activity. Ventricular activity is evidenced by wide, sine wave–like complexes where the QRS waveforms are not identifiable. The ventricular rate is extremely rapid.

### 7. INTERPRETATION

Ventricular tachycardia (flutter)

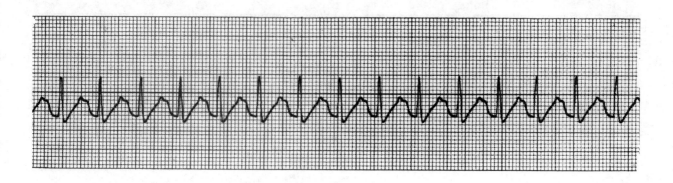

Figure 1-63A

# ECG RHYTHM STRIP #63

**1. RHYTHM**

    Atrial:

    Ventricular:

**2. RATE**

    Atrial:

    Ventricular:

**3. P WAVE**

    Presence:

    Appearance:

    Consistency:

    Relation to QRS:

**4. P-R INTERVAL**

    Duration:

    Consistency:

**5. QRS COMPLEX**

    Presence:

    Appearance:

    Consistency:

    Duration:

**6. DATA ANALYSIS**

**7. INTERPRETATION**

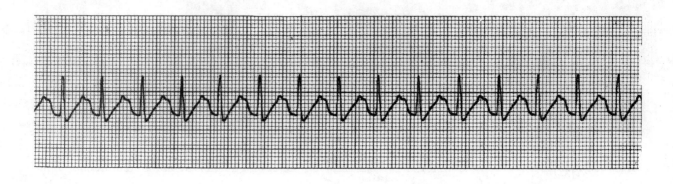

Figure 1-63B

# ECG RHYTHM STRIP #63

## 1. RHYTHM

Atrial: Regular

Ventricular: Regular

## 2. RATE

Atrial: 140

Ventricular: 140

## 3. P WAVE

Presence: Yes

Appearance: Normal—superimposed on preceding T wave

Consistency: Consistent

Relation to QRS: 1:1

## 4. P-R INTERVAL

Duration: 0.20 seconds

Consistency: Consistent

## 5. QRS COMPLEX

Presence: Yes

Appearance: Normal

Consistency: Consistent

Duration: 0.08 seconds

## 6. DATA ANALYSIS

The atrial and ventricular rates are the same, but very rapid. Other values are normal. The exact origin of the atrial mechanism is difficult to determine since P waves are somewhat obscured in the preceding T wave; a 12 lead ECG would be helpful to distinguish this. The QRS is 0.08 seconds in duration, indicating a supraventricular origin.

## 7. INTERPRETATION

Supraventricular tachycardia, probably sinus

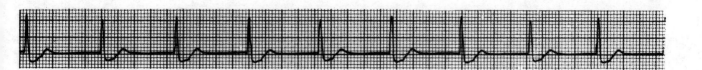

Figure 1-64A

# ECG RHYTHM STRIP #64

## 1. RHYTHM

Atrial:

Ventricular:

## 2. RATE

Atrial:

Ventricular:

## 3. P WAVE

Presence:

Appearance:

Consistency:

Relation to QRS:

## 4. P-R INTERVAL

Duration:

Consistency:

## 5. QRS COMPLEX

Presence:

Appearance:

Consistency:

Duration:

## 6. DATA ANALYSIS

## 7. INTERPRETATION

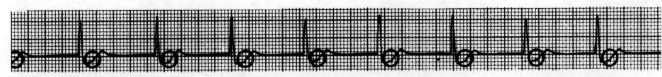

**RETROGRADE P WAVES**

Figure 1-64B

# ECG RHYTHM STRIP #64

## I. RHYTHM

Atrial: Essentially regular

Ventricular: Essentially regular

## 2. RATE

Atrial: 68

Ventricular: 68

## 3. P WAVE

Presence: Yes

Appearance: A negative deflection

Consistency: Consistent

Relation to QRS: 1:1 with P wave following QRS

## 4. P-R INTERVAL

Duration: (R-P) approximately 0.14 seconds

Consistency: Consistent

## 5. QRS COMPLEX

Presence: Yes

Appearance: Normal

Consistency: Consistent

Duration: 0.06 seconds

## 6. DATA ANALYSIS

Ventricular rate and rhythm are normal. Atrial activity is evidenced by P waves that follow the QRS complex with a constant R-P interval. These P waves are negative deflections in a lead (II) where they are normally positive, which further supports their retrograde conduction. The narrow QRS indicates a supraventricular origin.

## 7. INTERPRETATION

Junctional rhythm

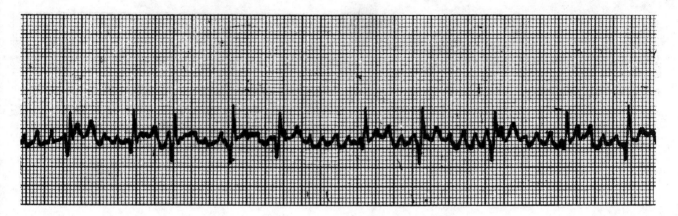

Figure 1-65A

# ECG RHYTHM STRIP #65

**I. RHYTHM**

    Atrial:

    Ventricular:

**2. RATE**

    Atrial:

    Ventricular:

**3. P WAVE**

    Presence:

    Appearance:

    Consistency:

    Relation to QRS:

**4. P-R INTERVAL**

    Duration:

    Consistency:

**5. QRS COMPLEX**

    Presence:

    Appearance:

    Consistency:

    Duration:

**6. DATA ANALYSIS**

**7. INTERPRETATION**

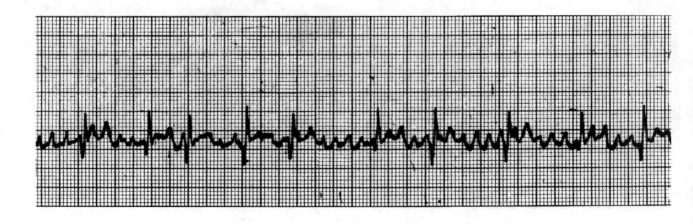

Figure 1-65B

## ECG RHYTHM STRIP #65

### I. RHYTHM

Atrial: Irregular

Ventricular: Irregularly irregular

### 2. RATE

Atrial: Unable to determine precisely

Ventricular: 90

### 3. P WAVE

Presence: Not as a distinct single waveform

Appearance: Coarse fibrillatory and flutter-like waves

Consistency: Vary in size, shape, and number

Relation to QRS: Unable to determine

### 4. P-R INTERVAL

Duration: Unable to determine

Consistency: —

### 5. QRS COMPLEX

Presence: Yes

Appearance: Distorted by fibrillatory waves

Consistency: Vary somewhat due to distortion by fibrillatory waves

Duration: 0.08 seconds

### 6. DATA ANALYSIS

Atrial activity is manifested as irregular waveforms resembling both fibrillatory and flutter waves; these waveforms distort the QRS complex. The atrial rate is rapid and its rhythm is irregular. The ventricular rhythm is irregularly irregular.

### 7. INTERPRETATION

Coarse atrial fibrillation with a controlled ventricular response (Some would refer to this pattern as atrial flutter-fibrillation).

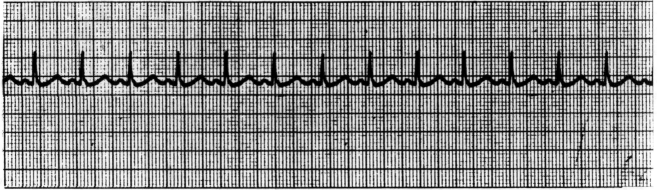

Figure 1-66A

# ECG RHYTHM STRIP #66

## 1. RHYTHM

Atrial:

Ventricular:

## 2. RATE

Atrial:

Ventricular:

## 3. P WAVE

Presence:

Appearance:

Consistency:

Relation to QRS:

## 4. P-R INTERVAL

Duration:

Consistency:

## 5. QRS COMPLEX

Presence:

Appearance:

Consistency:

Duration:

## 6. DATA ANALYSIS

## 7. INTERPRETATION

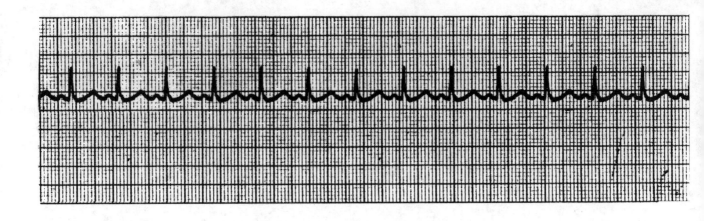

Figure 1-66B

# ECG RHYTHM STRIP #66

## I. RHYTHM

Atrial: Regular

Ventricular: Regular

## 2. RATE

Atrial: 120

Ventricular: 120

## 3. P WAVE

Presence: Yes

Appearance: Normal

Consistency: Consistent

Relation to QRS: 1:1

## 4. P-R INTERVAL

Duration: 0.12 seconds

Consistency: Consistent

## 5. QRS COMPLEX

Presence: Yes

Appearance: Normal

Consistency: Consistent

Duration: 0.06 seconds

## 6. DATA ANALYSIS

All values are within normal limits except the rates are rapid.

## 7. INTERPRETATION

Sinus tachycardia

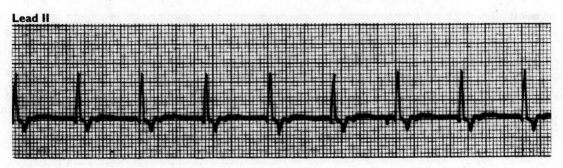

Lead II

Figure 1-67A

## ECG RHYTHM STRIP #67

**1. RHYTHM**

    Atrial:

    Ventricular:

**2. RATE**

    Atrial:

    Ventricular:

**3. P WAVE**

    Presence:

    Appearance:

    Consistency:

    Relation to QRS:

**4. P-R INTERVAL**

    Duration:

    Consistency:

**5. QRS COMPLEX**

    Presence:

    Appearance:

    Consistency:

    Duration:

**6. DATA ANALYSIS**

**7. INTERPRETATION**

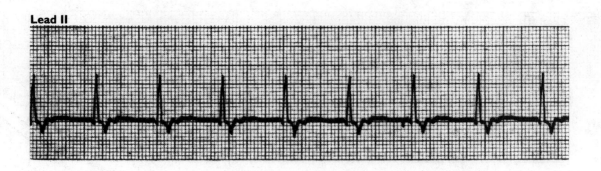

Lead II

Figure 1-67B

# ECG RHYTHM STRIP #67

## I. RHYTHM

Atrial: Regular

Ventricular: Regular

## 2. RATE

Atrial: 90

Ventricular: 90

## 3. P WAVE

Presence: Yes

Appearance: Negative deflection following the QRS complex

Consistency: Consistent

Relation to QRS: 1:1

## 4. P-R INTERVAL

Duration: (R-P interval) 0.12 seconds

Consistency: Consistent

## 5. QRS COMPLEX

Presence: Yes

Appearance: Normal

Consistency: Consistent

Duration: 0.08 seconds

## 6. DATA ANALYSIS

Atrial rate and rhythm are normal. P waves are negative deflections in a lead (II) where they are normally positive deflections; they follow rather than precede the QRS. Additionally, the R-P interval remains constant, confirming the relationship between P waves and the **preceding** QRS complex. These findings together with a QRS of normal duration are consistent with a rhythm of junctional origin. The rates exceed the normal intrinsic juntional rate.

## 7. INTERPRETATION

Junctional tachycardia (accelerated junctional rhythm)

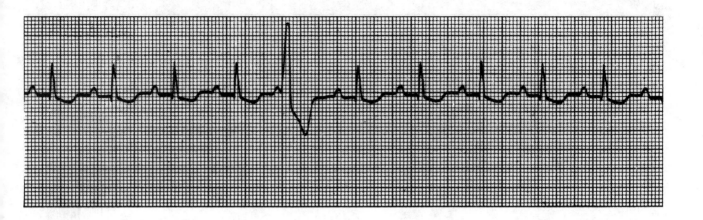

Figure 1-68A

# ECG RHYTHM STRIP #68

**1. RHYTHM**

Atrial:

Ventricular:

**2. RATE**

Atrial:

Ventricular:

**3. P WAVE**

Presence:

Appearance:

Consistency:

Relation to QRS:

**4. P-R INTERVAL**

Duration:

Consistency:

**5. QRS COMPLEX**

Presence:

Appearance:

Consistency:

Duration:

**6. DATA ANALYSIS**

**7. INTERPRETATION**

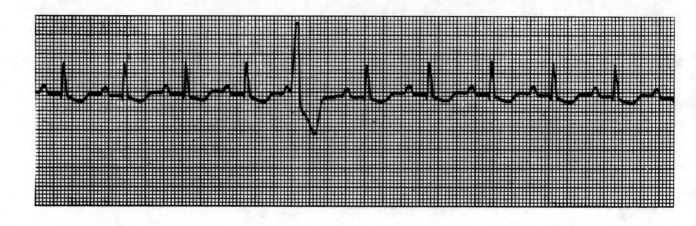

Figure 1-68B

# ECG RHYTHM STRIP #68

## I. RHYTHM

Atrial: Regular

Ventricular: Irregular

## 2. RATE

Atrial: 90

Ventricular: 90

## 3. P WAVE

Presence: Yes

Appearance: Normal

Consistency: Consistent

Relation to QRS: 1:1 except with premature QRS

## 4. P-R INTERVAL

Duration: 0.22 seconds

Consistency: Consistent, with conducted beats

## 5. QRS COMPLEX

Presence: Yes

Appearance: Normal—one is abnormal

Consistency: Consistent except for premature QRS

Duration: 0.08 seconds in normal QRS; 0.12 seconds in premature QRS

## 6. DATA ANALYSIS

Atrial rate and rhythm are normal. The P-R interval is prolonged, indicating delayed conduction through the AV junction. Ventricular rhythm is interrupted by a premature QRS complex that is wide and bizarre in appearance. A P wave precedes the premature QRS but bears no relationship to this QRS since the P-R interval here (0.06 seconds) is too short for the P wave to have been conducted.

## 7. INTERPRETATION

Sinus rhythm with first degree AV block and one PVC

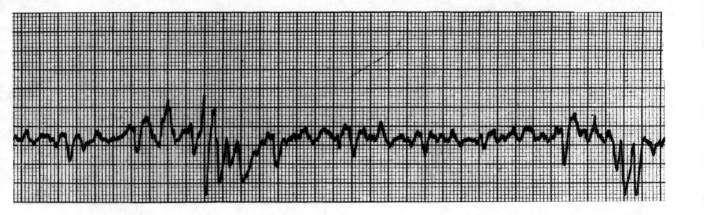

Figure 1-69A

# ECG RHYTHM STRIP #69

**I. RHYTHM**

Atrial:

Ventricular:

**2. RATE**

Atrial:

Ventricular:

**3. P WAVE**

Presence:

Appearance:

Consistency:

Relation to QRS:

**4. P-R INTERVAL**

Duration:

Consistency:

**5. QRS COMPLEX**

Presence:

Appearance:

Consistency:

Duration:

**6. DATA ANALYSIS**

**7. INTERPRETATION**

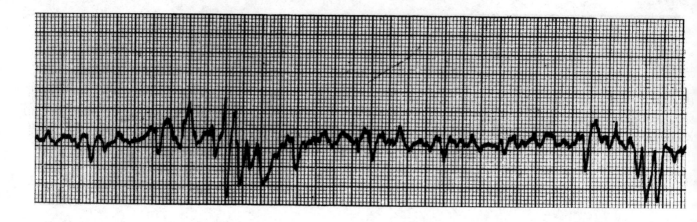

Figure 1-69B

# ECG RHYTHM STRIP #69

## I. RHYTHM

Atrial:  Unable to determine

Ventricular:  Irregular

## 2. RATE

Atrial:  Unable to determine

Ventricular:  Unable to calculate

## 3. P WAVE

Presence:  No evidence of

Appearance: —

Consistency: —

Relation to QRS: —

## 4. P-R INTERVAL

Duration: —

Consistency: —

## 5. QRS COMPLEX

Presence:  Not a distinguishable complex

Appearance:  Coarse, irregular waves of varying size and shape

Consistency:  Inconsistent

Duration:  Unable to calculate

## 6. DATA ANALYSIS

There is no identifiable evidence of atrial activity. Coarse fibrillatory waveforms of varying bizarre configurations appear as the ventricular activity.

## 7. INTERPRETATION

Ventricular fibrillation

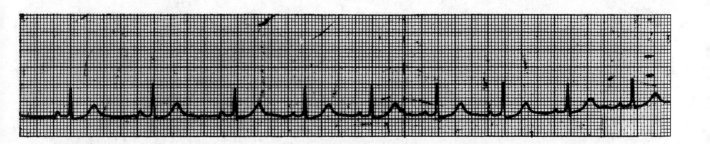

Figure 1-70A

## ECG RHYTHM STRIP #70

**1. RHYTHM**

Atrial:

Ventricular:

**2. RATE**

Atrial:

Ventricular:

**3. P WAVE**

Presence:

Appearance:

Consistency:

Relation to QRS:

**4. P-R INTERVAL**

Duration:

Consistency:

**5. QRS COMPLEX**

Presence:

Appearance:

Consistency:

Duration:

**6. DATA ANALYSIS**

**7. INTERPRETATION**

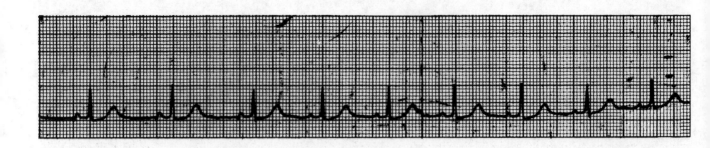

Figure 1-70B

# ECG RHYTHM STRIP #70

## I. RHYTHM

Atrial: Slightly irregular when rate increases

Ventricular: Slightly irregular when rate increases

## 2. RATE

Atrial: 70

Ventricular: 70 (both rates are initially slower then faster)

## 3. P WAVE

Presence: Yes

Appearance: Variants of normal

Consistency: Inconsistent appearance

Relation to QRS: 1:1

## 4. P-R INTERVAL

Duration: 0.16 seconds

Consistency: Consistent

## 5. QRS COMPLEX

Presence: Yes

Appearance: Normal

Consistency: Consistent

Duration: 0.04 seconds

## 6. DATA ANALYSIS

The rate increases slightly and causes the rhythm to be slightly irregular at that time. The P-R interval is normal, but the P waves vary in their configuration, suggesting a changing origin of atrial activity.

## 7. INTERPRETATION

Wandering atrial pacemaker

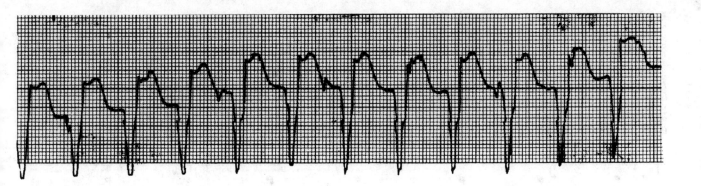

Figure 1-71A

# ECG RHYTHM STRIP #71

## 1. RHYTHM

Atrial:

Ventricular:

## 2. RATE

Atrial:

Ventricular:

## 3. P WAVE

Presence:

Appearance:

Consistency:

Relation to QRS:

## 4. P-R INTERVAL

Duration:

Consistency:

## 5. QRS COMPLEX

Presence:

Appearance:

Consistency:

Duration:

## 6. DATA ANALYSIS

## 7. INTERPRETATION

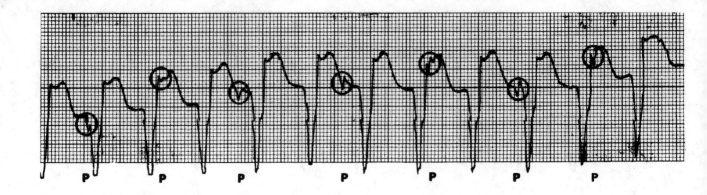

Figure 1-71B

# ECG RHYTHM STRIP #71

## 1. RHYTHM

Atrial: Slightly irregular

Ventricular: Regular

## 2. RATE

Atrial: 60

Ventricular: 100

## 3. P WAVE

Presence: Yes—obscured by QRS

Appearance: Obscured, distorted

Consistency: Generally consistent

Relation to QRS: Unrelated

## 4. P-R INTERVAL

Duration: Varies widely

Consistency: Inconsistent

## 5. QRS COMPLEX

Presence: Yes

Appearance: Prolonged, bizarre

Consistency: Consistent

Duration: 0.16 seconds

## 6. DATA ANALYSIS

Atrial rhythm is slow and slightly irregular; this may be due to a sinus arrhythmia. The ventricular rhythm is regular, however, and much faster that the atrial rate. P waves are difficult to distinguish since most are imbedded in various locations in the QRS complex. P-R intervals vary widely, further suggesting that the atrial and ventricular rhythms are independent of each other. QRS complexes are wide, bizarre, and unrelated to P waves.

## 7. INTERPRETATION

Ventricular tachycardia (accelerated idioventricular rhythm)

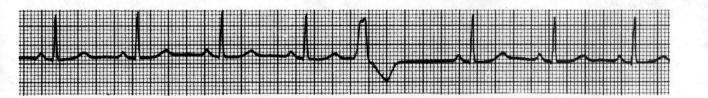

Figure 1-72A

# ECG RHYTHM STRIP #72

## 1. RHYTHM

Atrial:

Ventricular:

## 2. RATE

Atrial:

Ventricular:

## 3. P WAVE

Presence:

Appearance:

Consistency:

Relation to QRS:

## 4. P-R INTERVAL

Duration:

Consistency:

## 5. QRS COMPLEX

Presence:

Appearance:

Consistency:

Duration:

## 6. DATA ANALYSIS

## 7. INTERPRETATION

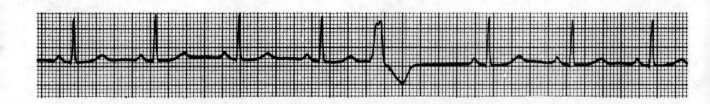

Figure 1-72B

# ECG RHYTHM STRIP #72

## I. RHYTHM

Atrial: Regular

Ventricular: Irregular

## 2. RATE

Atrial: 68

Ventricular: 68

## 3. P WAVE

Presence: Yes

Appearance: Normal

Consistency: Consistent

Relation to QRS: 1:1 (immediately follows premature QRS)

## 4. P-R INTERVAL

Duration: 0.17 seconds

Consistency: Consistent

## 5. QRS COMPLEX

Presence: Yes

Appearance: Normal—1 abnormal

Consistency: 1 inconsistency

Duration: 0.08 seconds in normal QRS; 0.16 seconds in premature QRS

## 6. DATA ANALYSIS

Atrial rate, rhythm, and P waves are normal, indicating a sinus rhythm. Ventricular rhythm is disrupted by a premature, wide, and bizarre QRS complex. A normal P wave exists in the S-T segment immediately following the premature QRS, indicating an undisturbed sinus rhythm.

## 7. INTERPRETATION

Sinus rhythm with one PVC

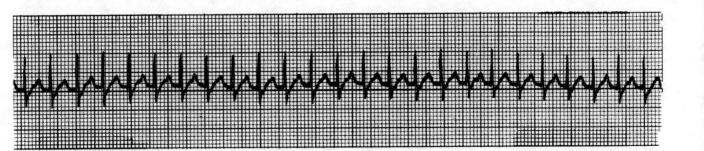

Figure 1-73A

# ECG RHYTHM STRIP #73

## I. RHYTHM

Atrial:

Ventricular:

## 2. RATE

Atrial:

Ventricular:

## 3. P WAVE

Presence:

Appearance:

Consistency:

Relation to QRS:

## 4. P-R INTERVAL

Duration:

Consistency:

## 5. QRS COMPLEX

Presence:

Appearance:

Consistency:

Duration:

## 6. DATA ANALYSIS

## 7. INTERPRETATION

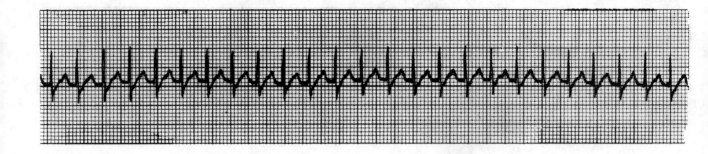

Figure 1-73B

# ECG RHYTHM STRIP #73

## I. RHYTHM

Atrial:  Unable to determine

Ventricular:  Regular

## 2. RATE

Atrial:  Unable to determine

Ventricular:  220

## 3. P WAVE

Presence:  Unable to identify

Appearance:  May be merged into T wave

Consistency: —

Relation to QRS: —

## 4. P-R INTERVAL

Duration: —

Consistency: —

## 5. QRS COMPLEX

Presence: Yes

Appearance: Normal

Consistency: Consistent

Duration: 0.05 seconds

## 6. DATA ANALYSIS

There is no clear evidence of atrial activity. The waveforms between consecutive QRS complexes are somewhat peaked and may represent a merging of T and P waves as often occurs with rapid rates. Ventricular activity is very rapid and regular. The ventricular rhythm originates above the ventricles since the QRS duration is normal. A 12 lead ECG would be necessary to determine the origin of this tachycardia; slowing the rate slightly might uncover P waves to assist in locating the site of origin.

## 7. INTERPRETATION

Supraventricular tachycardia

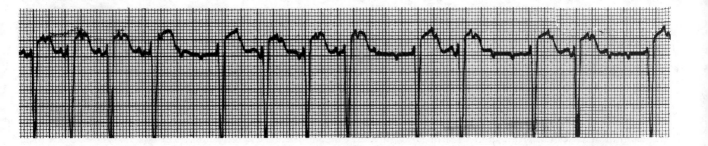

Figure 1-74A

# ECG RHYTHM STRIP #74

## 1. RHYTHM

Atrial:

Ventricular:

## 2. RATE

Atrial:

Ventricular:

## 3. P WAVE

Presence:

Appearance:

Consistency:

Relation to QRS:

## 4. P-R INTERVAL

Duration:

Consistency:

## 5. QRS COMPLEX

Presence:

Appearance:

Consistency:

Duration:

## 6. DATA ANALYSIS

## 7. INTERPRETATION

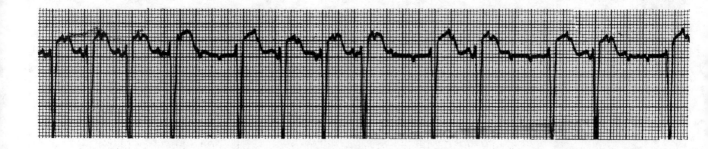

Figure 1-74B

# ECG RHYTHM STRIP #74

## 1. RHYTHM

Atrial: Regular

Ventricular: Irregular

## 2. RATE

Atrial: 250

Ventricular: 100

## 3. P WAVE

Presence: Yes

Appearance: Sharpened appearance

Consistency: Consistent

Relation to QRS: Varies between 2:1 and 4:1

## 4. P-R INTERVAL

Duration: Appears to vary

Consistency: —

## 5. QRS COMPLEX

Presence: Yes

Appearance: Normal

Consistency: Consistent

Duration: 0.10 seconds

## 6. DATA ANALYSIS

The atrial rate is extremely rapid but regular. These waveforms are different from normal P waves and also from classical flutter waves, yet the atrial rate is consistent with rates for atrial flutter. The ventricular rhythm is irregular. QRS complexes are of normal duration but are preceded by 2 to 4 flutter waves. The interval between the flutter wave and the QRS complex varies, suggesting that several levels of block may be present. The irregularity of the ventricular rhythm is attributable to varying AV conduction ratios.

## 7. INTERPRETATION

Atrial flutter with 2:1 and 4:1 AV conduction ratios

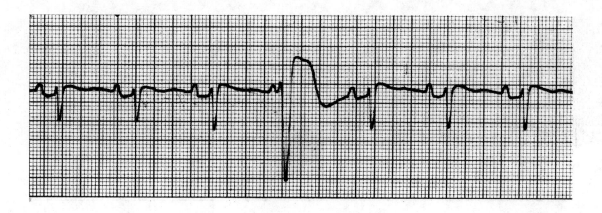

Figure 1-75A

# ECG RHYTHM STRIP #75

## 1. RHYTHM

Atrial:

Ventricular:

## 2. RATE

Atrial:

Ventricular:

## 3. P WAVE

Presence:

Appearance:

Consistency:

Relation to QRS:

## 4. P-R INTERVAL

Duration:

Consistency:

## 5. QRS COMPLEX

Presence:

Appearance:

Consistency:

Duration:

## 6. DATA ANALYSIS

## 7. INTERPRETATION

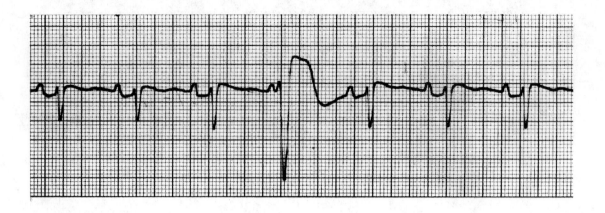

Figure 1-75B

# ECG RHYTHM STRIP #75

## I. RHYTHM

**Atrial:** Regular

**Ventricular:** Slightly irregular

## 2. RATE

**Atrial:** 70

**Ventricular:** 70

## 3. P WAVE

**Presence:** Yes

**Appearance:** Normal

**Consistency:** Consistent except one partially obscured by 4th QRS

**Relation to QRS:** 1:1 except with premature QRS

## 4. P-R INTERVAL

**Duration:** 0.20 seconds

**Consistency:** Consistent with conducted beats

## 5. QRS COMPLEX

**Presence:** Yes

**Appearance:** Normal—one abnormal

**Consistency:** Consistent except for premature QRS

**Duration:** 0.08 seconds in normal QRS; 0.16 seconds in premature QRS

## 6. DATA ANALYSIS

The atrial rate and rhythm are normal. The ventricular rhythm is interrupted by a slightly premature QRS complex, which is wide and bizarre in appearance. A normal P wave precedes the premature QRS but bears no relationship to this QRS, since the P-R interval here (0.06 seconds) is too short for the P wave to have been conducted.

## 7. INTERPRETATION

Sinus rhythm with one PVC

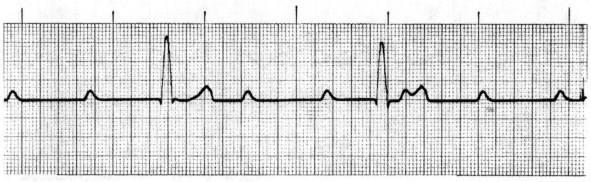

Figure 1-76A

# ECG RHYTHM STRIP #76

## 1. RHYTHM

Atrial:

Ventricular:

## 2. RATE

Atrial:

Ventricular:

## 3. P WAVE

Presence:

Appearance:

Consistency:

Relation to QRS:

## 4. P-R INTERVAL

Duration:

Consistency:

## 5. QRS COMPLEX

Presence:

Appearance:

Consistency:

Duration:

## 6. DATA ANALYSIS

## 7. INTERPRETATION

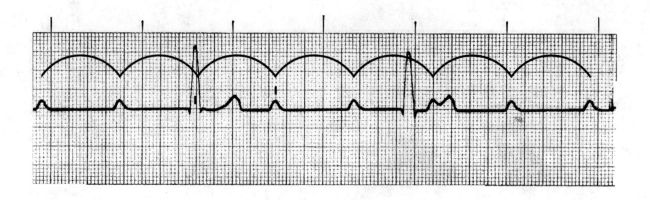

Figure 1-76B

# ECG RHYTHM STRIP #76

## I. RHYTHM

Atrial: Regular

Ventricular: Unable to determine—only one R-R interval

## 2. RATE

Atrial: 70

Ventricular: 20

## 3. P WAVE

Presence: Yes

Appearance: Normal

Consistency: Consistent

Relation to QRS: Variable

## 4. P-R INTERVAL

Duration: Variable

Consistency: No, the two P-QRS intervals differ

## 5. QRS COMPLEX

Presence: Yes

Appearance: Widened

Consistency: Consistent

Duration: 0.16 seconds

## 6. DATA ANALYSIS

The atrial rate, rhythm, and P waves are normal, indicating an underlying sinus rhythm. The ventricular rate is slower that the atrial rate due to nonconducted P waves. The P waves are unrelated to the QRS complex reflecting AV dissociation. The wide QRS complex and slow ventricular rate are consistent with an idioventriculer escape rhythm.

## 7. INTERPRETATION

Sinus rhythm with third degree (complete) AV block and a ventricular escape rhythm (or idioventricular rhythm).

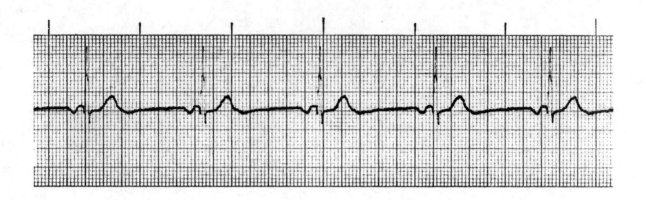

Figure 1-77A

# ECG RHYTHM STRIP #77
## Monitor Lead II

**I. RHYTHM**

    Atrial:

    Ventricular:

**2. RATE**

    Atrial:

    Ventricular:

**3. P WAVE**

    Presence:

    Appearance:

    Consistency:

    Relation to QRS:

**4. P-R INTERVAL**

    Duration:

    Consistency:

**5. QRS COMPLEX**

    Presence:

    Appearance:

    Consistency:

    Duration:

**6. DATA ANALYSIS**

**7. INTERPRETATION**

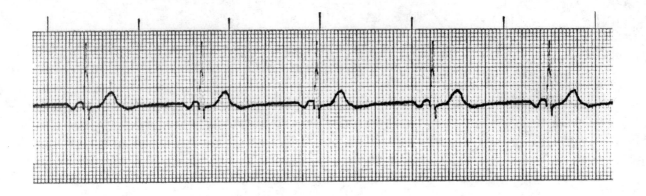

Figure 1-77B

# ECG RHYTHM STRIP #77
## Monitor Lead II

## 1. RHYTHM

Atrial: Regular

Ventricular: Regular

## 2. RATE

Atrial: 48

Ventricular: 48

## 3. P WAVE

Presence: Yes

Appearance: Negative deflection in Lead II

Consistency: Consistent

Relation to QRS: 1:1

## 4. P-R INTERVAL

Duration: 0.18 seconds

Consistency: Consistent

## 5. QRS COMPLEX

Presence: Yes

Appearance: Normal

Consistency: Consistent

Duration: 0.06 seconds

## 6. DATA ANALYSIS

Atrial and ventricular rates are both slow at 50 per minute. Atrial activity is evidenced by negative P waves in a lead where they are normally positive. This suggests retrograde atrial depolarization. It is probably due to a pacemaker site low in the atria near the AV junction, since the P-R interval is greater than 0.12 seconds. Ectopic atrial rhythms often occur in the area of the coronary sinus in the lower right atrium. The QRS of normal duration indicates the rhythm has a supraventricular origin.

## 7. INTERPRETATION

Coronary sinus rhythm

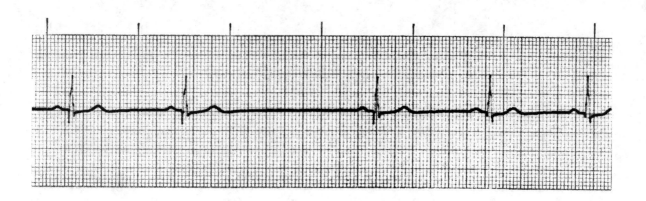

Figure 1-78A

# ECG RHYTHM STRIP #78

## I. RHYTHM

Atrial:

Ventricular:

## 2. RATE

Atrial:

Ventricular:

## 3. P WAVE

Presence:

Appearance:

Consistency:

Relation to QRS:

## 4. P-R INTERVAL

Duration:

Consistency:

## 5. QRS COMPLEX

Presence:

Appearance:

Consistency:

Duration:

## 6. DATA ANALYSIS

## 7. INTERPRETATION

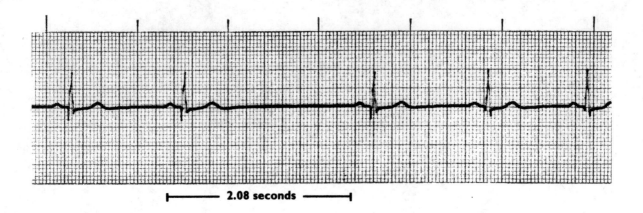

<— 2.08 seconds —>

Figure 1-78B

# ECG RHYTHM STRIP #78

## I. RHYTHM

Atrial: Irregular

Ventricular: Irregular

## 2. RATE

Atrial: 50

Ventricular: 50

## 3. P WAVE

Presence: Yes

Appearance: Normal

Consistency: Consistent

Relation to QRS: 1:1

## 4. P-R INTERVAL

Duration: 0.18 seconds

Consistency: Consistent

## 5. QRS COMPLEX

Presence: Yes

Appearance: Normal

Consistency: Consistent

Duration: 0.06 seconds

## 6. DATA ANALYSIS

All values are normal, except the rate is slow and the rhythm is irregular. There is a 2.08 second pause in sinus activity, which is not a multiple of the preceding sinus cycle.

## 7. INTERPRETATION

Sinus bradyarrhythmia with sinus arrest

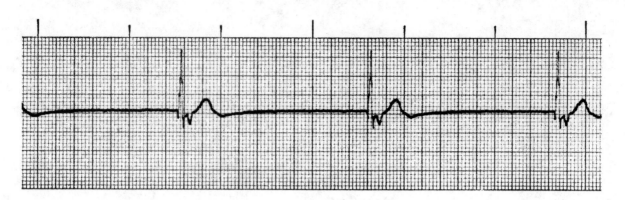

Figure 1-79A

# ECG RHYTHM STRIP #79
## Lead II

**I. RHYTHM**

   Atrial:

   Ventricular:

**2. RATE**

   Atrial:

   Ventricular:

**3. P WAVE**

   Presence:

   Appearance:

   Consistency:

   Relation to QRS:

**4. P-R INTERVAL**

   Duration:

   Consistency:

**5. QRS COMPLEX**

   Presence:

   Appearance:

   Consistency:

   Duration:

**6. DATA ANALYSIS**

**7. INTERPRETATION**

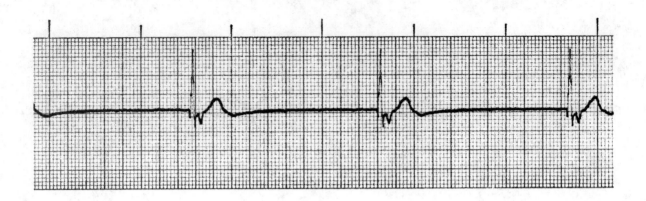

Figure 1-79B

# ECG RHYTHM STRIP #79
## Lead II

### I. RHYTHM

Atrial: Regular

Ventricular: Regular

### 2. RATE

Atrial: 30

Ventricular: 30

### 3. P WAVE

Presence: Yes

Appearance: Negative deflection following the QRS complex

Consistency: Consistent

Relation to QRS: 1:1

### 4. P-R INTERVAL

Duration: (R-P interval) 0.12 seconds

Consistency: Consistent

### 5. QRS COMPLEX

Presence: Yes

Appearance: Normal

Consistency: Consistent

Duration: 0.06 seconds

### 6. DATA ANALYSIS

The atrial rate is slow and the rhythm is regular. P waves are negative deflections in a lead (II) where they are normally positive deflections. They follow rather than precede the QRS. Additionally, the R-P interval remains constant, confirming the relationship between P waves and the preceding QRS complex. These findings together with a QRS of normal duration are consistent with a rhythm of junctional origin. The rates are slower than the normal intrinsic junctional rate.

### 7. INTERPRETATION

Junctional rhythm at a slow rate

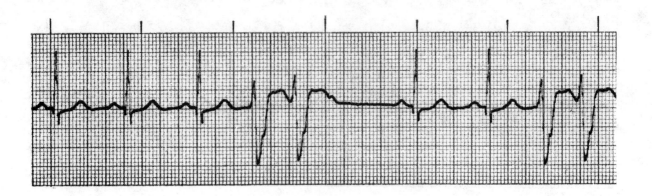

Figure 1-80A

# ECG RHYTHM STRIP #80

**1. RHYTHM**

   Atrial:

   Ventricular:

**2. RATE**

   Atrial:

   Ventricular:

**3. P WAVE**

   Presence:

   Appearance:

   Consistency:

   Relation to QRS:

**4. P-R INTERVAL**

   Duration:

   Consistency:

**5. QRS COMPLEX**

   Presence:

   Appearance:

   Consistency:

   Duration:

**6. DATA ANALYSIS**

**7. INTERPRETATION**

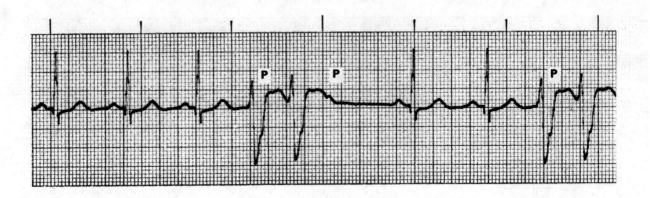

Figure 1-80B

## ECG RHYTHM STRIP #80

### I. RHYTHM

Atrial: Regular

Ventricular: Irregular

### 2. RATE

Atrial: 80

Ventricular: 80 to 90

### 3. P WAVE

Presence: Yes

Appearance: Normal

Consistency: Consistent

Relation to QRS: 1:1 with normal QRS; P
waves obscured by wide QRS
complexes

### 4. P-R INTERVAL

Duration: 0.18 seconds

Consistency: Consistent

### 5. QRS COMPLEX

Presence: Yes

Appearance: Some normal; premature QRS
complexes are abnormal and wide

Consistency: Inconsistent

Duration: 0.06 seconds in normal QRS; 0.18
seconds in abnormal QRS

### 6. DATA ANALYSIS

The underlying rhythm is normal. There are 4
premature QRS complexes that are wide and
abnormal but uniform in appearance; they
occur in pairs of 2 consecutive beats. The P-P
interval remains constant through the premature
beats, with some of the P waves being obscured
by the wide abnormal QRS complexes.

### 7. INTERPRETATION

Sinus rhythm with 2 pairs of consecutive uniform
(unifocal) PVCs

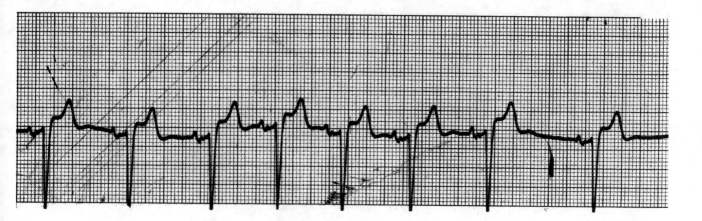

Figure 1-81A

# ECG RHYTHM STRIP #81
## Lead MCI₁

**1. RHYTHM**

    Atrial:

    Ventricular:

**2. RATE**

    Atrial:

    Ventricular:

**3. P WAVE**

    Presence:

    Appearance:

    Consistency:

    Relation to QRS:

**4. P-R INTERVAL**

    Duration:

    Consistency:

**5. QRS COMPLEX**

    Presence:

    Appearance:

    Consistency:

    Duration:

**6. DATA ANALYSIS**

**7. INTERPRETATION**

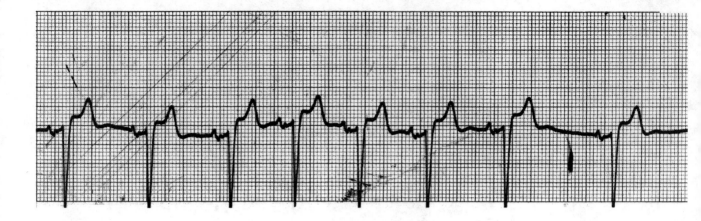

Figure 1-81B

# ECG RHYTHM STRIP #81
## Lead MCI₁

### 1. RHYTHM

Atrial: Irregular

Ventricular: Irregular

### 2. RATE

Atrial: 70

Ventricular: 70

### 3. P WAVE

Presence: Yes

Appearance: Normal

Consistency: Consistent

Relation to QRS: 1:1

### 4. P-R INTERVAL

Duration: 0.16 seconds

Consistency: Consistent

### 5. QRS COMPLEX

Presence: Yes

Appearance: Normal

Consistency: Consistent

Duration: 0.10 seconds

### 6. DATA ANALYSIS

All values are within normal limits except the rhythm is irregular

### 7. INTERPRETATION

Sinus arrhythmia

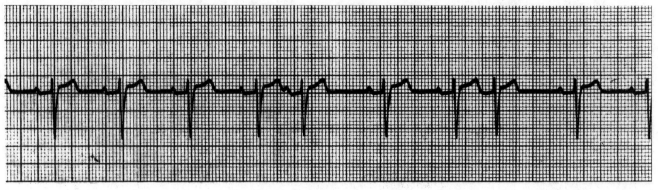

Figure 1-82A

# ECG RHYTHM STRIP #82
## Lead MCL₁

### 1. RHYTHM

Atrial:

Ventricular:

### 2. RATE

Atrial:

Ventricular:

### 3. P WAVE

Presence:

Appearance:

Consistency:

Relation to QRS:

### 4. P-R INTERVAL

Duration:

Consistency:

### 5. QRS COMPLEX

Presence:

Appearance:

Consistency:

Duration:

### 6. DATA ANALYSIS

### 7. INTERPRETATION

165

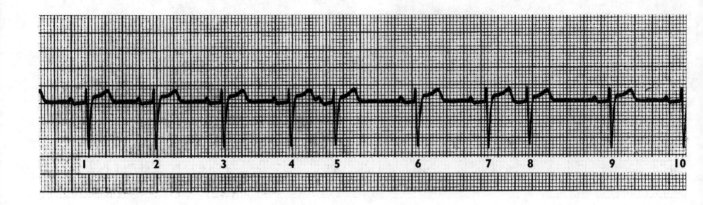

Figure 1-82B

# ECG RHYTHM STRIP #82
## Lead MCL₁

## I. RHYTHM

Atrial: Irregular

Ventricular: Irregular

## 2. RATE

Atrial: 80 (P on T after $QRS_7$)

Ventricular: 80

## 3. P WAVE

Presence: Yes

Appearance: Normal

Consistency: Consistent except for 5th and 8th beats

Relation to QRS: 1:1

## 4. P-R INTERVAL

Duration: 0.20 seconds

Consistency: Consistent; unable to determine with 8th beat

## 5. QRS COMPLEX

Presence: Yes

Appearance: Normal

Consistency: Consistent

Duration: 0.09 seconds

## 6. DATA ANALYSIS

The T wave following $QRS_7$ is unusually pointed, suggesting a superimposed P wave. This P wave along with the 5th P wave, interrupt the underlying rhythm and are premature in the basic sinus cycle. The QRS complexes in the premature beats are identical to those in the sinus beats. These findings are consistent with PACs.

## 7. INTERPRETATION

Sinus rhythm with two PACs

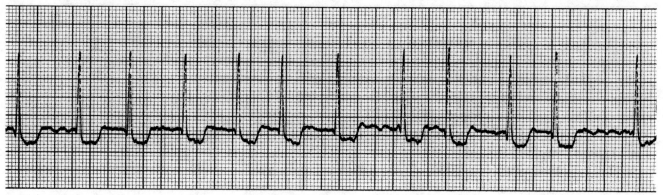

Figure 1-83A

# ECG RHYTHM STRIP #83

## 1. RHYTHM

Atrial:

Ventricular:

## 2. RATE

Atrial:

Ventricular:

## 3. P WAVE

Presence:

Appearance:

Consistency:

Relation to QRS:

## 4. P-R INTERVAL

Duration:

Consistency:

## 5. QRS COMPLEX

Presence:

Appearance:

Consistency:

Duration:

## 6. DATA ANALYSIS

## 7. INTERPRETATION

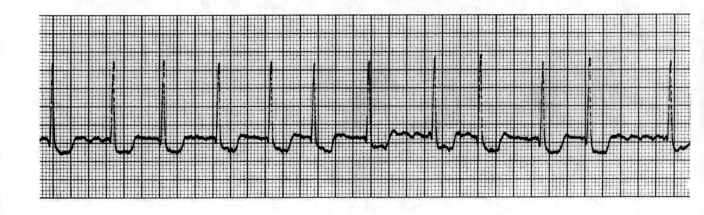

Figure 1-83B

# ECG RHYTHM STRIP #83

## I. RHYTHM

**Atrial:** Unable to determine

**Ventricular:** Irregularly irregular

## 2. RATE

**Atrial:** Unable to determine

**Ventricular:** 100

## 3. P WAVE

**Presence:** Not as a discrete waveform

**Appearance:** Replaced by fibrillatory waves

**Consistency:** Inconsistent

**Relation to QRS:** Unable to determine

## 4. P-R INTERVAL

**Duration:** Unable to calculate

**Consistency:** —

## 5. QRS COMPLEX

**Presence:** Yes

**Appearance:** Normal

**Consistency:** Consistent

**Duration:** 0.08 seconds

## 6. DATA ANALYSIS

P waves are not clearly identifiable, but atrial activity is manifested by irregular undulations of the baseline. These findings along with an irregularly irregular ventricular rhythm suggests a fibrillatory mechanism in the atria as the origin of the rhythm.

## 7. INTERPRETATION

Atrial fibrillation with a controlled ventricular response

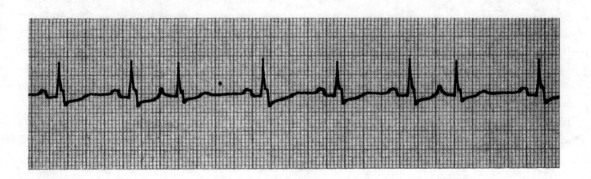

Figure 1-84A

# ECG RHYTHM STRIP #84
## Lead II

**1. RHYTHM**

Atrial:

Ventricular:

**2. RATE**

Atrial:

Ventricular:

**3. P WAVE**

Presence:

Appearance:

Consistency:

Relation to QRS:

**4. P-R INTERVAL**

Duration:

Consistency:

**5. QRS COMPLEX**

Presence:

Appearance:

Consistency:

Duration:

**6. DATA ANALYSIS**

**7. INTERPRETATION**

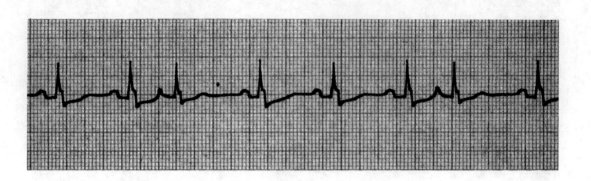

Figure 1-84B

# ECG RHYTHM STRIP #84
## Lead II

## 1. RHYTHM

Atrial: Approximately 80

Ventricular: Approximately 80

## 2. RATE

Atrial: Irregular

Ventricular: Irregular

## 3. P WAVE

Presence: Yes

Appearance: Two types; normal with underlying rhythm and a variant with
early beats

Consistency: Inconsistent

Relation to QRS: 1:1

## 4. P-R INTERVAL

Duration: 0.20 seconds

Consistency: Consistent

## 5. QRS COMPLEX

Presence: Yes

Appearance: Normal

Consistency: Consistent

Duration: 0.09 seconds

## 6. DATA ANALYSIS

The basic underlying rhythm is disrupted by
premature P-QRS cycles where the P wave differs from the sinus P wave. These early P waves
suggest ectopic atrial activity.

## 7. INTERPRETATION

Sinus rhythm with PACs

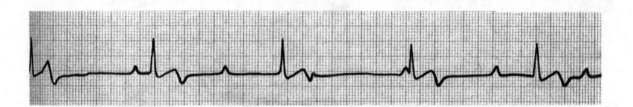

Figure 1-85A

# ECG RHYTHM STRIP #85
## Lead II

**1. RHYTHM**

    Atrial:

    Ventricular:

**2. RATE**

    Atrial:

    Ventricular:

**3. P WAVE**

    Presence:

    Appearance:

    Consistency:

    Relation to QRS:

**4. P-R INTERVAL**

    Duration:

    Consistency:

**5. QRS COMPLEX**

    Presence:

    Appearance:

    Consistency:

    Duration:

**6. DATA ANALYSIS**

**7. INTERPRETATION**

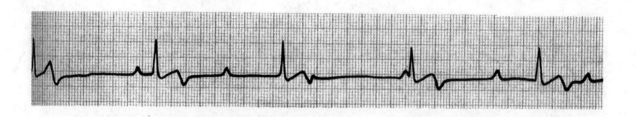

Figure 1-85B

# ECG RHYTHM STRIP #85
## Lead II

## 1. RHYTHM

Atrial: Regular

Ventricular: Regular

## 2. RATE

Atrial: 50

Ventricular: 35

## 3. P WAVE

Presence: Yes

Appearance: Normal

Consistency: Consistent

Relation to QRS: Variable

## 4. P-R INTERVAL

Duration: Variable

Consistency: Inconsistent

## 5. QRS COMPLEX

Presence: Yes

Appearance: Normal

Consistency: Consistent

Duration: 0.08 seconds

## 6. DATA ANALYSIS

Both the atrial and ventricular rhythms are slow and regular but are unrelated to each other. The normal P wave indicates sinus activity. The QRS of normal duration indicates that the pacemaking site for the ventricles is located in the AV junction. The variable P-R intervals support the presence of AV dissociation, while the slower ventricular rate suggests that the dissociation is caused by an AV block.

## 7. INTERPRETATION

Sinus bradycardia with third degree (complete) AV block and a junctional escape rhythm

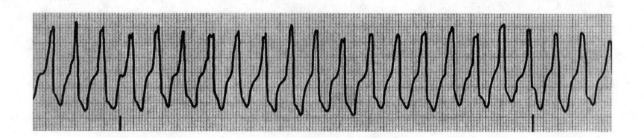

Figure 1-86A

# ECG RHYTHM STRIP #86
## Lead MCL₁

### 1. RHYTHM

Atrial:

Ventricular:

### 2. RATE

Atrial:

Ventricular:

### 3. P WAVE

Presence:

Appearance:

Consistency:

Relation to QRS:

### 4. P-R INTERVAL

Duration:

Consistency:

### 5. QRS COMPLEX

Presence:

Appearance:

Consistency:

Duration:

### 6. DATA ANALYSIS

### 7. INTERPRETATION

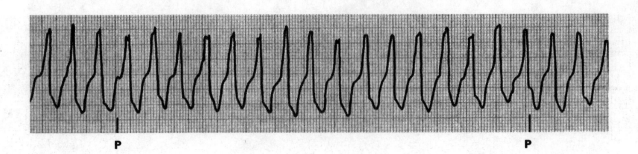

P                                                                    P

Figure 1-86B

# ECG RHYTHM STRIP #86
## Lead MCL₁

## I. RHYTHM

Atrial: Unable to determine

Ventricular: Regular

## 2. RATE

Atrial: Unable to determine

Ventricular: Approximately 164

## 3. P WAVE

Presence: Obscured by QRS

Appearance: —

Consistency: —

Relation to QRS: —

## 4. P-R INTERVAL

Duration: —

Consistency: —

## 5. QRS COMPLEX

Presence: Yes

Appearance: Abnormal

Consistency: Consistent

Duration: 0.12 seconds

## 6. DATA ANALYSIS

There is some evidence of atrial activity before beat 4 and following beat 19, but it is inconsistent and unrelated to the ventricular activity. The ventricular rate is rapid with wide, abnormal QRS complexes.

## 7. INTERPRETATION

Ventricular tachycardia

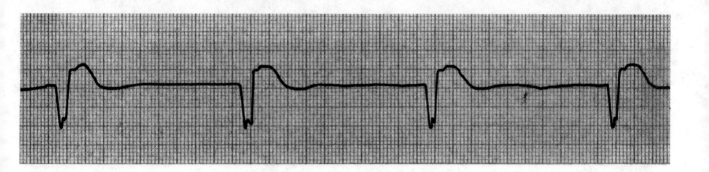

Figure 1-87A

# ECG RHYTHM STRIP #87
## Lead II

**1. RHYTHM**

  Atrial:

  Ventricular:

**2. RATE**

  Atrial:

  Ventricular:

**3. P WAVE**

  Presence:

  Appearance:

  Consistency:

  Relation to QRS:

**4. P-R INTERVAL**

  Duration:

  Consistency:

**5. QRS COMPLEX**

  Presence:

  Appearance:

  Consistency:

  Duration:

**6. DATA ANALYSIS**

**7. INTERPRETATION**

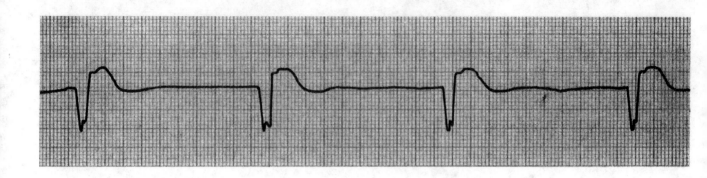

Figure 1-87B

# ECG RHYTHM STRIP #87
## Lead II

## I. RHYTHM

Atrial: Unable to determine

Ventricular: Regular

## 2. RATE

Atrial: —

Ventricular: 30

## 3. P WAVE

Presence: No

Appearance: —

Consistency: —

Relation to QRS: —

## 4. P-R INTERVAL

Duration: —

Consistency: —

## 5. QRS COMPLEX

Presence: Yes

Appearance: Abnormal

Consistency: Consistent

Duration: 0.14 seconds

## 6. DATA ANALYSIS

There is no identifiable atrial activity. QRS complexes are wide and bizarre in appearance. The ventricular rate is slow (ventricles firing at own inherent rate of impulse formation) and the rhythm is regular.

## 7. INTERPRETATION

Idioventricular rhythm

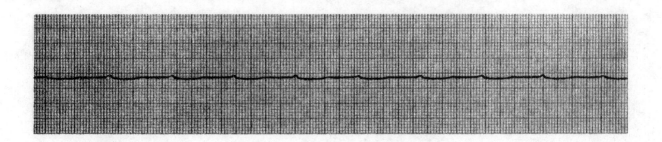

Figure 1-88A

# ECG RHYTHM STRIP #88
## Lead II

**1. RHYTHM**

Atrial:

Ventricular:

**2. RATE**

Atrial:

Ventricular:

**3. P WAVE**

Presence:

Appearance:

Consistency:

Relation to QRS:

**4. P-R INTERVAL**

Duration:

Consistency:

**5. QRS COMPLEX**

Presence:

Appearance:

Consistency:

Duration:

**6. DATA ANALYSIS**

**7. INTERPRETATION**

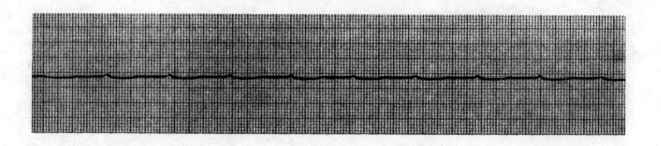

Figure 1-88B

# ECG RHYTHM STRIP #88
## Lead II

### 1. RHYTHM

Atrial: Regular

Ventricular: —

### 2. RATE

Atrial: 70

Ventricular: —

### 3. P WAVE

Presence: Yes

Appearance: Normal

Consistency: Consistent

Relation to QRS: N/A

### 4. P-R INTERVAL

Duration: —

Consistency: —

### 5. QRS COMPLEX

Presence: Absent

Appearance: —

Consistency: —

Duration: —

### 6. DATA ANALYSIS

There is no evidence of ventricular activity. The atrial rate, rhythm, and P waves are normal indicating a sinus rhythm in the atria.

### 7. INTERPRETATION

Sinus rhythm with ventricular standstill

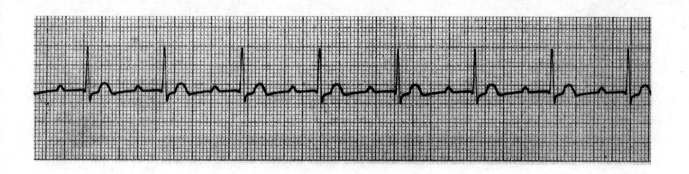

Figure 1-89A

# ECG RHYTHM STRIP #89
## Lead II

**1. RHYTHM**

Atrial:

Ventricular:

**2. RATE**

Atrial:

Ventricular:

**3. P WAVE**

Presence:

Appearance:

Consistency:

Relation to QRS:

**4. P-R INTERVAL**

Duration:

Consistency:

**5. QRS COMPLEX**

Presence:

Appearance:

Consistency:

Duration:

**6. DATA ANALYSIS**

**7. INTERPRETATION**

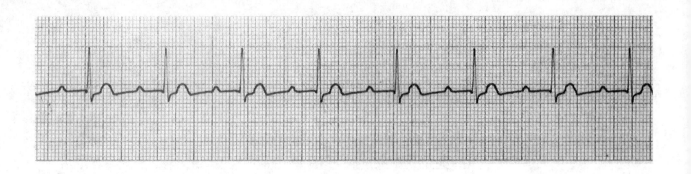

Figure 1-89B

# ECG RHYTHM STRIP #89
## Lead II

### 1. RHYTHM

Atrial: Regular

Ventricular: Regular

### 2. RATE

Atrial: 70

Ventricular: 70

### 3. P WAVE

Presence: Yes

Appearance: Normal

Consistency: Consistent

Relation to QRS: 1:1

### 4. P-R INTERVAL

Duration: 0.32 seconds

Consistency: Consistent

### 5. QRS COMPLEX

Presence: Yes

Appearance: Normal

Consistency: Consistent

Duration: 0.08 seconds

### 6. DATA ANALYSIS

The atrial rate and rhythm are normal. The P-R interval is prolonged, indicating delayed conduction through the AV junction.

### 7. INTERPRETATION

Sinus rhythm with first degree AV block

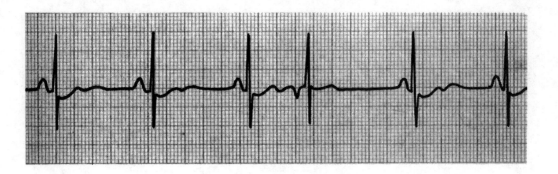

Figure 1-90A

# ECG RHYTHM STRIP #90
## Lead II

### 1. RHYTHM

Atrial:

Ventricular:

### 2. RATE

Atrial:

Ventricular:

### 3. P WAVE

Presence:

Appearance:

Consistency:

Relation to QRS:

### 4. P-R INTERVAL

Duration:

Consistency:

### 5. QRS COMPLEX

Presence:

Appearance:

Consistency:

Duration:

### 6. DATA ANALYSIS

### 7. INTERPRETATION

181

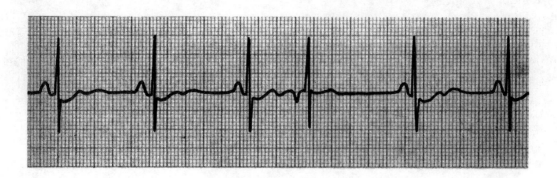

Figure 1-90B

# ECG RHYTHM STRIP #90
## Lead II

### I. RHYTHM

Atrial: Irregular

Ventricular: Irregular

### 2. RATE

Atrial: 60

Ventricular: 60

### 3. P WAVE

Presence: Yes

Appearance: Normal except in 4th beat
(inverted/negative)

Consistency: Consistent, except in 4th beat

Relation to QRS: 1:1

### 4. P-R INTERVAL

Duration: 0.14 seconds except 0.10 seconds in
4th beat

Consistency: Consistent except shorter when P
wave is negative

### 5. QRS COMPLEX

Presence: Yes

Appearance: Normal

Consistency: Consistent

Duration: 0.08 seconds

### 6. DATA ANALYSIS

The normal underlying rhythm is interrupted by
one premature cycle in which the P wave
becomes a negative deflection. P wave inversion
suggests retrograde atrial conduction in lead II.
The shortened P-R interval that occurs with the
negative P wave is consistent with an AV junctional pacemaker site.

### 7. INTERPRETATION

Sinus rhythm with one premature junctional
beat (PJC)

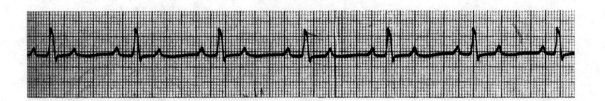

Figure 1-91A

## ECG RHYTHM STRIP #91
### Lead II

**1. RHYTHM**

Atrial:

Ventricular:

**2. RATE**

Atrial:

Ventricular:

**3. P WAVE**

Presence:

Appearance:

Consistency:

Relation to QRS:

**4. P-R INTERVAL**

Duration:

Consistency:

**5. QRS COMPLEX**

Presence:

Appearance:

Consistency:

Duration:

**6. DATA ANALYSIS**

**7. INTERPRETATION**

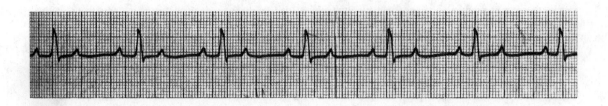

Figure 1-91B

# ECG RHYTHM STRIP #91
## Lead II

## 1. RHYTHM

Atrial: Regular

Ventricular: Regular

## 2. RATE

Atrial: 100

Ventricular: 50

## 3. P WAVE

Presence: Yes

Appearance: Normal

Consistency: Consistent

Relation to QRS: 2:1

## 4. P-R INTERVAL

Duration: 0.24 seconds

Consistency: Consistent

## 5. QRS COMPLEX

Presence: Yes

Appearance: Widened

Consistency: Consistent

Duration: 0.12 seconds

## 6. DATA ANALYSIS

The normal P waves, regular atrial rhythm, and atrial rate of 100 are consistent with sinus tachycardia. The ventricular rate is half the atrial rate, indicating an AV block. On the conducted beats, the prolonged P-R interval remains constant. Since there are no instances of two consecutively conducted beats, the ability to distinguish between the forms of second degree AV block is limited. The QRS duration is prolonged, suggesting the block is located below the level of the AV junction.

## 7. INTERPRETATION

Sinus tachycardia with first degree and second degree AV block with 2:1 AV conduction ratios and an intraventricular conduction delay

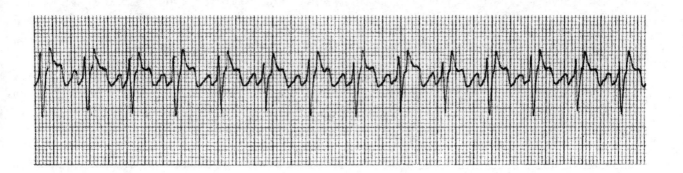

Figure 1-92A

# ECG RHYTHM STRIP #92
## Monitor Lead III

### 1. RHYTHM

Atrial:

Ventricular:

### 2. RATE

Atrial:

Ventricular:

### 3. P WAVE

Presence:

Appearance:

Consistency:

Relation to QRS:

### 4. P-R INTERVAL

Duration:

Consistency:

### 5. QRS COMPLEX

Presence:

Appearance:

Consistency:

Duration:

### 6. DATA ANALYSIS

### 7. INTERPRETATION

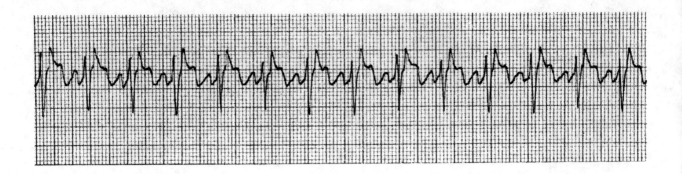

Figure 1-92B

# ECG RHYTHM STRIP #92
## Monitor Lead III

## I. RHYTHM

Atrial: Regular

Ventricular: Regular

## 2. RATE

Atrial: 125

Ventricular: 125

## 3. P WAVE

Presence: Yes

Appearance: Normal

Consistency: Consistent

Relation to QRS: 1:1

## 4. P-R INTERVAL

Duration: 0.18 seconds

Consistency: Consistent

## 5. QRS COMPLEX

Presence: Yes

Appearance: Abnormal (rSR[1] pattern)

Consistency: Consistent

Duration: 0.16 seconds

## 6. DATA ANALYSIS

The atrial and ventricular rates are both rapid. The QRS complexes are abnormal and wide, indicating an intraventricular conduction delay. A 12 lead ECG is necessary to determine the specific type of bundle branch block.

## 7. INTERPRETATION

Sinus tachycardia with an intraventricular conduction delay

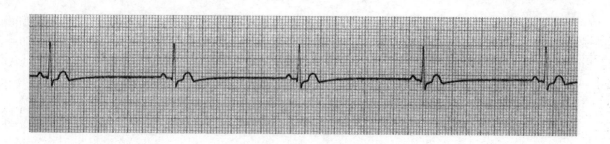

Figure 1-93A

# ECG RHYTHM STRIP #93
## Lead II

**1. RHYTHM**

Atrial:

Ventricular:

**2. RATE**

Atrial:

Ventricular:

**3. P WAVE**

Presence:

Appearance:

Consistency:

Relation to QRS:

**4. P-R INTERVAL**

Duration:

Consistency:

**5. QRS COMPLEX**

Presence:

Appearance:

Consistency:

Duration:

**6. DATA ANALYSIS**

**7. INTERPRETATION**

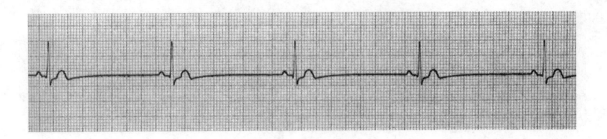

Figure 1-93B

# ECG RHYTHM STRIP #93
## Lead II

## 1. RHYTHM

Atrial: Regular

Ventricular: Regular

## 2. RATE

Atrial: 35

Ventricular: 35

## 3. P WAVE

Presence: Yes

Appearance: Normal

Consistency: Consistent

Relation to QRS: 1:1

## 4. P-R INTERVAL

Duration: 0.14 seconds

Consistency: Consistent

## 5. QRS COMPLEX

Presence: Yes

Appearance: Normal

Consistency: Consistent

Duration: 0.08 seconds

## 6. DATA ANALYSIS

All values are normal, except that the rates are 35 per minute.

## 7. INTERPRETATION

Sinus bradycardia

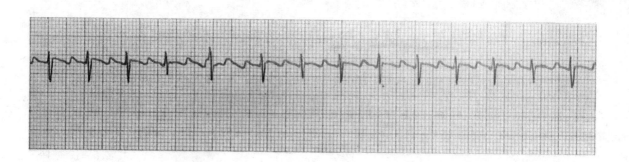

Figure 1-94A

# ECG RHYTHM STRIP #94
## Lead II

**I. RHYTHM**

Atrial:

Ventricular:

**2. RATE**

Atrial:

Ventricular:

**3. P WAVE**

Presence:

Appearance:

Consistency:

Relation to QRS:

**4. P-R INTERVAL**

Duration:

Consistency:

**5. QRS COMPLEX**

Presence:

Appearance:

Consistency:

Duration:

**6. DATA ANALYSIS**

**7. INTERPRETATION**

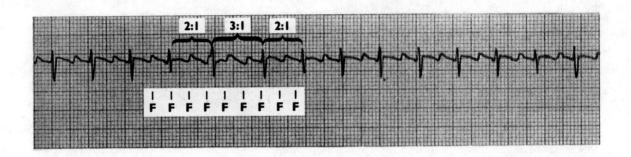

Figure 1-94B

# ECG RHYTHM STRIP #94
## Lead II

## I. RHYTHM

Atrial: Regular

Ventricular: Slightly irregular

## 2. RATE

Atrial: 300

Ventricular: 140

## 3. P WAVE

Presence: Yes

Appearance: Sawtooth waves

Consistency: Consistent

Relation to QRS: 2:1 except with 6th QRS
complex—3:1

## 4. P-R INTERVAL

Duration: Unable to determine

Consistency: —

## 5. QRS COMPLEX

Presence: Yes

Appearance: Normal

Consistency: Consistent when not distorted by
sawtooth waves

Duration: 0.06 seconds

## 6. DATA ANALYSIS

The atrial rate is extremely rapid and is more
than twice the ventricular rate. P waves are
replaced by sawtooth flutter waves that partially
merge with the QRS complexes. The AV junction physiologically blocks every 2nd or 3rd atrial
impulse due to the rapidity of the atrial rate.

## 7. INTERPRETATION

Atrial flutter with variable (2:1 and 3:1) AV conduction ratios

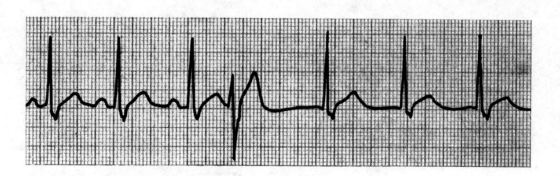

Figure 1-95A

# ECG RHYTHM STRIP #95
## Lead II

**1. RHYTHM**

   Atrial:

   Ventricular:

**2. RATE**

   Atrial:

   Ventricular:

**3. P WAVE**

   Presence:

   Appearance:

   Consistency:

   Relation to QRS:

**4. P-R INTERVAL**

   Duration:

   Consistency:

**5. QRS COMPLEX**

   Presence:

   Appearance:

   Consistency:

   Duration:

**6. DATA ANALYSIS**

**7. INTERPRETATION**

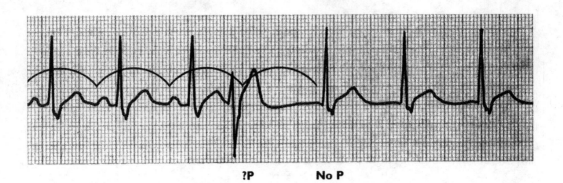

?P          No P

Figure 1-95B

# ECG RHYTHM STRIP #95
## Lead II

## I. RHYTHM

Atrial: Regular with visible P waves

Ventricular: Irregular

## 2. RATE

Atrial: 75 with identifiable P waves

Ventricular: Approximately 70

## 3. P WAVE

Presence: 3 identifiable at beginning

Appearance: Normal

Consistency: Consistent, when visible

Relation to QRS: 1:1 with first 3 beats

## 4. P-R INTERVAL

Duration: 0.22 seconds

Consistency: Consistent, when measurable

## 5. QRS COMPLEX

Presence: Yes

Appearance: Normal and wide, except 4th
              QRS—abnormal

Consistency: Inconsistent

Duration: Normal—0.14 seconds
          Abnormal—0.16 seconds

## 6. DATA ANALYSIS

The first 3 beats in this strip are normal, establishing a sinus rhythm at 75 beats per minute. The P-R interval with the sinus beats is prolonged at 0.22 seconds.

The fourth QRS complex is abnormal, wide, and premature in the underlying rhythm. This is consistent with an ectopic ventricular beat.

The QRS (beat 5) terminating the pause is identical to the normally conducted impulses but is not preceded by a P wave and is consistent with a junctional origin. This beat occurs after the expected sinus P wave fails to occur, making it an escape mechanism. Beats 5, 6, and 7 represent an accelerated junctional rhythm at approximately 75 per minute.

## 7. INTERPRETATION

Sinus rhythm with first degree AV block, one PVC, and accelerated junctional escape rhythm

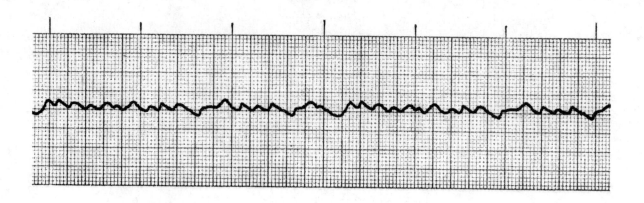

Figure 1-96A

# ECG RHYTHM STRIP #96

**1. RHYTHM**

    Atrial:

    Ventricular:

**2. RATE**

    Atrial:

    Ventricular:

**3. P WAVE**

    Presence:

    Appearance:

    Consistency:

    Relation to QRS:

**4. P-R INTERVAL**

    Duration:

    Consistency:

**5. QRS COMPLEX**

    Presence:

    Appearance:

    Consistency:

    Duration:

**6. DATA ANALYSIS**

**7. INTERPRETATION**

193

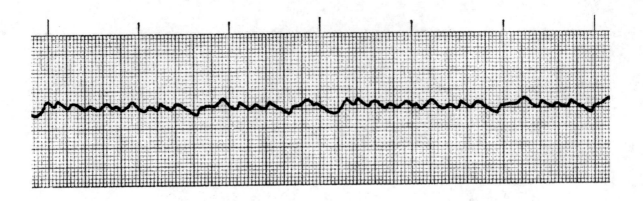

Figure 1-96B

## ECG RHYTHM STRIP #96

## I. RHYTHM

Atrial:  Unable to determine

Ventricular:  Irregular

## 2. RATE

Atrial:  Unable to determine

Ventricular:  Unable to determine

## 3. P WAVE

Presence:  No evidence of

Appearance:  —

Consistency:  —

Relation to QRS:  —

## 4. P-R INTERVAL

Duration:  —

Consistency:  —

## 5. QRS COMPLEX

Presence:  Not a distinguishable complex

Appearance:  Irregular waves of varying size and shape

Consistency:  Inconsistent

Duration:  Unable to determine

## 6. DATA ANALYSIS

There is no identifiable evidence of atrial activity. Fibrillatory waveforms of varying configurations appear as the ventricular activity.

## 7. INTERPRETATION

Ventricular fibrillation

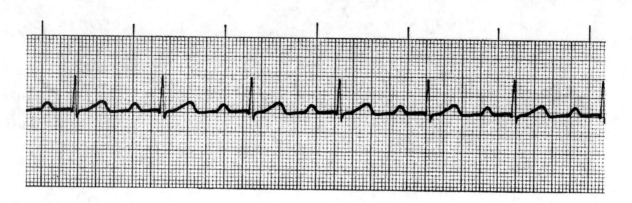

Figure 1-97A

# ECG RHYTHM STRIP #97

## 1. RHYTHM

Atrial:

Ventricular:

## 2. RATE

Atrial:

Ventricular:

## 3. P WAVE

Presence:

Appearance:

Consistency:

Relation to QRS:

## 4. P-R INTERVAL

Duration:

Consistency:

## 5. QRS COMPLEX

Presence:

Appearance:

Consistency:

Duration:

## 6. DATA ANALYSIS

## 7. INTERPRETATION

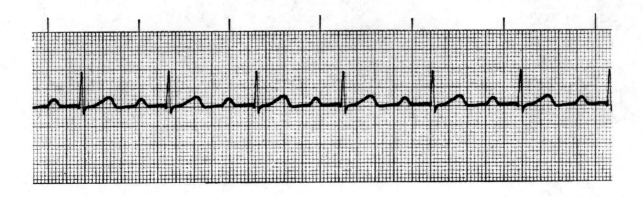

Figure 1-97B

# ECG RHYTHM STRIP #97

## 1. RHYTHM

Atrial: Regular

Ventricular: Regular

## 2. RATE

Atrial: 60

Ventricular: 60

## 3. P WAVE

Presence: Yes

Appearance: Normal

Consistency: Consistent

Relation to QRS: 1:1

## 4. P-R INTERVAL

Duration: 0.32 seconds

Consistency: Consistent

## 5. QRS COMPLEX

Presence: Yes

Appearance: Normal

Consistency: Consistent

Duration: 0.06 seconds

## 6. DATA ANALYSIS

All values are within normal limits except the P-R interval is prolonged, indicating delayed conduction through the AV junction.

## 7. INTERPRETATION

Sinus rhythm with first degree AV block

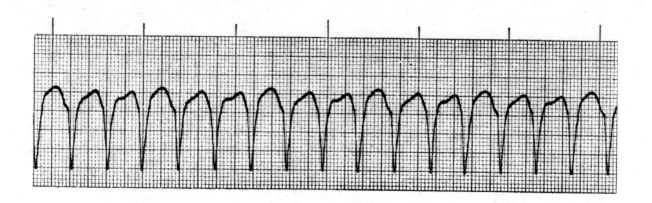

Figure 1-98A

# ECG RHYTHM STRIP #98

## 1. RHYTHM

Atrial:

Ventricular:

## 2. RATE

Atrial:

Ventricular:

## 3. P WAVE

Presence:

Appearance:

Consistency:

Relation to QRS:

## 4. P-R INTERVAL

Duration:

Consistency:

## 5. QRS COMPLEX

Presence:

Appearance:

Consistency:

Duration:

## 6. DATA ANALYSIS

## 7. INTERPRETATION

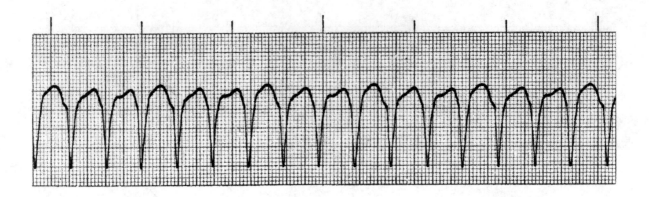

Figure 1-98B

# ECG RHYTHM STRIP #98

## I. RHYTHM

Atrial:  Unable to determine

Ventricular:  Regular

## 2. RATE

Atrial:  Unable to determine

Ventricular:  150

## 3. P WAVE

Presence:  Unable to determine

Appearance:  —

Consistency:  —

Relation to QRS:  —

## 4. P-R INTERVAL

Duration:  —

Consistency:  —

## 5. QRS COMPLEX

Presence:  Yes

Appearance:  Widened, bizarre

Consistency:  Consistent

Duration:  0.12 seconds

## 6. DATA ANALYSIS

There is no clear evidence of atrial activity. The ventricular rate is rapid with wide, abnormal QRS complexes. This is consistent with rapid ventricular ectopy.

## 7. INTERPRETATION

Ventricular tachycardia

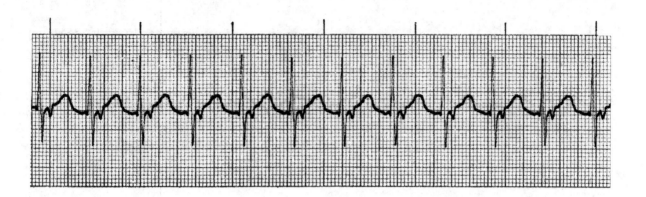

Figure 1-99A

# ECG RHYTHM STRIP #99
## Lead II

**1. RHYTHM**

    Atrial:

    Ventricular:

**2. RATE**

    Atrial:

    Ventricular:

**3. P WAVE**

    Presence:

    Appearance:

    Consistency:

    Relation to QRS:

**4. P-R INTERVAL**

    Duration:

    Consistency:

**5. QRS COMPLEX**

    Presence:

    Appearance:

    Consistency:

    Duration:

**6. DATA ANALYSIS**

**7. INTERPRETATION**

199

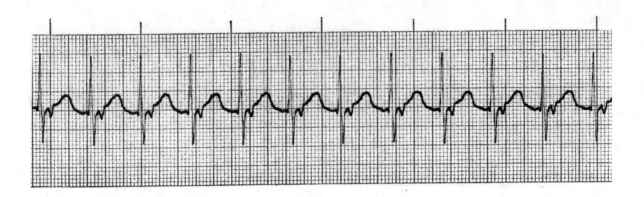

Figure 1-99B

# ECG RHYTHM STRIP #99
## Lead II

## I. RHYTHM

Atrial: Regular

Ventricular: Regular

## 2. RATE

Atrial: 107

Ventricular: 107

## 3. P WAVE

Presence: Yes

Appearance: Negative

Consistency: Consistent

Relation to QRS: 1:1 with P wave following QRS

## 4. P-R INTERVAL

Duration: (R-P) approximately 0.12 seconds

Consistency: Consistent

## 5. QRS COMPLEX

Presence: Yes

Appearance: Normal

Consistency: Consistent

Duration: 0.08 seconds

## 6. DATA ANALYSIS

The rhythm is regular, but the rates are over 100 per minute. P waves are negative deflections in lead II where they are normally positive, which supports retrograde conduction in the atria. The constant R-P interval confirms the relationship between P waves and the preceding QRS complex. These findings together with a QRS of normal duration are consistent with ectopic junctional activity.

## 7. INTERPRETATION

Junctional tachycardia

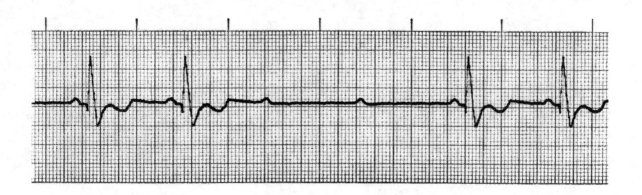

Figure 1-100A

# ECG RHYTHM STRIP #100

### 1. RHYTHM

Atrial:

Ventricular:

### 2. RATE

Atrial:

Ventricular:

### 3. P WAVE

Presence:

Appearance:

Consistency:

Relation to QRS:

### 4. P-R INTERVAL

Duration:

Consistency:

### 5. QRS COMPLEX

Presence:

Appearance:

Consistency:

Duration:

### 6. DATA ANALYSIS

### 7. INTERPRETATION

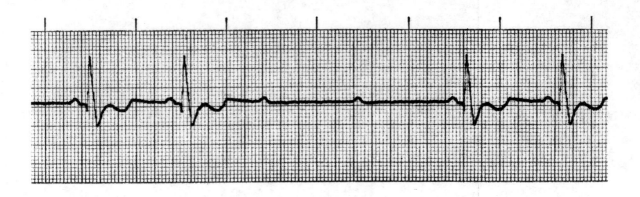

Figure 1-100B

## ECG RHYTHM STRIP #100

### I. RHYTHM

Atrial: Regular

Ventricular: Irregular

### 2. RATE

Atrial: 60

Ventricular: 40

### 3. P WAVE

Presence: Yes

Appearance: Normal

Consistency: Consistent

Relation to QRS: Varies 1:1 and 3:1

### 4. P-R INTERVAL

Duration: 0.16 seconds

Consistency: Consistent

### 5. QRS COMPLEX

Presence: Yes

Appearance: Normal, widened

Consistency: Consistent

Duration: 0.18 seconds

### 6. DATA ANALYSIS

The atrial rate, rhythm, and normal P waves are consistent with a sinus rhythm. The atrial rate exceeds the ventricular rate, suggesting some form of AV block. The 3rd and 4th P waves are not followed by a QRS complex, indicating these P waves were not conducted. Prior to the nonconducted P waves, the P-R interval remains constant. The QRS duration is prolonged indicating an intraventricular conduction delay.

### 7. INTERPRETATION

Sinus rhythm with second degree AV block Mobitz Type II and an intraventricular conduction delay

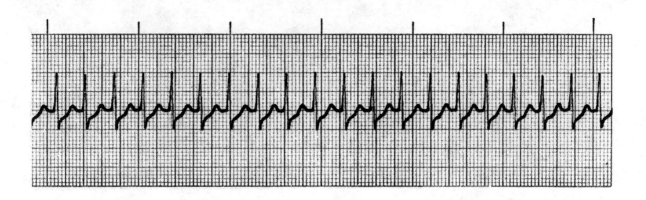

Figure 1-101A

# ECG RHYTHM STRIP #101

## I. RHYTHM

Atrial:

Ventricular:

## 2. RATE

Atrial:

Ventricular:

## 3. P WAVE

Presence:

Appearance:

Consistency:

Relation to QRS:

## 4. P-R INTERVAL

Duration:

Consistency:

## 5. QRS COMPLEX

Presence:

Appearance:

Consistency:

Duration:

## 6. DATA ANALYSIS

## 7. INTERPRETATION

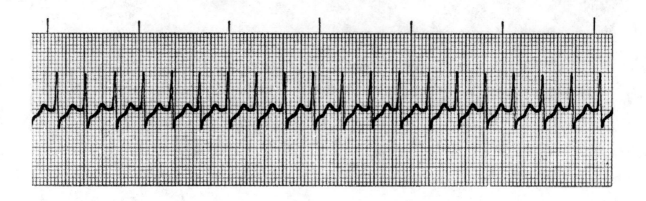

Figure 1-101B

# ECG RHYTHM STRIP #101

## I. RHYTHM

Atrial: Unable to determine

Ventricular: Regular

## 2. RATE

Atrial: Unable to determine

Ventricular: 190

## 3. P WAVE

Presence: Unable to identify

Appearance: May be merged into T wave

Consistency: —

Relation —

## 4. P-R INTERVAL

Duration: —

Consistency: —

## 5. QRS COMPLEX

Presence: Yes

Appearance: Normal

Consistency: Consistent

Duration: 0.06 seconds

## 6. DATA ANALYSIS

There is no clear evidence of atrial activity. The P wave may be merged with the T wave between QRS complexes, since this often occurs with rapid rates. A 12 lead ECG would be helpful in identifying atrial activity; slowing the rate slightly might uncover P waves to assist in locating the site of origin.

The ventricular rate is rapid and the rhythm is regular. Since the QRS duration is normal, the ventricular rhythm originates above the ventricles.

## 7. INTERPRETATION

Supraventricular tachycardia

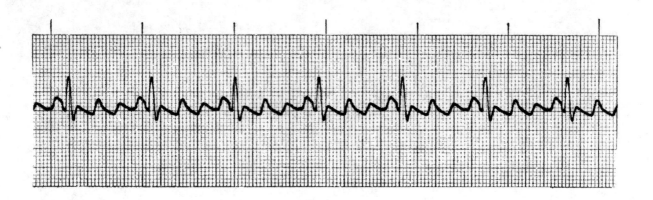

Figure 1-102A

# ECG RHYTHM STRIP #102

## 1. RHYTHM

Atrial:

Ventricular:

## 2. RATE

Atrial:

Ventricular:

## 3. P WAVE

Presence:

Appearance:

Consistency:

Relation to QRS:

## 4. P-R INTERVAL

Duration:

Consistency:

## 5. QRS COMPLEX

Presence:

Appearance:

Consistency:

Duration:

## 6. DATA ANALYSIS

## 7. INTERPRETATION

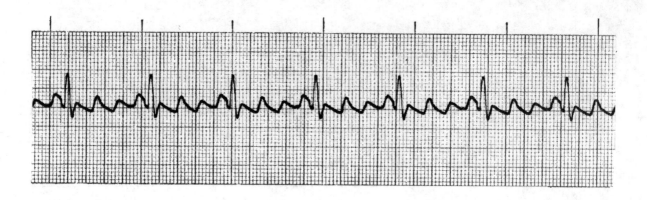

Figure 1-102B

# ECG RHYTHM STRIP #102

## I. RHYTHM

Atrial: Regular

Ventricular: Regular

## 2. RATE

Atrial: Approximately 280

Ventricular: Approximately 70

## 3. P WAVE

Presence: Yes

Appearance: Sawtooth flutter waves rather than discrete P waves

Consistency: Consistent

Relation to QRS: 4:1

## 4. P-R INTERVAL

Duration: Unable to determine

Consistency: —

## 5. QRS COMPLEX

Presence: Yes

Appearance: Normal

Consistency: Consistent

Duration: 0.12 seconds

## 6. DATA ANALYSIS

The atrial activity is characterized by regular sawtooth flutter waves at a rate of approximately 280 per minute. The ventricular rate is one fourth of the atrial rate, indicating a 4:1 conduction ratio with a controlled ventricular response. The QRS complex is prolonged in duration.

## 7. INTERPRETATION

Atrial flutter with 4:1 conduction ratio and an intraventricular conduction delay

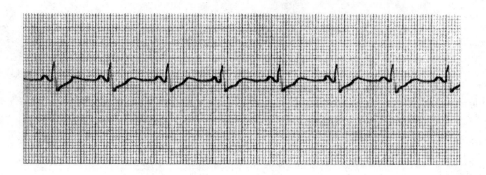

Figure 1-103A

# ECG RHYTHM STRIP #103
## Lead II

### I. RHYTHM

Atrial:

Ventricular:

### 2. RATE

Atrial:

Ventricular:

### 3. P WAVE

Presence:

Appearance:

Consistency:

Relation to QRS:

### 4. P-R INTERVAL

Duration:

Consistency:

### 5. QRS COMPLEX

Presence:

Appearance:

Consistency:

Duration:

### 6. DATA ANALYSIS

### 7. INTERPRETATION

207

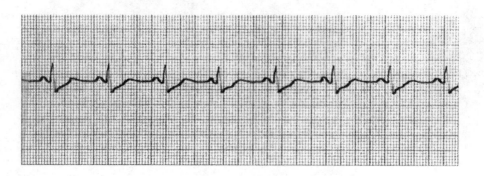

Figure 1-103B

# ECG RHYTHM STRIP #103
## Lead II

### 1. RHYTHM

Atrial: Regular

Ventricular: Regular

### 2. RATE

Atrial: 75

Ventricular: 75

### 3. P WAVE

Presence: Yes

Appearance: Normal

Consistency: Consistent

Relation to QRS: 1:1

### 4. P-R INTERVAL

Duration: 0.14 seconds

Consistency: Consistent

### 5. QRS COMPLEX

Presence: Yes

Appearance: Normal

Consistency: Consistent

Duration: 0.10 seconds

### 6. DATA ANALYSIS

All values are normal. The ST segment is depressed.

### 7. INTERPRETATION

(Normal) sinus rhythm

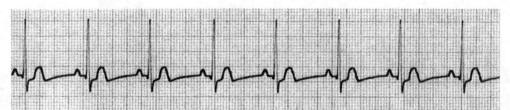

Figure 1-104A

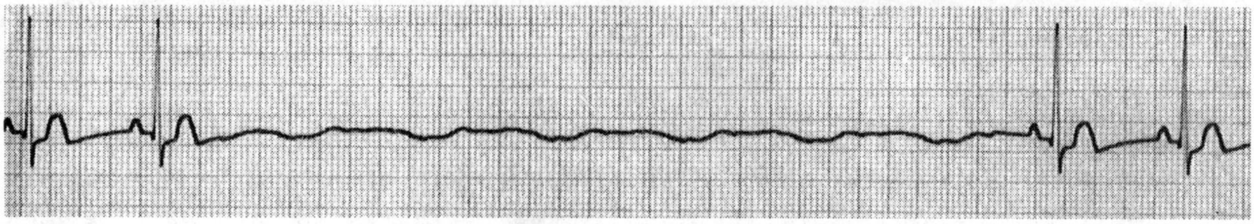

Figure 1-104B

# ECG RHYTHM STRIP #104
## Lead II

**1. RHYTHM**

Atrial:

Ventricular:

**2. RATE**

Atrial:

Ventricular:

**3. P WAVE**

Presence:

Appearance:

Consistency:

Relation to QRS:

**4. P-R INTERVAL**

Duration:

Consistency:

**5. QRS COMPLEX**

Presence:

Appearance:

Consistency:

Duration:

**6. DATA ANALYSIS**

**7. INTERPRETATION**

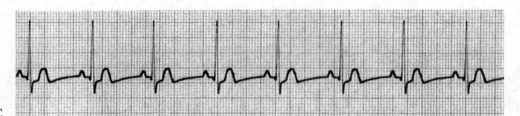

Figure 1-104C

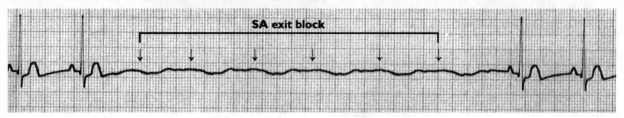

Figure 1-104D

# ECG RHYTHM STRIP #104
## Lead II

## 1. RHYTHM

Atrial: Regular; irregular with long pause

Ventricular: Regular; irregular with long pause

## 2. RATE

Atrial: 70 top; 20 bottom

Ventricular: Same as atrial rate

## 3. P WAVE

Presence: Yes

Appearance: Normal

Consistency: Consistent

Relation to QRS: 1:1

## 4. P-R INTERVAL

Duration: 0.14 seconds

Consistency: Consistent

## 5. QRS COMPLEX

Presence: Yes

Appearance: Normal

Consistency: Consistent

Duration: 0.08 seconds

## 6. DATA ANALYSIS

There is a 6 second interruption in the sinus cycle. When the P wave returns, it is a 7:1 multiple of the regular P-P cycle. (The arrows indicate blocked sinus impulses.) This is consistent with a Mobitz Type II SA exit block.

## 7. INTERPRETATION

Normal sinus rhythm with SA exit block, Type II

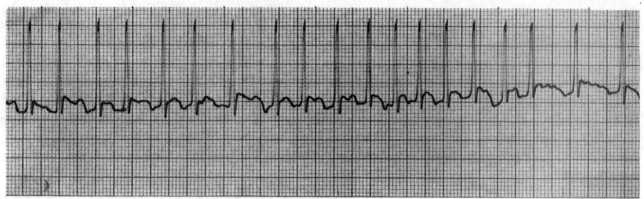

Figure 1-105A

# ECG RHYTHM STRIP #105
## Lead II

### 1. RHYTHM

Atrial:

Ventricular:

### 2. RATE

Atrial:

Ventricular:

### 3. P WAVE

Presence:

Appearance:

Consistency:

Relation to QRS:

### 4. P-R INTERVAL

Duration:

Consistency:

### 5. QRS COMPLEX

Presence:

Appearance:

Consistency:

Duration:

### 6. DATA ANALYSIS

### 7. INTERPRETATION

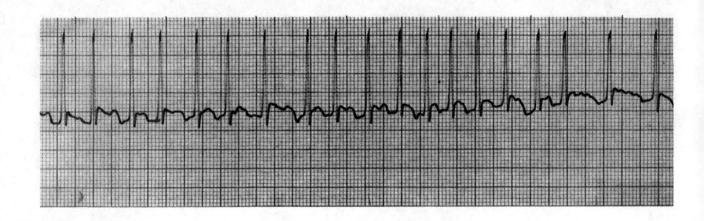

Figure 1-105B

# ECG RHYTHM STRIP #105
## Lead II

### 1. RHYTHM

Atrial: Irregular

Ventricular: Irregular

### 2. RATE

Atrial: Indeterminable

Ventricular: 170

### 3. P WAVE

Presence: No—unable to identify discrete
P waves

Appearance: Fine fibrillatory waves

Consistency: Inconsistent

Relation to QRS: Unable to determine without
distinct P waves

### 4. P-R INTERVAL

Duration: Unable to calculate

Consistency: —

### 5. QRS COMPLEX

Presence: Yes

Appearance: Normal

Consistency: Consistent

Duration: 0.06 seconds

### 6. DATA ANALYSIS

Discrete P waves are not present. Fine, fibrillatory waves are visible between the last two complexes. The ventricular rhythm is irregularly irregular.

### 7. INTERPRETATION

Atrial fibrillation with an uncontrolled ventricular response (ventricular rate greater than 100)

# • Part II •

## Complex Dysrhythmias

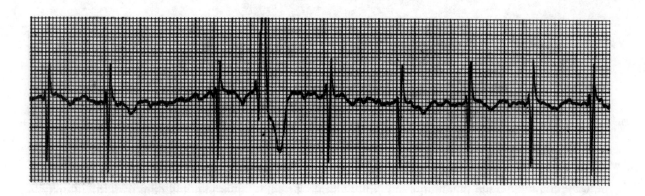

Figure 2-1A

# ECG RHYTHM STRIP #1
## Lead V₁

**I. RHYTHM**

    Atrial:

    Ventricular:

**2. RATE**

    Atrial:

    Ventricular:

**3. P WAVE**

    Present:

    Configuration:

    Consistency:

    Relation to QRS:

**4. P-R INTERVAL**

    Duration:

    Consistency:

**5. QRS COMPLEX**

    Present:

    Configuration:

    Consistency:

    Duration:

**6. DATA ANALYSIS**

**7. RHYTHM INTERPRETATION**

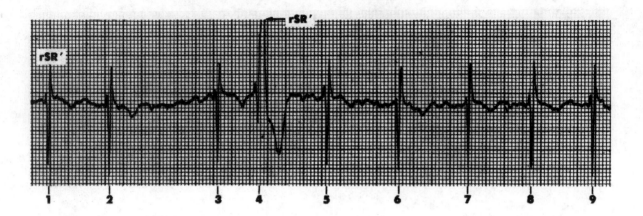

Figure 2-1B

# ECG RHYTHM STRIP #1
## Lead V₁

## 1. RHYTHM

Atrial:  Irregular

Ventricular:  Irregular

## 2. RATE

Atrial:  Indeterminable

Ventricular:  80

## 3. P WAVE

Present:  Variable atrial activity

Configuration:  Abnormal, fibrillatory waves

Consistency:  Inconsistent; varies in size, shape, and width

Relation to QRS:  Indeterminable

## 4. P-R INTERVAL  Undefined

Duration: —

Consistency: —

## 5. QRS COMPLEX

Present:  Yes

Configuration:  All abnormal —rSR'; beat 4 is more bizarre

Consistency:  Consistent, except for beat 4

Duration:  0.10 seconds except in beat 4 (0.16 seconds)

## 6. DATA ANALYSIS

The abnormal values include fibrillatory waves that make the atrial rate, P-R interval, and P to QRS relation indeterminable. In addition, the ventricular rhythm is irregular and the morphology of the QRS complex is abnormal in lead V₁. The QRS complex changes in beat 4—wider, shorter S wave, and taller, more slurred R wave.

The morphology of the QRS complexes (rSR') is consistent with RBBB in lead V₁. The width of the QRS is normal at 0.10 seconds making it an incomplete RBBB. The QRS complex in beat 4 is an extension of the same morphology but wider (0.16 seconds). Beat 4 is a classic example of an aberrantly conducted impulse. It follows a long preceding R-R interval (beat 2 to beat 3) and is of RBBB morphology. The long R-R interval (beat 2-3) gives beat 3 a long refractory period. The descending atrial impulse (leading to beat 4) finds the ventricles partially refractory and hence ventricular aberrancy results. 80% of aberrantly conducted impulses are conducted with RBBB morphology.

## 7. RHYTHM INTERPRETATION

Atrial fibrillation with a controlled ventricular response, incomplete RBBB, and one aberrantly conducted beat

216

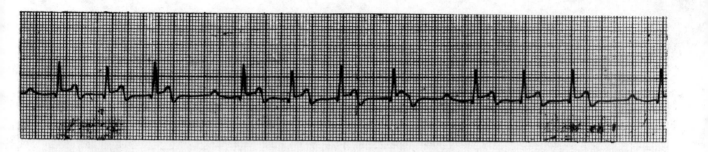

Figure 2-2A

# ECG RHYTHM STRIP #2
## Lead II

### 1. RHYTHM

Atrial:

Ventricular:

### 2. RATE

Atrial:

Ventricular:

### 3. P WAVE

Present:

Configuration:

Consistency:

Relation to QRS:

### 4. P-R INTERVAL

Duration:

Consistency:

### 5. QRS COMPLEX

Present:

Configuration:

Consistency:

Duration:

### 6. DATA ANALYSIS

### 7. RHYTHM INTERPRETATION

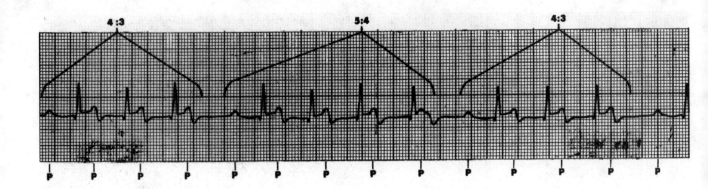

Figure 2-2B

# ECG RHYTHM STRIP #2
## Lead II

### 1. RHYTHM

Atrial: Regular

Ventricular: Irregular

### 2. RATE

Atrial: 100 (most P's obscure on ST-T waves)

Ventricular: 80

### 3. P WAVE

Present: Yes

Configuration: Normal, most P's on top of ST-T waves

Consistency: Consistent

Relation to QRS: Varies, 5:4 and 4:3

### 4. P-R INTERVAL

Duration: 0.38-0.52 seconds

Consistency: Inconsistent, progressively lengthens before pause

### 5. QRS COMPLEX

Present: Yes

Configuration: Normal

Consistency: Consistent

Duration: 0.08 seconds

### 6. DATA ANALYSIS

The abnormal values include:
- an irregular ventricular rhythm
- a slower ventricular versus atrial rate
- a variable P to QRS relation
- a variable and prolonged P-R interval

Several nonconducted P waves account for the slower ventricular rate and the pauses in the rhythm. Since the atrial rhythm is regular, the nonconducted P waves are of sinus origin indicating second degree AV block. There is a progressive increase in the P-R intervals consistent with Wenckebach phenomenon. In addition, the R-R interval containing the pause is less than two shorter R-R intervals. Variable AV conduction ratios are present (5:4, 4:3).

### 7. RHYTHM INTERPRETATION

Sinus rhythm with second degree AV block–Mobitz I (Wenckebach)

218

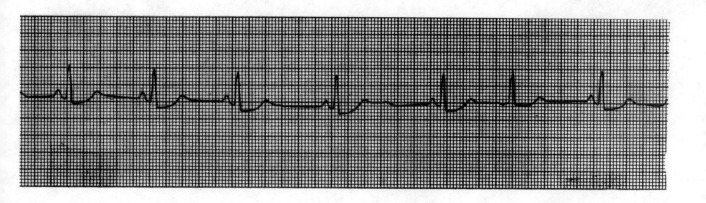

Figure 2-3A

# ECG RHYTHM STRIP #3
## Lead II

**I. RHYTHM**

   Atrial:

   Ventricular:

**2. RATE**

   Atrial:

   Ventricular:

**3. P WAVE**

   Present:

   Configuration:

   Consistency:

   Relation to QRS:

**4. P-R INTERVAL**

   Duration:

   Consistency:

**5. QRS COMPLEX**

   Present:

   Configuration:

   Consistency:

   Duration:

**6. DATA ANALYSIS**

**7. RHYTHM INTERPRETATION**

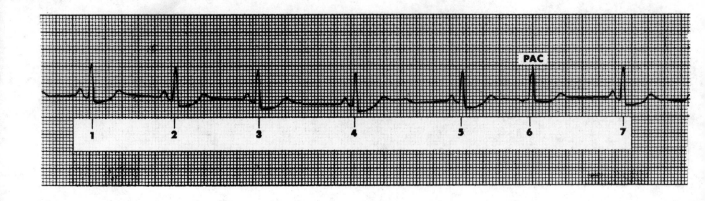

Figure 2-3B

# ECG RHYTHM STRIP #3
## Lead II

### I. RHYTHM

Atrial: Irregular

Ventricular: Irregular

### 2. RATE

Atrial: 60

Ventricular: 60

### 3. P WAVE

Present: Yes

Configuration: Normal—positive;
1 abnormal—negative

Consistency: Consistent, except for $P_6$

Relation to QRS: 1:1

### 4. P-R INTERVAL

Duration: 0.14 seconds

Consistency: Consistent

### 5. QRS COMPLEX

Present: Yes

Configuration: Normal

Consistency: Consistent

Duration: 0.08 seconds

### 6. DATA ANALYSIS

The abnormal values include:
- an irregular rhythm
- an abnormal P wave in beat 6

The shortest P-P interval ($P_1$-$P_2$) occurs at a rate slightly less than 60, indicating a basic sinus bradycardia.

$P_6$ is different in configuration and premature in the basic sinus cycle. The remaining P waves are identical in configuration; however, the P-P intervals vary by as much as 0.24 seconds. This most likely is secondary to sinus arrhythmia. Short periods of sinus arrest in an appropriate clinical setting is an additional consideration.

### 7. RHYTHM INTERPRETATION

Sinus bradycardia and arrhythmia with one PAC

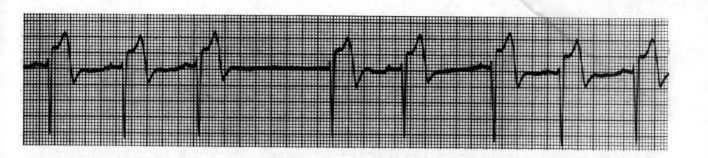

Figure 2-4A

# ECG RHYTHM STRIP #4
## Lead V₁

**I. RHYTHM**

  Atrial:

  Ventricular:

**2. RATE**

  Atrial:

  Ventricular:

**3. P WAVE**

  Present:

  Configuration:

  Consistency:

  Relation to QRS:

**4. P-R INTERVAL**

  Duration:

  Consistency:

**5. QRS COMPLEX**

  Present:

  Configuration:

  Consistency:

  Duration:

**6. DATA ANALYSIS**

**7. RHYTHM INTERPRETATION**

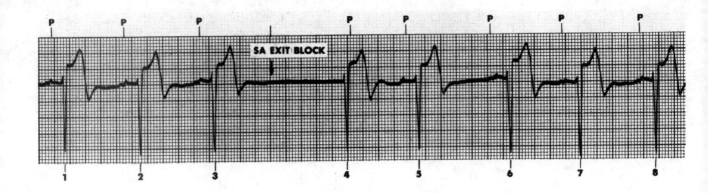

Figure 2-4B

# ECG RHYTHM STRIP #4
## Lead V₁

## 1. RHYTHM

Atrial: Irregular

Ventricular: Irregular

## 2. RATE

Atrial: 60

Ventricular: 60

## 3. P WAVE

Present: Yes (P wave obscure in ST segment of beat 4)

Configuration: Notched

Consistency: Inconsistent; P wave before QRS complexes 5 and 6 is slightly different

Relation to QRS: 1:1 (except with beat 4)

## 4. P-R INTERVAL

Duration: 0.22 seconds

Consistency: Consistent

## 5. QRS COMPLEX

Present: Yes

Configuration: Normal

Consistency: Consistent

Duration: 0.08 seconds

## 6. DATA ANALYSIS

The abnormal values include:
- an irregular ventricular rhythm
- a notched and slightly variable P wave configuration
- a prolonged P-R interval (0.22 seconds)

The first three P waves are regular and identical and establish a sinus rhythm at 65 per minute. The notched P wave could be normal for the lead but raises the possibility of an atrial abnormality. However, a 12 lead ECG is necessary to accurately assess this. No P wave is identifiable in the pause (QRS₃-QRS₄); however, a portion of the sinus P wave is seen in the ST segment immediately following QRS₄. The P-P interval (P preceding QRS₃-P following QRS₄) is equivalent to two full sinus cycles and indicates an SA exit block (sinus pause). (The sinus node can arrest for any period of time but pauses for precise intervals.) The P wave preceding QRS₅ falls premature in the basic sinus cycle and appears to be of slightly different morphology. The P wave preceding QRS₆ is similar to that preceding QRS₂, while those preceding QRS complexes 7 and 8 are identical to the sinus P waves. The findings are most consistent with ectopic atrial beats, although exaggerated sinus arrhythmia cannot be excluded. The P waves are conducted with slight first degree AV block.

QRS₄, which terminates the period of ventricular asystole induced by the SA exit block, is identical to the other QRS complexes and is of junctional origin. This junctional escape beat occurs slightly later (equivalent to a rate of 35) than expected for the AV junction, whose intrinsic rate is 40 to 60.

## 7. RHYTHM INTERPRETATION

Sinus rhythm with SA exit block, junctional escape beat, ectopic atrial beats ( versus exaggerated sinus arrhythmia), and first degree AV block

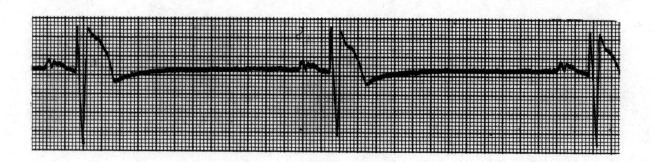

Figure 2-5A

# ECG RHYTHM STRIP #5
## Lead V₁

**I. RHYTHM**

   Atrial:

   Ventricular:

**2. RATE**

   Atrial:

   Ventricular:

**3. P WAVE**

   Present:

   Configuration:

   Consistency:

   Relation to QRS:

**4. P-R INTERVAL**

   Duration:

   Consistency:

**5. QRS COMPLEX**

   Present:

   Configuration:

   Consistency:

   Duration:

**6. DATA ANALYSIS**

**7. RHYTHM INTERPRETATION**

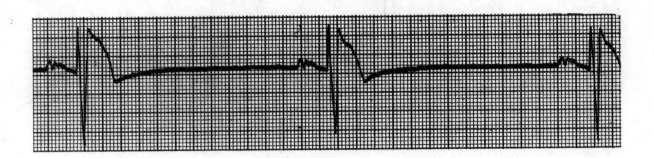

Figure 2-5B

# ECG RHYTHM STRIP #5
## Lead V₁

## I. RHYTHM

Atrial: Slightly irregular

Ventricular: Slightly irregular

## 2. RATE

Atrial: 20

Ventricular: 20

## 3. P WAVE

Present: Yes

Configuration: Notched, prolonged duration

Consistency: Consistent

Relation to QRS: 1:1

## 4. P-R INTERVAL

Duration: 0.34 seconds

Consistency: Consistent

## 5. QRS COMPLEX

Present: Yes

Configuration: Abnormal RSR'

Consistency: Consistent

Duration: 0.16 seconds

## 6. DATA ANALYSIS

The abnormal values include:
- a rate of 20 beats per minute
- a prolonged P-R interval at 0.34 seconds
- a wide, abnormal QRS complex

The P wave may originate from the sinus node with an atrial abnormality or from an ectopic atrial focus. A 12 lead ECG is needed to assess this.

An atrial rate of 20 is unusually slow for either pacemaker site. The possibility of a 2:1 or 3:1 SA or atrial exit block exists, but it is impossible to identify in this strip.

The morphology of the QRS complex (RSR') is consistent with RBBB in lead V₁.

## 7. RHYTHM INTERPRETATION

Marked sinus/atrial bradycardia with first degree AV block (rule out SA or atrial exit block) and RBBB

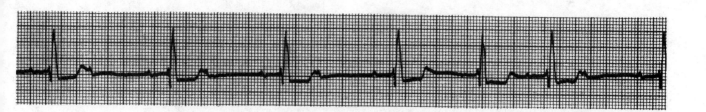

Figure 2-6A

# ECG RHYTHM STRIP #6
## Lead V₁

### 1. RHYTHM

Atrial:

Ventricular:

### 2. RATE

Atrial:

Ventricular:

### 3. P WAVE

Present:

Configuration:

Consistency:

Relation to QRS:

### 4. P-R INTERVAL

Duration:

Consistency:

### 5. QRS COMPLEX

Present:

Configuration:

Consistency:

Duration:

### 6. DATA ANALYSIS

### 7. RHYTHM INTERPRETATION

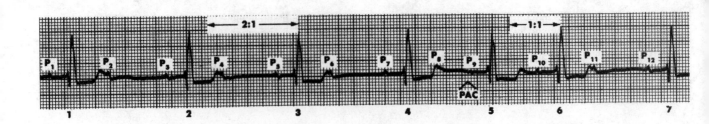

Figure 2-6B

# ECG RHYTHM STRIP #6
## Lead V₁

## I. RHYTHM

Atrial: Slightly irregular

Ventricular: Irregular

## 2. RATE

Atrial: 90 (Obscure P's in downslope of 1st, 2nd, 3rd, and 6th T wave and upstroke/peak of 4th T wave

Ventricular: 45

## 3. P WAVE

Present: Yes

Configuration: Sinus—diphasic; 1 ectopic—flattened

Consistency: Consistent, except preceding QRS₅

Relation to QRS: Varies, predominantly 2:1

## 4. P-R INTERVAL

Duration: 0.24 seconds

Consistency: Consistent

## 5. QRS COMPLEX

Present: Yes

Configuration: Abnormal, slurred rSR'

Consistency: Consistent

Duration: 0.12 seconds

## 6. DATA ANALYSIS

The abnormal values include:
- a ventricular rate of 45 (due to nonconducted P waves)
- an irregular rhythm
- a slight variation in P waves
- a variable P to QRS relation (2:1 except with beat 6)
- a prolonged P-R interval at 0.24 seconds
- an abnormal and wide (0.12 seconds) QRS complex

In examining the atrial rhythm, there is some variability in the P-P interval. P waves 1 through 8 are sinus since they march out fairly regularly. The diphasic P waves could be normal for the lead, but a 12 lead ECG is needed to rule out atrial abnormality. P wave 9 is premature in the sinus cycle (P-P interval between $P_8$ and $P_9$ is significantly shorter) and has a different P wave configuration, indicating a PAC. There is a greater pause (in the atrial rhythm) between $P_9$ (PAC) and $P_{10}$ (sinus). This pause permits the diseased conduction tissue to "rest" a little longer so that it conducts the next sinus impulse, hence 1:1 conduction occurs with the 6th beat.

The morphology of the QRS complex (rSR') is consistent with RBBB in lead $V_1$.

The second degree AV block is probable Mobitz II because of the presence of the bundle branch block.

## 7. RHYTHM INTERPRETATION

Sinus rhythm with one PAC, first degree and second degree AV block with 2:1 conduction ratios (probably Mobitz II) and RBBB

226

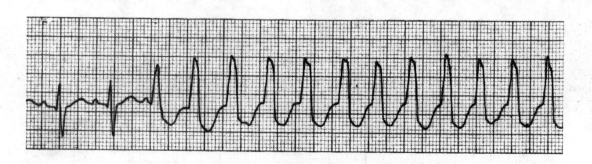

Figure 2-7A

# ECG RHYTHM STRIP #7
## Lead V₁

**1. RHYTHM**

Atrial:

Ventricular:

**2. RATE**

Atrial:

Ventricular:

**3. P WAVE**

Present:

Configuration:

Consistency:

Relation to QRS:

**4. P-R INTERVAL**

Duration:

Consistency:

**5. QRS COMPLEX**

Present:

Configuration:

Consistency:

Duration:

**6. DATA ANALYSIS**

**7. RHYTHM INTERPRETATION**

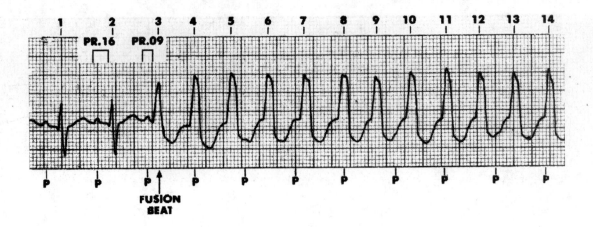

Figure 2-7B

## ECG RHYTHM STRIP #7
### Lead V₁

## I. RHYTHM

Atrial:  Regular with visible P waves

Ventricular:  Predominantly regular after beat 2

## 2. RATE

Atrial:  110 with identifiable P waves

Ventricular:  110 to 160

## 3. P WAVE

Present:  3 identifiable at beginning then variably seen deforming ST-T complex

Configuration:  Normal

Consistency:  Consistent, when visible

Relation to QRS:  1:1 with first 3 beats

## 4. P-R INTERVAL

Duration:  0.09-0.16 seconds

Consistency:  Consistent, with first 2 beats; beat 3 P-R shortens

## 5. QRS COMPLEX

Present:  Yes

Configuration:  Normal to abnormal

Consistency:  Inconsistent

Duration:  Normal—0.10 seconds
Abnormal—0.14 seconds

## 6. DATA ANALYSIS

The abnormal values include:
- a rapid atrial rate (110 beats per minute)
- a rapid ventricular rate (initially 110 then increases to 160)
- unidentifiable P waves after 3rd beat
- a shortened P-R interval in the 3rd cycle
- a change in the QRS complex from normal to abnormal and wide

The first 2 beats in this strip are normal, except that the cycle length indicates a rate of 110 beats per minute. The 3rd beat is immediately preceded by a normal P wave and has an abnormal QRS, which is slightly different from those that follow. The P-R interval (0.09 seconds) is too short to allow for normal conduction; however, some degree of ventricular fusion occurs (descending sinus impulse with ectopic ventricular beat). Note that the QRS here is slightly premature in the basic cycle length (initial R-R interval).

Following the 3rd beat, it is difficult to identify P waves due to the wide, abnormal QRS-T sequences. There appears to be a P wave following QRS 5, 6, 9 and 12. This would make the atrial rhythm a dissociated sinus rhythm, since those obscure P waves measure out in the basic sinus cycle. Furthermore, the wide QRS complexes are consistent with a ventricular focus.

## 7. RHYTHM INTERPRETATION

Sinus tachycardia with a fusion beat and ventricular tachycardia

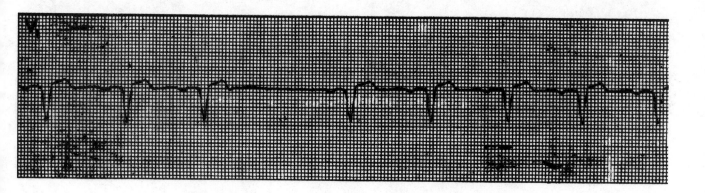

Figure 2-8A

# ECG RHYTHM STRIP #8
## Lead V₁

**I. RHYTHM**

Atrial:

Ventricular:

**2. RATE**

Atrial:

Ventricular:

**3. P WAVE**

Present:

Configuration:

Consistency:

Relation to QRS:

**4. P-R INTERVAL**

Duration:

Consistency:

**5. QRS COMPLEX**

Present:

Configuration:

Consistency:

Duration:

**6. DATA ANALYSIS**

**7. RHYTHM INTERPRETATION**

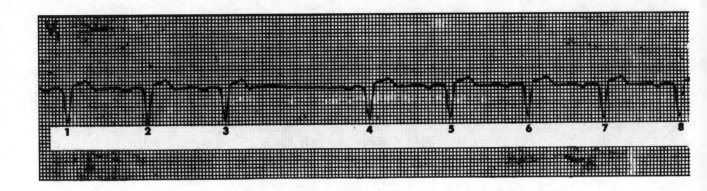

Figure 2-8B

# ECG RHYTHM STRIP #8
## Lead V₁

## I. RHYTHM

Atrial: Irregular

Ventricular: Irregular

## 2. RATE

Atrial: 60

Ventricular: 60

## 3. P WAVE

Present: Yes

Configuration: Negative polarity

Consistency: Consistent

Relation to QRS: 1:1

## 4. P-R INTERVAL

Duration: 0.24 seconds

Consistency: Consistent

## 5. QRS COMPLEX

Present: Yes

Configuration: Negative, slightly notched

Consistency: Consistent

Duration: 0.12 seconds

## 6. DATA ANALYSIS

All values are normal except:
- the rhythm is irregular (due primarily to a pause following beat 3)
- the P-R interval is prolonged at 0.24 seconds
- the QRS complex is wide

Although the polarity of the P wave is negative, a sinus rhythm is probable since the P wave is often negative in polarity in lead V₁. A 12 lead ECG is needed to assess the presence of a left atrial abnormality.

The pause in the ventricular rhythm is due to the absence of a P wave following beat 3. Careful measurement of R-R intervals (and hence the P-P intervals) shows a progressive decrease prior to the "dropped P wave." Following the pause the "P-P intervals" again show a progressive decrease. The findings are consistent with SA Wenckebach.

The wide QRS complex is related to an IV conduction delay. The configuration of the QRS complex in lead V₁—monophasic slurred QS—is consistent with left bundle branch block.

## 7. RHYTHM INTERPRETATION

Sinus rhythm with SA Wenckebach, first degree AV block, and an intraventricular conduction delay (probable LBBB)

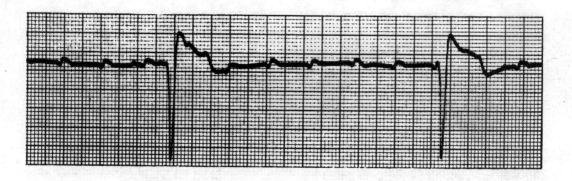

Figure 2-9A

# ECG RHYTHM STRIP #9
## Lead V₁

**1. RHYTHM**

    Atrial:

    Ventricular:

**2. RATE**

    Atrial:

    Ventricular:

**3. P WAVE**

    Present:

    Configuration:

    Consistency:

    Relation to QRS:

**4. P-R INTERVAL**

    Duration:

    Consistency:

**5. QRS COMPLEX**

    Present:

    Configuration:

    Consistency:

    Duration:

**6. DATA ANALYSIS**

**7. RHYTHM INTERPRETATION**

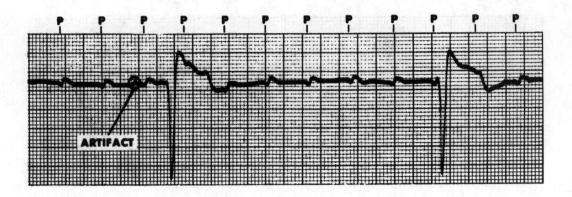

Figure 2-9B

# ECG RHYTHM STRIP #9
## Lead V₁

### 1. RHYTHM

Atrial: Regular

Ventricular: Indeterminable—only 1 R-R interval

### 2. RATE

Atrial: 140 (P's obscure on ST segment of both QRS complexes)

Ventricular: 20

### 3. P WAVE

Present: Yes

Configuration: Diphasic and wide

Consistency: Consistent

Relation to QRS: Probably none—P to QRS relation changes with 2 beats

### 4. P-R INTERVAL

Duration: Variable

Consistency: Inconsistent; the two P-QRS intervals differ

### 5. QRS COMPLEX

Present: Yes

Configuration: Unusual QR pattern

Consistency: Consistent

Duration: 0.12 seconds

### 6. DATA ANALYSIS

The abnormal values include:
- an atrial rate of 140 and ventricular rate of 20
- P waves unrelated to the QRS complex
- wide (0.12 seconds) QRS complexes

The origin of the P wave is difficult to determine without a 12 lead ECG. It may be sinus with an atrial abnormality, or an ectopic atrial rhythm.

The P's are unrelated to the QRS complex reflecting AV dissociation. The wide QRS complex and slow ventricular rate are consistent with an idioventricular escape rhythm.

### 7. RHYTHM INTERPRETATION

Supraventricular tachycardia with complete heart block and a ventricular escape pacemaker (or idioventricular rhythm)

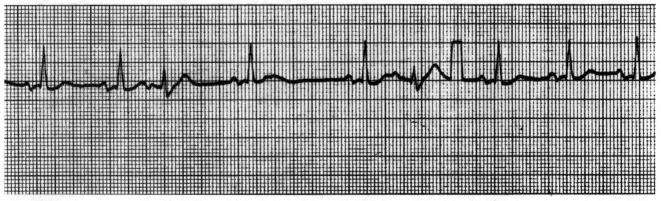

Figure 2-10A

# ECG RHYTHM STRIP #10
## Monitor Lead II

**I. RHYTHM**

    Atrial:

    Ventricular:

**2. RATE**

    Atrial:

    Ventricular:

**3. P WAVE**

    Present:

    Configuration:

    Consistency:

    Relation to QRS:

**4. P-R INTERVAL**

    Duration:

    Consistency:

**5. QRS COMPLEX**

    Present:

    Configuration:

    Consistency:

    Duration:

**6. DATA ANALYSIS**

**7. RHYTHM INTERPRETATION**

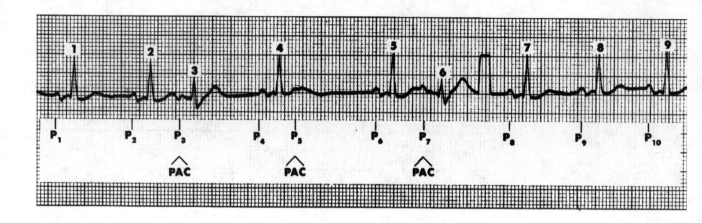

Figure 2-10B

# ECG RHYTHM STRIP #10
## Monitor Lead II

### 1. RHYTHM

Atrial: Irregular

Ventricular: Irregular

### 2. RATE

Atrial: 80 (P obscure in T following beat 4)

Ventricular: 70 (ECG standard marking between beats 6 and 7)

### 3. P WAVE

Present: Yes

Configuration: Sinus—diphasic; ectopic—positive

Consistency: Inconsistent

Relation to QRS: 1:1 except for nonconducted P wave

### 4. P-R INTERVAL

Duration: 0.18 seconds

Consistency: Consistent

### 5. QRS COMPLEX

Present: Yes

Configuration: Normal—positive
Abnormal—diphasic

Consistency: Inconsistent

Duration: Normal—0.08 seconds
Abnormal—0.12 seconds

### 6. DATA ANALYSIS

The abnormal values include:
- a slower ventricular versus atrial rate (due to nonconducted P wave after 4th beat)
- an irregular rhythm
- an inconsistent P wave
- two abnormal QRS complexes

Similar P waves precede QRS complexes 1, 2, 4, 5, and 7 to 9, representing the underlying rhythm. The first P-P interval represents the basic cycle length and it is consistent when 2 similar P's conduct consecutively (i.e., last 2 cycles). The atrial rate is consistent with underlying sinus rhythm. The diphasic P waves in Lead II may be related to monitor lead placement or an atrial abnormality. A 12 lead ECG is needed to accurately assess this.

P waves 3, 5 (distorts T wave), and 7 appear different in configuration and are premature in the basic rhythm. Two PAC's (P waves 3 and 7) are followed by QRS complexes that are different in configuration from the normally conducted QRS complexes. These represent aberrant ventricular conduction due to the descending impulse arriving at the ventricles during the relative refractory period. The nonconducted PAC ($P_5$) arrives at the ventricles during the absolute refractory period.

### 7. RHYTHM INTERPRETATION

Sinus rhythm with 2 aberrantly conducted PAC's and 1 nonconducted PAC

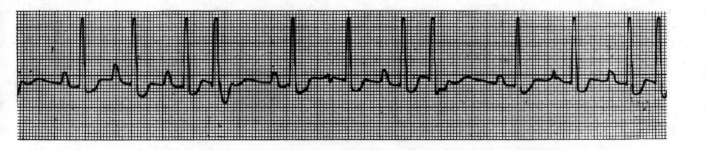

Figure 2-11A

# ECG RHYTHM STRIP #11
## Monitor Lead II

**1. RHYTHM**

    Atrial:

    Ventricular:

**2. RATE**

    Atrial:

    Ventricular:

**3. P WAVE**

    Present:

    Configuration:

    Consistency:

    Relation to QRS:

**4. P-R INTERVAL**

    Duration:

    Consistency:

**5. QRS COMPLEX**

    Present:

    Configuration:

    Consistency:

    Duration:

**6. DATA ANALYSIS**

**7. RHYTHM INTERPRETATION**

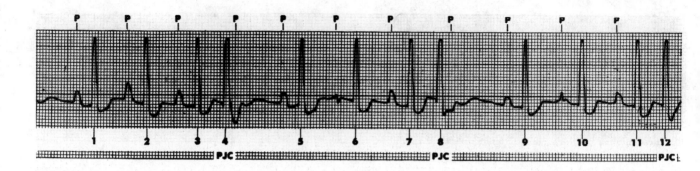

Figure 2-11B

# ECG RHYTHM STRIP #11
## Monitored Lead II

## 1. RHYTHM

Atrial: Slightly irregular

Ventricular: Irregular

## 2. RATE

Atrial: 80 (some obscure, distorting ST segment of beats 4 and 8)

Ventricular: 80

## 3. P WAVE

Present: Yes

Configuration: Some peaked, some diphasic

Consistency: Inconsistent; varies in configuration and polarity

Relation to QRS: 1:1 except for premature beats

## 4. P-R INTERVAL

Duration: 0.24 seconds

Consistency: Consistent

## 5. QRS COMPLEX

Present: Yes

Configuration: Positive

Consistency: Consistent

Duration: 0.12 seconds
0.14 seconds (beat 4, 8, 12)

## 6. DATA ANALYSIS

The abnormal values include:
- an irregular ventricular rhythm
- a variable P wave morphology
- an abnormal P to QRS relation with the premature beats
- a prolonged P-R interval at 0.24 seconds
- a wide QRS complex

There is clearly a P wave before every QRS complex except for the premature beats—beats 4, 8, and 12. The ST segments of beats 4 and 8 appear distorted, probably due to a P wave. Since the distortion in the ST segment changes and the "obscure" P waves almost measure out in the atrial rhythm (P-P only slightly irregular), they are consistent with dissociated P waves falling in or after the QRS complex of the premature beats. Retrograde P waves, however, cannot be totally excluded.

The irregular ventricular rhythm is caused primarily by the premature beats. The premature QRS complexes have basically the same configuration as the remaining QRS complexes consistent with a supraventricular origin. They may be conducting with slight aberrancy since they are slightly wider. The "normal" QRS complexes are prolonged in duration, indicating an intraventricular conduction delay.

## 7. RHYTHM INTERPRETATION

Wandering atrial pacemaker with premature junctional contractions (PJC's), first degree AV block, and an intraventricular conduction delay

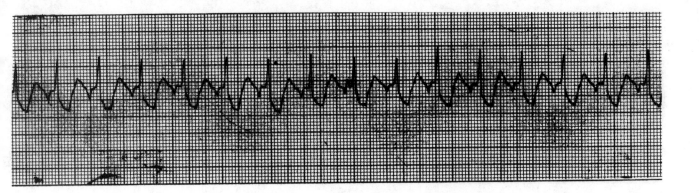

Figure 2-12A

# ECG RHYTHM STRIP #12
## Lead II

**1. RHYTHM**

　　Atrial:

　　Ventricular:

**2. RATE**

　　Atrial:

　　Ventricular:

**3. P WAVE**

　　Present:

　　Configuration:

　　Consistency:

　　Relation to QRS:

**4. P-R INTERVAL**

　　Duration:

　　Consistency:

**5. QRS COMPLEX**

　　Present:

　　Configuration:

　　Consistency:

　　Duration:

**6. DATA ANALYSIS**

**7. RHYTHM INTERPRETATION**

237

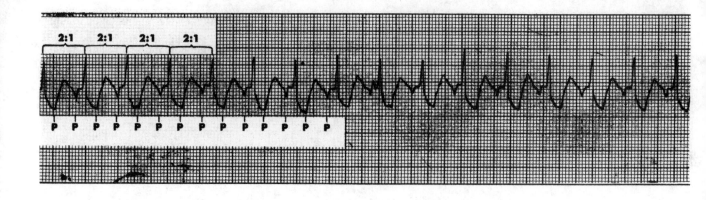

Figure 2-12B

# ECG RHYTHM STRIP #12
## Lead II

### 1. RHYTHM

Atrial: Regular

Ventricular: Regular

### 2. RATE

Atrial: 230 (every other P obscure in ST segment, just prior to upstroke of T wave)

Ventricular: 115

### 3. P WAVE

Present: Yes

Configuration: Abnormal—peaked and negative

Consistency: Consistent when visible

Relation to QRS: 2:1

### 4. P-R INTERVAL

Duration: Difficult to determine—approximately 0.14 seconds

Consistency: Consistent

### 5. QRS COMPLEX

Present: Yes

Configuration: Normal

Consistency: Consistent

Duration: 0.04 seconds

### 6. DATA ANALYSIS

The abnormal values include:
- an atrial rate of 230 and a ventricular rate of 115 beats per minute
- an abnormal P wave with 2:1 conduction to the ventricles

The atrial rate does not give us precise help in identifying the rhythm's origin since it is faster than a typical paroxysmal SVT (150-220) and slower than a typical atrial flutter (250-350). Quinidine-like drug effect can slow the atrial rate of atrial flutter. Clinical correlation is necessary.

### 7. RHYTHM INTERPRETATION

Supraventricular tachycardia (probably atrial flutter) with 2:1 AV conduction ratios

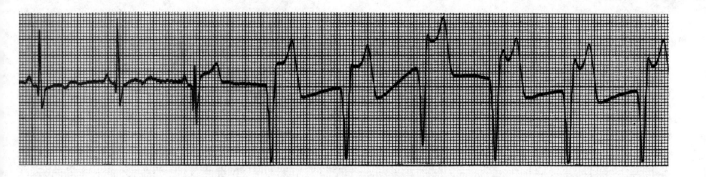

Figure 2-13A

# ECG RHYTHM STRIP #13
## Lead II

### 1. RHYTHM

Atrial:

Ventricular:

### 2. RATE

Atrial:

Ventricular:

### 3. P WAVE

Present:

Configuration:

Consistency:

Relation to QRS:

### 4. P-R INTERVAL

Duration:

Consistency:

### 5. QRS COMPLEX

Present:

Configuration:

Consistency:

Duration:

### 6. DATA ANALYSIS

### 7. RHYTHM INTERPRETATION

239

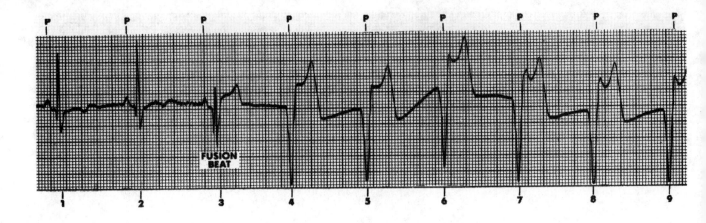

Figure 2-13B

# ECG RHYTHM STRIP #13
## Lead II

### 1. RHYTHM

**Atrial:** Slightly irregular

**Ventricular:** Slightly irregular

### 2. RATE

**Atrial:** 58 (P's probably hidden in beats 4 and 5. Obscure in beginning of ST segment in beats 6-9)

**Ventricular:** 62

### 3. P WAVE

**Present:** Yes

**Configuration:** Normal

**Consistency:** Consistent when identifiable

**Relation to QRS:** Varies, 1:1 to none

### 4. P-R INTERVAL

**Duration:** 0.14 seconds

**Consistency:** Slightly shorter in beat 3 (0.12 seconds)

### 5. QRS COMPLEX

**Present:** Yes

**Configuration:** Most are abnormal

**Consistency:** Inconsistent; varies in configuration and polarity

**Duration:** 0.12 to 0.14 seconds

### 6. DATA ANALYSIS

The abnormal values include:
- a slightly irregular rhythm and slow atrial rate
- a variable P to QRS relation
- a change in the P-R interval with beat 3
- an inconsistent QRS complex, which lengthens as the rhythm progresses

The atrial rhythm is characterized by P waves that measure out at a rate of 58. The P's are probably buried in QRS complexes 4 and 5. They appear in the beginning of the ST segments of beats 6 through 9. The origin of the P's is probably sinus.

The *slightly* irregular ventricular rhythm is due to the slight premature occurrence of QRS 4, where a change in the primary pacemaker occurs.

The third beat, with a QRS complex different from the sinus conducted and ectopic beats, is a fusion beat (shorter P-R interval) and represents a transition in pacemaker control.

The P to QRS relationship varies from 1:1 in the first 3 beats to isorhythmic AV dissociation with onset of the ectopic rhythm (sinus P's fall in or at slightly irregular intervals after QRS complexes). Note the sinus and ectopic rhythms are at approximately the same rate, hence the term isorhythmic AV dissociation.

The wide QRS complexes associated with the sinus conducted beats are probably related to an intraventricular conduction delay. The wide, abnormal, and negative QRS complexes following beat 3 are consistent with an ectopic ventricular rhythm.

### 7. RHYTHM INTERPRETATION

Mild sinus bradycardia and arrhythmia with an intraventricular conduction delay, a fusion beat, and accelerated idioventricular rhythm with isorhythmic AV dissociation

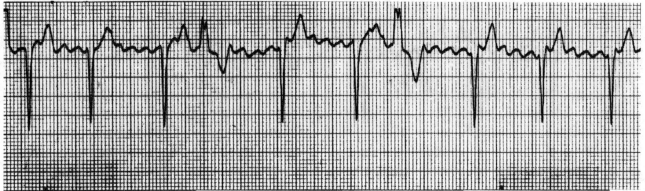

Figure 2-14A

## ECG RHYTHM STRIP #14
### Lead V₁

**1. RHYTHM**

  Atrial:

  Ventricular:

**2. RATE**

  Atrial:

  Ventricular:

**3. P WAVE**

  Present:

  Configuration:

  Consistency:

  Relation to QRS:

**4. P-R INTERVAL**

  Duration:

  Consistency:

**5. QRS COMPLEX**

  Present:

  Configuration:

  Consistency:

  Duration:

**6. DATA ANALYSIS**

**7. RHYTHM INTERPRETATION**

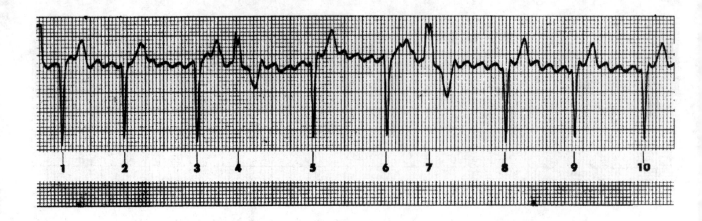

Figure 2-14B

# ECG RHYTHM STRIP #14
## Lead V₁

## 1. RHYTHM

Atrial: Regular

Ventricular: Irregular

## 2. RATE

Atrial: 375

Ventricular: 90

## 3. P WAVE

Present: Yes

Configuration: Abnormal—zig-zag, diphasic in polarity

Consistency: Consistent

Relation to QRS: Varies

## 4. P-R INTERVAL  Indeterminable

Duration: —

Consistency: —

## 5. QRS COMPLEX

Present: Yes

Configuration: Normal—negative
Abnormal—positive, notched

Consistency: Inconsistent

Duration: Normal—0.08 seconds
Abnormal—0.10 seconds

## 6. DATA ANALYSIS

The abnormal values include:
- an atrial rate of 375 with abnormal atrial activity that marches out regularly through the QRS and T waves
- an irregular ventricular rhythm
- two abnormal QRS complexes

The atrial activity (or P wave morphology) is slightly atypical for flutter and the rate is slightly faster than the usual flutter range (250-350), but the "flutter waves" do consistently repeat themselves. The variable flutter-R interval, the variable AV conduction ratios, and the ectopic beats account for the irregular ventricular rhythm. The overall ventricular rate, however, is controlled.

Two abnormal, wide QRS complexes (4 and 7) fall "premature" and most likely represent ectopic ventricular beats. However, because they both follow the longest R-R intervals and show RBBB configuration, aberrantly conducted impulses cannot be excluded. The fact that fixed coupling to the antecedant QRS is present and because the 1st rabbit ear is equal to or greater than the 2nd rabbit ear favors an ectopic ventricular origin.

## 7. RHYTHM INTERPRETATION

Atrial flutter with variable AV conduction ratios, a controlled ventricular rate, and 2 ectopic ventricular beats (rule out aberrantly conducted impulse)

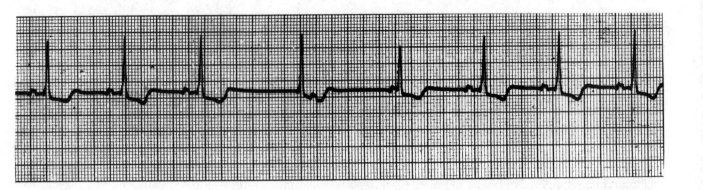

Figure 2-15A

# ECG RHYTHM STRIP #15
## Lead II

**1. RHYTHM**

    Atrial:

    Ventricular:

**2. RATE**

    Atrial:

    Ventricular:

**3. P WAVE**

    Present:

    Configuration:

    Consistency:

    Relation to QRS:

**4. P-R INTERVAL**

    Duration:

    Consistency:

**5. QRS COMPLEX**

    Present:

    Configuration:

    Consistency:

    Duration:

**6. DATA ANALYSIS**

**7. RHYTHM INTERPRETATION**

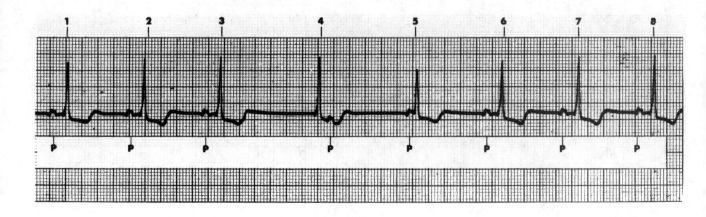

Figure 2-15B

# ECG RHYTHM STRIP #15
## Lead II

## 1. RHYTHM

Atrial: Irregular

Ventricular: Irregular

## 2. RATE

Atrial: 60

Ventricular: 60

## 3. P WAVE

Present: Yes

Configuration: Predominantly positive; slightly notched

Consistency: Consistent; one obscure at onset of $QRS_5$, but measures out in atrial rhythm

Relation to QRS: Varies, 1:1 except for beats 4 and 5 (P's not related)

## 4. P-R INTERVAL

Duration: 0.18 seconds

Consistency: Consistent except with beat 5

## 5. QRS COMPLEX

Present: Yes

Configuration: Normal

Consistency: Consistent

Duration: 0.08 seconds

## 6. DATA ANALYSIS

The abnormal values include:
- an irregular rhythm
- a variable P to QRS relation
- a shortened P-R interval with beat 5

Other than the pause in the atrial rhythm following beat 3, the P-P interval measures out regularly. The origin of the P waves is the same. $P_4$ (in ST segment) is identical in configuration to others and $P_5$ (partly hidden in QRS) measures out in the atrial rhythm and the initial deflection resembles the remaining P waves. Because the P waves in beats 4 and 5 are part of the underlying atrial rhythm, they are dissociated from the QRS complexes due to their respective locations—beat 4 after QRS; beat 5 immediately preceding QRS with P-R interval too short to conduct. The P waves are probably sinus in origin, although a 12 lead ECG is necessary to rule out atrial abnormality since the P waves are slightly notched.

The slowing of the atrial rate is probably due to a sinus arrest. The ventricular rhythm is restored following the sinus arrest with a junctional escape rhythm (QRS complexes 4 and 5). The sinus node captures the ventricles again starting with beat 6.

## 7. RHYTHM INTERPRETATION

Sinus rhythm with sinus arrest and 2 junctional escape beats

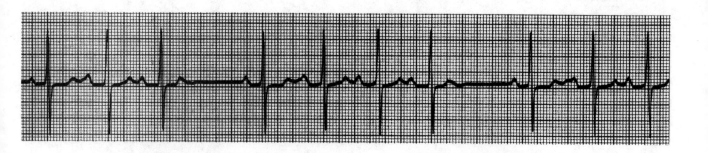

Figure 2-16A

# ECG RHYTHM STRIP #16
## Lead II

### 1. RHYTHM

Atrial:

Ventricular:

### 2. RATE

Atrial:

Ventricular:

### 3. P WAVE

Present:

Configuration:

Consistency:

Relation to QRS:

### 4. P-R INTERVAL

Duration:

Consistency:

### 5. QRS COMPLEX

Present:

Configuration:

Consistency:

Duration:

### 6. DATA ANALYSIS

### 7. RHYTHM INTERPRETATION

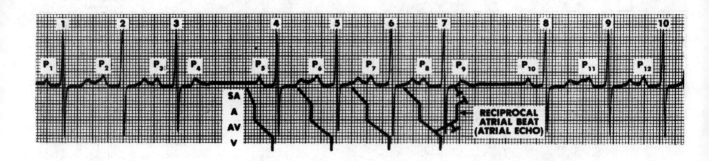

Figure 2-16B

# ECG RHYTHM STRIP #16
## Lead II

## I. RHYTHM

Atrial:  Irregular

Ventricular:  Irregular (Note: P-P and R-R intervals shorten after pauses)

## 2. RATE

Atrial:  90 (2 P waves obscured on ST-T waves after QRS 3 and 7)

Ventricular:  70

## 3. P WAVE

Present:  Yes

Configuration:  Normal, when visible

Consistency:  Consistent

Relation to QRS:  1:1 except P waves 4 and 9

## 4. P-R INTERVAL

Duration:  Beats 1, 4, 8: 0.22 seconds
Other beats: 0.28 seconds

Consistency:  Inconsistent

## 5. QRS COMPLEX

Present:  Yes

Configuration:  Normal

Consistency:  Consistent

Duration:  0.08 seconds

## 6. DATA ANALYSIS

The abnormal values include:
- a ventricular rate (70) that is less than the atrial rate (90), due to nonconducted P waves 4 and 9
- an irregular rhythm
- a prolonged (0.22-0.28 seconds) and inconsistent P-R interval
- a variable P to QRS relation

The atrial and ventricular rhythm is characterized by group beating separated by pauses in the rhythm. The shortening of the P-P intervals in the groups, and a pause that is less than twice the shortest P-P interval, suggest a Mobitz Type 1 (Wenckebach) conduction defect in the SA node.

The prolonged P-R intervals indicate an AV block. The shorter P-R intervals (0.22 versus 0.28 seconds) are probably related to the preceding pauses in the rhythm, allowing the AV node to "rest" or regain its nonrefractoriness.

Careful inspection of the ST-T wave following QRS 3 and 7 reveals a deformity consistent with a P wave. These P waves occur too premature to be sinus P waves. They could be nonconducted PAC's but more likely represent retrograde atrial conduction (atrial echo beat) via dissociated AV nodal pathways as they occur following a long P-R interval (see diagram).

## 7. RHYTHM INTERPRETATION

Sinus rhythm with probable SA exit block (Wenckebach), atrial echo beats, and first degree AV block

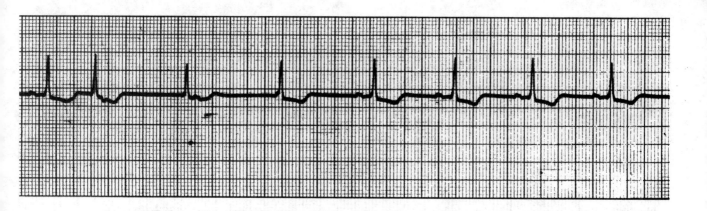

Figure 2-17A

## ECG RHYTHM STRIP #17
### Monitor Lead II

**1. RHYTHM**

    Atrial:

    Ventricular:

**2. RATE**

    Atrial:

    Ventricular:

**3. P WAVE**

    Present:

    Configuration:

    Consistency:

    Relation to QRS:

**4. P-R INTERVAL**

    Duration:

    Consistency:

**5. QRS COMPLEX**

    Present:

    Configuration:

    Consistency:

    Duration:

**6. DATA ANALYSIS**

**7. RHYTHM INTERPRETATION**

247

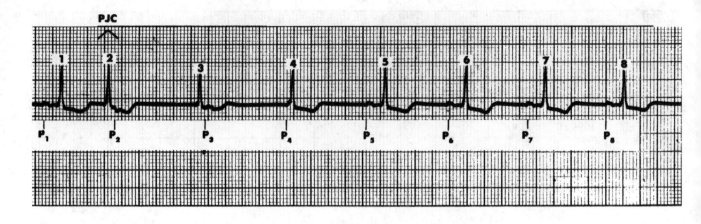

Figure 2-17B

# ECG RHYTHM STRIP #17
## Monitor Lead II

## 1. RHYTHM

Atrial: Irregular

Ventricular: Irregular

## 2. RATE

Atrial: 60 (P wave obscure in beat 4—distorts onset of QRS)

Ventricular: 60

## 3. P WAVE

Present: Yes

Configuration: Sinus—notched; ectopic—negative($P_2$)

Consistency: Consistent except following $QRS_2$ where P is negative

Relation to QRS: Varies

## 4. P-R INTERVAL

Duration: 0.16 seconds

Consistency: Consistent with conducted beats (1, 5, 6, 7, 8)

R-P Interval 0.14 seconds in beat 2

## 5. QRS COMPLEX

Present: Yes

Configuration: Normal

Consistency: Consistent

Duration: 0.08 seconds

## 6. DATA ANALYSIS

All values are normal except:
- the rhythm is irregular
- the P wave changes polarity after $QRS_2$
- the P to QRS relation varies

The atrial rhythm is characterized by positive notched P waves that march out regularly (after $QRS_3$ and onset of $QRS_4$) except after the premature beat. The notching of these P waves raises the possibility of an atrial abnormality; however, a 12 lead ECG is necessary to accurately diagnose this. The second negative P wave represents retrograde conduction to the atria from the premature ectopic focus since it is also premature in the otherwise consistent P-P intervals.

Since the P waves occurring with QRS complexes 3 and 4 are sinus, they are dissociated beats. In each case, a junctional pacemaker fired before the sinus impulse could conduct to the ventricles. Similarly, the sinus node depolarized the atria before retrograde conduction from the junctional impulse occurred. This is known as interference AV dissociation.

Note that the pause in the rhythm after the 2nd beat permitted the occurrence of the junctional escape beat.

## 7. RHYTHM INTERPRETATION

Sinus rhythm with one PJC followed by two junctional escape beats

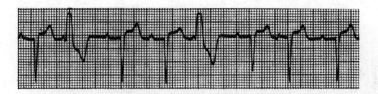

Figure 2-18A

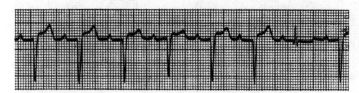

Figure 2-18B

# ECG RHYTHM STRIP #18 (Continuous Strip)
## Lead V₁

**I. RHYTHM**

Atrial:

Ventricular:

**2. RATE**

Atrial:

Ventricular:

**3. P WAVE**

Present:

Configuration:

Consistency:

Relation to QRS:

**4. P-R INTERVAL**

Duration:

Consistency:

**5. QRS COMPLEX**

Present:

Configuration:

Consistency:

Duration:

**6. DATA ANALYSIS**

**7. RHYTHM INTERPRETATION**

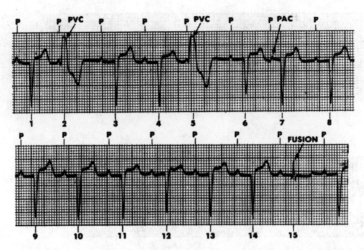

Figure 2-18C

Figure 2-18D

# ECG RHYTHM STRIP #18 (Continuous Strip)
## Lead V₁

## 1. RHYTHM

**Atrial:** Regular

**Ventricular:** Irregular

## 2. RATE

**Atrial:** 90

**Ventricular:** 90

## 3. P WAVE

**Present:** Yes

**Configuration:** Normal—positive; one diphasic—beat 7

**Consistency:** Consistent except in beat 7

**Relation to QRS:** Varies, 1:1 and none (beats 2 and 5)

## 4. P-R INTERVAL

**Duration:** 0.24 seconds (sinus beats)

**Consistency:** Consistent in sinus beats, varies in beat 7 (PAC 0.18 seconds) and in beat 15 (Fusion beat 0.20 seconds)

## 5. QRS COMPLEX

**Present:** Yes

**Configuration:** Normal and abnormal

**Consistency:** Inconsistent; varies in configuration and polarity

**Duration:** 0.08 to 0.12 seconds

## 6. DATA ANALYSIS

The abnormal values include:
- an irregular ventricular rhythm
- a change in the polarity of the P wave in beat 7
- an inconsistent P to QRS relation
- a variation in the P-R interval
- an inconsistent QRS configuration
- a wide (0.12 seconds) and abnormal QRS complex in beats 2 and 5

QRS complexes 2 and 5 are abnormal, wide, and premature in the underlying ventricular rhythm. Although a normal P wave appears before them, the P-R interval is too short to conduct, making them dissociated sinus P's.

QRS complex 7 is premature in the underlying ventricular rhythm. It is preceded by an ectopic P wave (different from sinus P) and is slightly early in the basic atrial rhythm. It conducts with a shorter P-R interval (approximately 0.18 seconds) than the sinus conducted beats and is probably of low atrial origin.

Beat 15 is characterized by a change in the configuration of the QRS complex and a shortened P-R interval (0.20 versus 0.24 seconds). The preceding sinus P rules out a junctional or atrial ectopic beat. The shorter P-R interval and the existence of ventricular ectopy indicate a ventricular fusion beat.

The prolonged P-R intervals (0.24 seconds) with the sinus conducted P waves indicate first degree AV block.

## 7. RHYTHM INTERPRETATION

Sinus rhythm with first degree AV block, 2 PVC's, 1 PAC, and 1 ventricular fusion beat

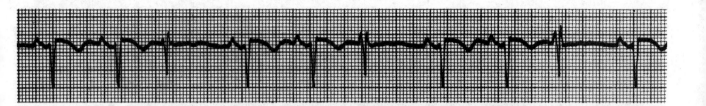

Figure 2-19A

# ECG RHYTHM STRIP #19
## MCL₁

## I. RHYTHM

    Atrial:

    Ventricular:

## 2. RATE

    Atrial:

    Ventricular:

## 3. P WAVE

    Present:

    Configuration:

    Consistency:

    Relation to QRS:

## 4. P-R INTERVAL

    Duration:

    Consistency:

## 5. QRS COMPLEX

    Present:

    Configuration:

    Consistency:

    Duration:

## 6. DATA ANALYSIS

## 7. RHYTHM INTERPRETATION

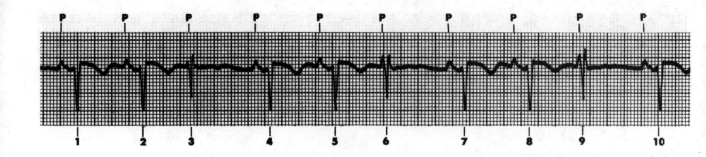

Figure 2-19B

# ECG RHYTHM STRIP #19
## MCL₁

### I. RHYTHM

Atrial: Regular

Ventricular: Irregular (regularly irregular or cyclic)

### 2. RATE

Atrial: 80 (obscure in initial R wave of premature beats)

Ventricular: 80

### 3. P WAVE

Present: Yes

Configuration: Notched, prolonged duration

Consistency: Consistent

Relation to QRS: 1:1 except with premature beats

### 4. P-R INTERVAL

Duration: 0.18 seconds

Consistency: Consistent

### 5. QRS COMPLEX

Present: Yes

Configuration: Normal and abnormal

Consistency: Inconsistent

Duration: 0.08 seconds (appears wider in premature beats due to superimposed P waves)

### 6. DATA ANALYSIS

The abnormal values include:
• an irregular ventricular rhythm
• a change in the P to QRS relation and QRS configuration with the premature beats (3, 6, 9)

The P waves march out regularly and appear to distort the initial deflection of the premature beats except in beat 3. Since they measure out in the atrial rhythm, they are dissociated from the QRS complexes in the premature beats. The atrial rate and rhythm are consistent with sinus origin. Since the P wave is notched and prolonged in duration, a 12 lead ECG is needed to rule out left atrial abnormality.

The ectopic beats are probably of ventricular origin. A 12 lead ECG may reveal they are "wider" in another lead. Because the ectopic beats show and rSR' configuration, junctional beats with aberrancy is an alternative consideration. However, the fact that these beats do not follow a long R-R interval is against this explanation.

### 7. RHYTHM INTERPRETATION

Sinus rhythm with PVC's (ventricular trigeminy)

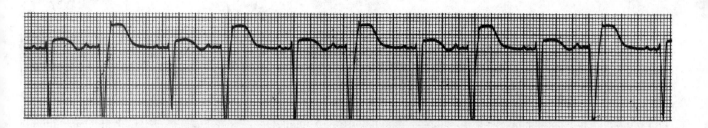

Figure 2-20A

# ECG RHYTHM STRIP #20
## Lead V₁

**1. RHYTHM**

    Atrial:

    Ventricular:

**2. RATE**

    Atrial:

    Ventricular:

**3. P WAVE**

    Present:

    Configuration:

    Consistency:

    Relation to QRS:

**4. P-R INTERVAL**

    Duration:

    Consistency:

**5. QRS COMPLEX**

    Present:

    Configuration:

    Consistency:

    Duration:

**6. DATA ANALYSIS**

**7. RHYTHM INTERPRETATION**

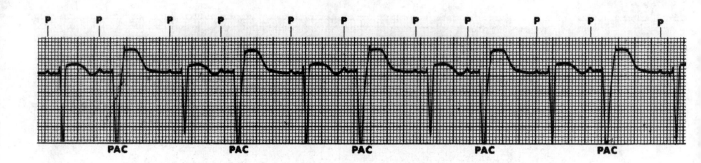

Figure 2-20B

# ECG RHYTHM STRIP #20
## Lead V₁

## I. RHYTHM

Atrial: Irregular—cyclic

Ventricular: Irregular—cyclic

## 2. RATE

Atrial: 80

Ventricular: 80

## 3. P WAVE

Present: Yes

Configuration: Notched

Consistency: Inconsistent; varies slightly with alternating P's

Relation to QRS: 1:1

## 4. P-R INTERVAL

Duration: 0.16 seconds

Consistency: Consistent

## 5. QRS COMPLEX

Present: Yes

Configuration: Normal and abnormal

Consistency: Inconsistent; alternating variation

Duration: Normal—0.09 seconds
Abnormal—0.16 seconds

## 6. DATA ANALYSIS

The abnormal values include:
- an irregular (cyclic) rhythm
- a notched and inconsistent P wave
- an alternating change in the QRS complex from normal and narrow to abnormal and wide

The cyclic rhythm is due to the alternating occurrence of premature atrial beats. All the P waves appear notched but change slightly with the premature beats (i.e., initial peak taller). This indicates a change in pacemaker site. The underlying rhythm is probably sinus, since the atrial rate is normal. The notched P wave in V₁ could be normal for the lead, however, a 12 lead ECG is needed to rule out atrial abnormality.

The abnormal and wide QRS complexes with the premature beats are due to aberrancy secondary to a change in cycle length—that is, shortening of immediate cycle after preceding cycle was lengthened. Expressing it another way, the PACs follow longer R-R intervals. Since the rhythm strip is V₁ the PAC's are conducted with LBBB aberrancy. This is unusual, occurring in only 20% of aberrantly conducted impulses.

## 7. RHYTHM INTERPRETATION

Sinus rhythm with frequent PAC's (atrial bigeminy) conducted with LBBB aberrancy

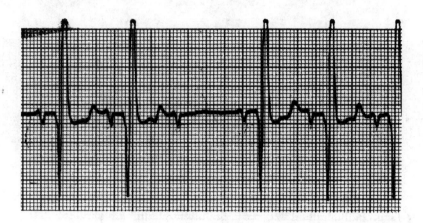

Figure 2-21A

# ECG RHYTHM STRIP #21
## Lead MCL₁

**1. RHYTHM**

    Atrial:

    Ventricular:

**2. RATE**

    Atrial:

    Ventricular:

**3. P WAVE**

    Present:

    Configuration:

    Consistency:

    Relation to QRS:

**4. P-R INTERVAL**

    Duration:

    Consistency:

**5. QRS COMPLEX**

    Present:

    Configuration:

    Consistency:

    Duration:

**6. DATA ANALYSIS**

**7. RHYTHM INTERPRETATION**

255

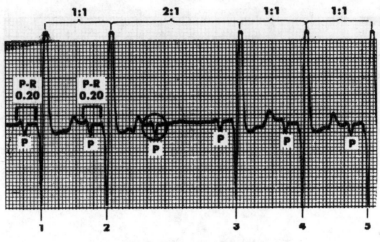

Figure 2-21B

# ECG RHYTHM STRIP #21
## Lead MCL₁

## 1. RHYTHM

Atrial: Regular

Ventricular: Irregular

## 2. RATE

Atrial: 80

Ventricular: 70

## 3. P WAVE

Present: Yes

Configuration: Diphasic with large terminal negative deflection

Consistency: Consistent

Relation to QRS: Varies 1:1 and 2:1

## 4. P-R INTERVAL

Duration: 0.20 seconds

Consistency: Consistent

## 5. QRS COMPLEX

Present: Yes

Configuration: Abnormal—slurred R wave

Consistency: Consistent

Duration: 0.16 seconds

## 6. DATA ANALYSIS

The abnormal values include:
- a slower ventricular versus atrial rate
- an irregular ventricular rhythm (due to pause)
- a variation in the P to QRS relation from 1:1 to 2:1

All of these abnormal values can be attributed to the nonconducted P wave following beat 2. In addition, the QRS complex is wide and abnormal.

The nonconducted P wave is identical to the other P waves and is on time in the sinus cycle (regular P-P intervals). The configuration of the P wave (diphasic with large terminal negative deflection) in MCL₁ raises the possibility of left atrial abnormality; however, a 12 lead ECG is needed to accurately assess this. The P-R intervals preceding the nonconducted sinus impulse are identical. The QRS is wide and abnormal, indicating an intraventricular conduction delay. The findings are consistent with infranodal second degree Av block (Mobitz II).

## 7. RHYTHM INTERPRETATION

Sinus rhythm with second degree AV block-Mobitz Type II and an intraventricular conduction delay

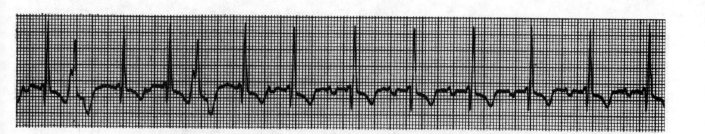

Figure 2-22A

# ECG RHYTHM STRIP #22
## Lead V₁

**I. RHYTHM**

Atrial:

Ventricular:

**2. RATE**

Atrial:

Ventricular:

**3. P WAVE**

Present:

Configuration:

Consistency:

Relation to QRS:

**4. P-R INTERVAL**

Duration:

Consistency:

**5. QRS COMPLEX**

Present:

Configuration:

Consistency:

Duration:

**6. DATA ANALYSIS**

**7. RHYTHM INTERPRETATION**

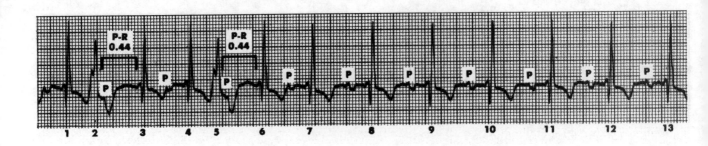

Figure 2-22B

## ECG RHYTHM STRIP #22
### Lead V₁

### I. RHYTHM

Atrial: Regular

Ventricular: Irregular

### 2. RATE

Atrial: 80 (Obscure P waves in ST-T sequence of QRS complexes 2 and 5)

Ventricular: 100

### 3. P WAVE

Present: Yes

Configuration: Disphasic, large terminal negative deflection

Consistency: Consistent when visible

Relation to QRS: 1:1 except with QRS complexes 2 and 5

### 4. P-R INTERVAL

Duration: 0.24 seconds; approximately 0.44 seconds in beats 3 and 6

Consistency: Consistent except for beats 3 and 6

### 5. QRS COMPLEX

Present: Yes

Configuration: Abnormal, varies—rSR' and double-peaked R

Consistency: Inconsistent

Duration: 0.12 seconds

### 6. DATA ANALYSIS

The abnormal values include:
- a ventricular rate of 100-faster than atrial rate due to extra beats
- an irregular ventricular rhythm
- a variable P to QRS relation
- a prolonged and inconsistent P-R interval
- an abnormal, wide QRS complex that varies in configuration

The P waves, sometimes distorted slightly by artifact, do march out regularly despite the irregularity in the ventricular rhythm. They are probably sinus in origin, since the atrial rate and rhythm are normal. The morphology of the P wave in V₁—large terminal negative deflection—raises the possibility of left atrial abnormality; however, a 12 lead ECG is needed to accurately access this.

QRS complexes 2 and 5 are wide, abnormal, and different from the sinus conducted beats. They are premature in the basic sinus cycle (fall on preceding T wave) and dissociated from the atrial rhythm— sinus P wave follows the QRS. These beats are most likely ventricular in origin. The PVC's are interpolated—interposed between two sinus conducted beats.

The prolonged P-R interval (0.24 seconds) is related to an AV block. Beats 3 and 6 are sinus conducted, since a sinus P wave can be found preceding these QRS complexes—in the ST-T sequence of the PVC's. The reason for the prolonged P-R interval (0.44 seconds) with these beats is concealed AV conduction from the PVC's.

The abnormal, wide QRS complexes with the sinus conducted beats are due to an intraventricular conduction delay. An rSR' configuration is consistent with RBBB in V₁.

### 7. RHYTHM INTERPRETATION

Sinus rhythm with interpolated PVC's (R on T, evidence for concealed conduction), first degree AV block and RBBB

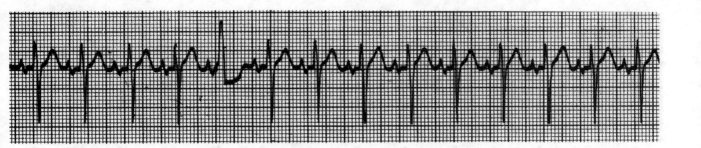

Figure 2-23A

# ECG RHYTHM STRIP #23
## Lead V₁

**I. RHYTHM**

    Atrial:

    Ventricular:

**2. RATE**

    Atrial:

    Ventricular:

**3. P WAVE**

    Present:

    Configuration:

    Consistency:

    Relation to QRS:

**4. P-R INTERVAL**

    Duration:

    Consistency:

**5. QRS COMPLEX**

    Present:

    Configuration:

    Consistency:

    Duration:

**6. DATA ANALYSIS**

**7. RHYTHM INTERPRETATION**

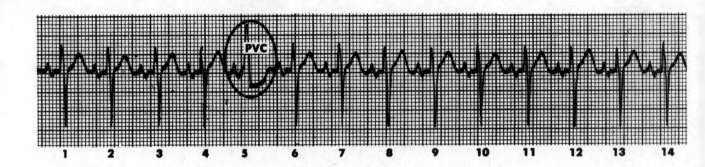

Figure 2-23B

## ECG RHYTHM STRIP 23
### Lead V₁

### 1. RHYTHM

Atrial: Regular

Ventricular: Slightly irregular (QRS₅ slightly early in R-R interval)

### 2. RATE

Atrial: 120

Ventricular: 120

### 3. P WAVE

Present: Yes

Configuration: Diphasic

Consistency: Consistent

Relation to QRS: 1:1

### 4. P-R INTERVAL

Duration: 0.16 seconds

Consistency: Consistent, except in beat 5 where P-R is slightly less at 0.13 seconds

### 5. QRS COMPLEX

Present: Yes

Configuration: Normal—diphasic; one abnormal and positive

Consistency: Consistent, except in beat 5

Duration: 0.08 seconds; 0.09 seconds in beat 5

### 6. DATA ANALYSIS

The abnormal values include:
- a rate of 120 beats per minute
- a slightly irregular ventricular rhythm
- a change in the P-R interval and the configuration of QRS complex 5

The diphasic P wave in V₁ could be normal for the lead, but a 12 lead ECG is needed to rule out atrial abnormality.

Beat 5 stands out in the basic rhythm. Although it is preceded by a sinus P wave, the P-R interval is shortened and the QRS is abnormal in configuration. Since the R wave is slightly premature in the basic R-R interval and the QRS is different from the normally conducted beats, it must be a type of PVC—end-diastolic (ventricular ectopic beat occurring late in diastole). End-diastolic PVC's are frequently fusion beats, since the ventricular ectopic focus merges with the sinus impulse in the ventricles. This is probably the case here, since the width of the QRS is 0.09 seconds and the P-R interval is only 0.03 seconds shorter than the normally conducted beats.

### 7. RHYTHM INTERPRETATION

Sinus tachycardia with end-diastolic PVC (probable fusion beat)

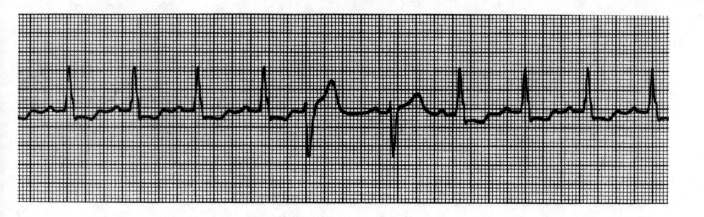

Figure 2-24A

# ECG RHYTHM STRIP #24
## Lead I

**1. RHYTHM**

Atrial:

Ventricular:

**2. RATE**

Atrial:

Ventricular:

**3. P WAVE**

Present:

Configuration:

Consistency:

Relation to QRS:

**4. P-R INTERVAL**

Duration:

Consistency:

**5. QRS COMPLEX**

Present:

Configuration:

Consistency:

Duration:

**6. DATA ANALYSIS**

**7. RHYTHM INTERPRETATION**

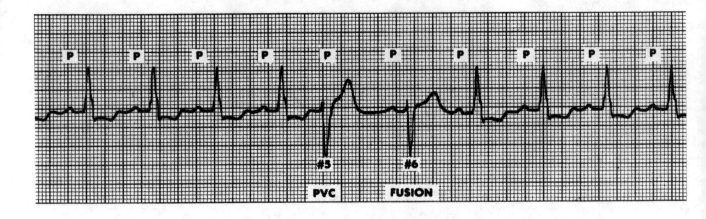

Figure 2-24B

# ECG RHYTHM STRIP #24
## Lead I

## I. RHYTHM

Atrial: Regular

Ventricular: Irregular

## 2. RATE

Atrial: 90 (P hidden in $QRS_5$)

Ventricular: 90

## 3. P WAVE

Present: Yes

Configuration: Normal

Consistency: Consistent

Relation to QRS: 1:1 except with beat 5

## 4. P-R INTERVAL

Duration: 0.21 seconds

Consistency: Consistent (may be slightly shorter with beat 6)

## 5. QRS COMPLEX

Present: Yes

Configuration: Positive beats: abnormal, slightly notched. QRS's 5 and 6: negative, slurred S

Consistency: Inconsistent; varies in configuration and polarity

Duration: 0.12 seconds except 0.09 seconds with beat 6

## 6. DATA ANALYSIS

The abnormal values include:
- an irregular ventricular rhythm
- an unrelated P to QRS in beat 5
- a prolonged P-R interval of 0.21 seconds
- an inconsistent and wide (except beat 6) QRS complex

The P wave hidden in beat 5 is dissociated from the QRS complex since it measures out in the atrial rhythm.

The basic rhythm conducts abnormally through the ventricles—positive, wide (0.12 seconds) QRS complexes. The 5th beat is premature, wide, and different in configuration from the preceding beats consistent with an ectopic ventricular origin. Beat 6, which is preceded by a normal P wave but with a different QRS complex, probably represents a ventricular fusion beat (ventricular depolarization due in part to descending sinus impulse plus simultaneous ectopic ventricular beat). Notice the P-R interval appears slightly shorter and the QRS complex resembles the ventricular ectopic beat but is narrower.

## 7. RHYTHM INTERPRETATION

Sinus rhythm with borderline first degree AV block, intraventricular conduction delay, and back to back ectopic ventricular beats including one ventricular fusion beat

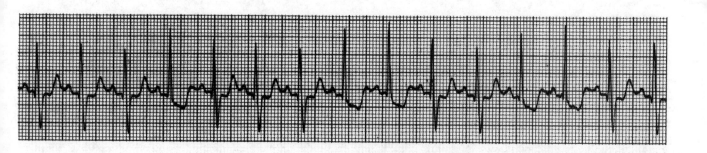

Figure 2-25A

# ECG RHYTHM STRIP #25
## Monitor Lead II

**1. RHYTHM**

Atrial:

Ventricular:

**2. RATE**

Atrial:

Ventricular:

**3. P WAVE**

Present:

Configuration:

Consistency:

Relation to QRS:

**4. P-R INTERVAL**

Duration:

Consistency:

**5. QRS COMPLEX**

Present:

Configuration:

Consistency:

Duration:

**6. DATA ANALYSIS**

**7. RHYTHM INTERPRETATION**

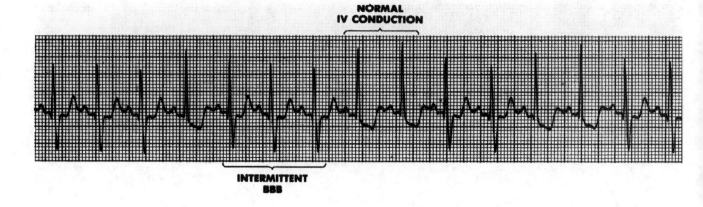

NORMAL
IV CONDUCTION

INTERMITTENT
BBB

Figure 2-25B

# ECG RHYTHM STRIP #25
## Monitor Lead II

## I. RHYTHM

Atrial: Regular

Ventricular: Regular

## 2. RATE

Atrial: 120

Ventricular: 120

## 3. P WAVE

Present: Yes

Configuration: Normal

Consistency: Consistent

Relation to QRS: 1:1

## 4. P-R INTERVAL

Duration: 0.14 seconds

Consistency: Consistent

## 5. QRS COMPLEX

Present: Yes

Configuration: Some normal, some abnormal
(wide, diphasic)

Consistency: Inconsistent; varies in configuration and polarity

Duration: Diphasic—0.12 seconds
Positive—0.07 seconds

## 6. DATA ANALYSIS

All values are normal, except that the rate is 120
beats per minute and the QRS complexes vary in
configuration, polarity, and width (from
abnormal, diphasic, and wide to normal, positive, and narrow). Since the P-R intervals of all
the QRS complexes are identical and since the
R-R intervals are essentially regular, an ectopic
ventricular focus or aberrant conduction can be
excluded. The abnormal QRS complexes must
be related to an intermittent intraventricular
conduction delay, i.e., intermittent bundle
branch block. A 12 lead ECG is needed to identify the specific type (left or right).

## 7. RHYTHM INTERPRETATION

Sinus tachycardia with intermittent bundle
branch block

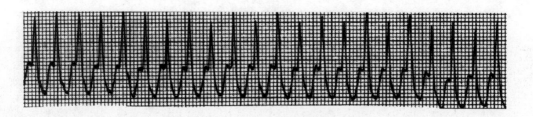

Figure 2-26A

# ECG RHYTHM STRIP #26
## Lead II

**I. RHYTHM**

Atrial:

Ventricular:

**2. RATE**

Atrial:

Ventricular:

**3. P WAVE**

Presence:

Appearance:

Consistency:

Relation to QRS:

**4. P-R INTERVAL**

Duration:

Consistency:

**5. QRS COMPLEX**

Present:

Configuration:

Consistency:

Duration:

**6. DATA ANALYSIS**

**7. RHYTHM INTERPRETATION**

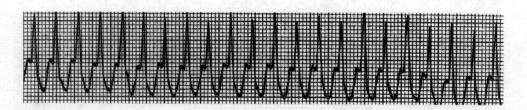

Figure 2-26B

# ECG RHYTHM STRIP #26
## Lead II

## 1. RHYTHM

Atrial: Indeterminable

Ventricular: Regular

## 2. RATE

Atrial: Indeterminable

Ventricular: 250

## 3. P WAVE  Not identifiable

Present: —

Configuration: —

Consistency: —

Relation to QRS: —

## 4. P-R INTERVAL  Indeterminable

Duration: —

Consistency: —

## 5. QRS COMPLEX

Present: Yes

Configuration: Normal

Consistency: Consistent

Duration: 0.06 seconds

## 6. DATA ANALYSIS

The abnormal values include:
- the absence of discernible atrial activity (therefore atrial rate, rhythm, and P-R interval indeterminable)
- a ventricular rate of 250 beats per minute

The origin of the tachycardia (rate > 100) must be supraventricular since the QRS complex is normal. Although we are unable to examine the morphology of the P wave, a ventricular rate of 250 makes atrial flutter with 1:1 conduction a good possibility.

## 7. RHYTHM INTERPRETATION

Supraventricular tachycardia (probable atrial flutter with 1:1 conduction)

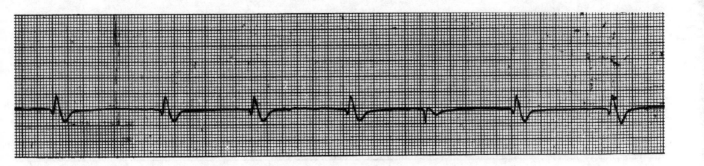

Figure 2-27A

# ECG RHYTHM STRIP #27
## Lead V₁

**1. RHYTHM**

    Atrial:

    Ventricular:

**2. RATE**

    Atrial:

    Ventricular:

**3. P WAVE**

    Present:

    Configuration:

    Consistency:

    Relation to QRS:

**4. P-R INTERVAL**

    Duration:

    Consistency:

**5. QRS COMPLEX**

    Present:

    Configuration:

    Consistency:

    Duration:

**6. DATA ANALYSIS**

**7. RHYTHM INTERPRETATION**

267

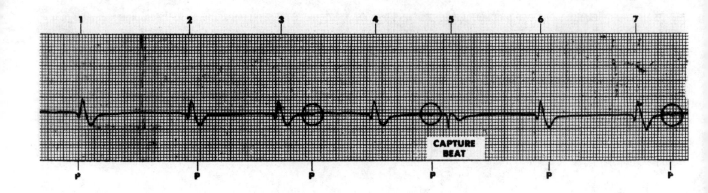

Figure 2-27B

# ECG RHYTHM STRIP #27
## Lead II

## I. RHYTHM

Atrial: Regular

Ventricular: Irregular

## 2. RATE

Atrial: 40—P's obscure (follow QRS complexes 3 and 7, before QRS$_5$)

Ventricular: 50

## 3. P WAVE

Present: Yes, hidden in QRS complexes 1, 2, and 6

Configuration: Negative, flattened

Consistency: Consistent

Relation to QRS: None except for beat 5 (1:1)

## 4. P-R INTERVAL

Duration: 0.22 seconds with one conducted beat (beat 5)

Consistency: —

## 5. QRS COMPLEX

Present: Yes

Configuration: Abnormal, 1 normal

Consistency: Consistent except for beat 5

Duration: Normal—0.08 seconds
Abnormal—0.12 seconds

## 6. DATA ANALYSIS

The abnormal values include:
- an atrial rate of 40 and a ventricular rate of 50
- an irregular ventricular rhythm
- obscure, flattened P waves with a variable P to QRS relation
- a prolonged P-R interval (0.22 seconds) with the conducted beat
- an inconsistent QRS complex

The atrial activity is difficult to identify. There is clearly a P wave before QRS$_5$ and also one appears following QRS$_3$. Using these two P waves as the basic P-P interval, one finds that there is probably a P in the negative T of beat 6 and a P appears after beat 7. Also, there may be a P in the Q wave of beat 1 and the T wave of beat 2. The presence of P waves at the rate of 40 would indicate some type of supraventricular bradycardia. The flattened negative P wave in lead V$_1$ may be normal for a sinus pacemaker. A 12 lead ECG may help make the differential diagnosis between sinus and an ectopic atrial rhythm.

There is no relation of P to QRS except with beat 5, indicating AV dissociation. Beat 5 is premature in the ventricular rhythm, shows normal conduction through the ventricles (normal QRS), and is preceded by a P wave. This is a capture beat—premature beat conducted from the atria, which interrupts AV dissociation. Hence the AV dissociation is incomplete.

Aside from the capture beat, the ventricular rhythm is characterized by wide, abnormal QRS complexes and a ventricular rate of 50. Although it is irregular initially, the last two R-R intervals (QRS$_{3-4}$, QRS$_{6-7}$) are regular. This most likely represents an accelerated idioventricular escape mechanism.

The P-R interval with the conducted beat is prolonged at 0.22 seconds. There is probably significant AV conduction problems, since the P wave after the 3rd QRS failed to conduct to the ventricles.

## 7. RHYTHM INTERPRETATION

Sinus bradycardia, incomplete AV dissociation (one capture beat conducted with first degree AV block), and accelerated idioventricular escape rhythm

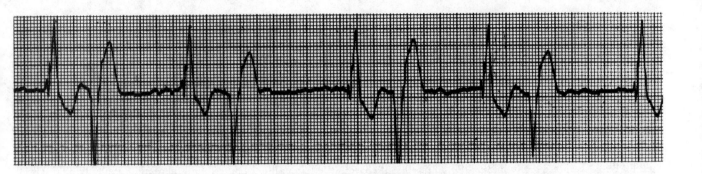

Figure 2-28A

# ECG RHYTHM STRIP #28
## Lead MCL₁

**1. RHYTHM**

    Atrial:

    Ventricular:

**2. RATE**

    Atrial:

    Ventricular:

**3. P WAVE**

    Present:

    Configuration:

    Consistency:

    Relation to QRS:

**4. P-R INTERVAL**

    Duration:

    Consistency:

**5. QRS COMPLEX**

    Present:

    Configuration:

    Consistency:

    Duration:

**6. DATA ANALYSIS**

**7. RHYTHM INTERPRETATION**

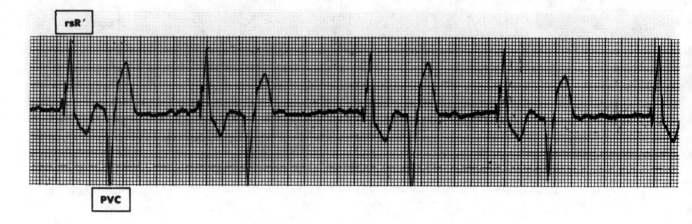

rsR'

PVC

Figure 2-28B

# ECG RHYTHM STRIP #28
## Lead MCL₁

## I. RHYTHM

Atrial: Irregular

Ventricular: Irregular

## 2. RATE

Atrial: Indeterminable

Ventricular: 70

## 3. P WAVE

Present: Variable atrial activity

Configuration: Abnormal, fibrillatory waves

Consistency: Inconsistent; varies in size, shape, width, and polarity

Relation to QRS: Indeterminable

## 4. P-R INTERVAL Undefined

Duration: —

Consistency: —

## 5. QRS COMPLEX

Present: Yes

Configuration: All abnormal

Consistency: Inconsistent; alternates in configuration and polarity

Duration: Positive QRS—0.16 seconds
Negative QRS—0.12 seconds

## 6. DATA ANALYSIS

The abnormal values include atrial fibrillatory waves (related to irregular atrial rhythm and multiple, varying P waves) which makes the atrial rate, P-R interval, and P to QRS relation indeterminable. In addition, the ventricular rhythm is irregular and the QRS complexes are abnormal, wide, and inconsistent in their morphology.

Every other QRS complex is premature—it ends a relatively short interval followed by a pause. These abnormal (negative) beats are ventricular in origin since the coupling intervals are regular and the configuration of the QRS complexes is identical despite the variation in preceding cycle lengths (pauses). The abnormal, positive, wide QRS complexes are conducted irregularly. The rsR' morphology in MCL₁ is consistent with RBBB.

## 7. RHYTHM INTERPRETATION

Atrial fibrillation with an intraventricular conduction delay (RBBB) and ventricular bigeminy (alternating ectopic ventricular beats)

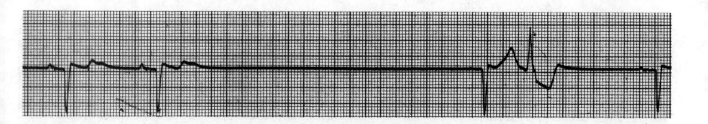

Figure 2-29A

# ECG RHYTHM STRIP #29
## Lead V₁

**1. RHYTHM**

    Atrial:

    Ventricular:

**2. RATE**

    Atrial:

    Ventricular:

**3. P WAVE**

    Present:

    Configuration:

    Consistency:

    Relation to QRS:

**4. P-R INTERVAL**

    Duration:

    Consistency:

**5. QRS COMPLEX**

    Present:

    Configuration:

    Consistency:

    Duration:

**6. DATA ANALYSIS**

**7. RHYTHM INTERPRETATION**

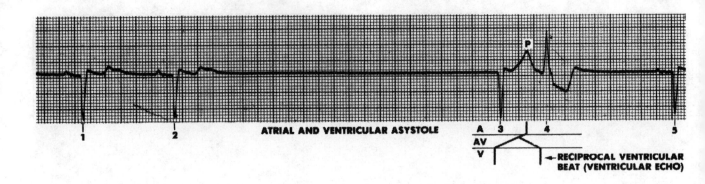

ATRIAL AND VENTRICULAR ASYSTOLE

← RECIPROCAL VENTRICULAR BEAT (VENTRICULAR ECHO)

Figure 2-29B

# ECG RHYTHM STRIP #29
## Lead V₁

## 1. RHYTHM

**Atrial:** Irregular

**Ventricular:** Irregular

## 2. RATE

**Atrial:** 20 (P wave absent in beat 3)

**Ventricular:** 30

## 3. P WAVE

**Present:** Yes, probable P on T after QRS$_3$

**Configuration:** Notched, prolonged duration

**Consistency:** Consistent when seen

**Relation to QRS:** 1:1 except for beat 3 and possibly beat 4

## 4. P-R INTERVAL

**Duration:** 0.22 seconds when measurable

**Consistency:** Consistent

## 5. QRS COMPLEX

**Present:** Yes

**Configuration:** Normal—negative
One abnormal—positive

**Consistency:** Consistent except for beat 4

**Duration:** Normal—0.08 seconds
Abnormal—0.12 seconds

## 6. DATA ANALYSIS

The abnormal values include:
- an atrial rate of 20 and ventricular rate of 30
- an irregular rhythm
- a long period of atrial and ventricular asystole
- notched P waves which are prolonged in duration
- an unidentifiable P wave before beat 3
- a P-R interval of 0.22 seconds
- one abnormal and wide QRS (beat 4)

The origin of the P waves is probably sinus; however, the notching of the P waves raises the possibility of an atrial abnormality. A 12 lead ECG is needed to confirm this.

QRS$_3$ is identical to the first two QRS complexes, is not preceded by a P wave, and terminates a long period (4.24 seconds) of ventricular asystole.

Beat 4 is characterized by a wide, abnormal QRS complex. There is probably a preceding P wave since the T wave of QRS$_3$ is distorted. The origin of the P wave may be sinus, atrial, or junctional (as a result of retrograde conduction to the atria from beat 3). If the P wave is the result of retrograde conduction then QRS complex 4 is most likely a reciprocal (ventricular echo) beat (see ladder diagram). The abnormal QRS is probably caused by aberrant conduction secondary to the shortening in the cycle length (QRS$_3$ to QRS$_4$) which immediately followed the long pause (QRS$_2$ to QRS$_3$). An ectopic ventricular beat cannot be completely excluded.

## 7. RHYTHM INTERPRETATION

Sinus bradycardia with first degree AV block, sinus arrest, prolonged ventricular asystole, late occurring junctional escape beat, and probable aberrantly conducted impulse

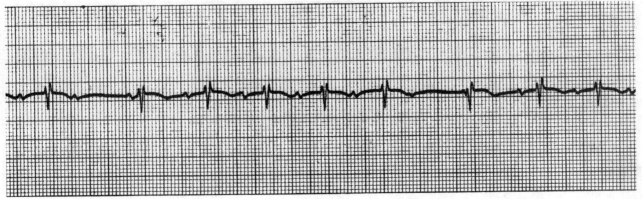

Figure 2-30A

# ECG RHYTHM STRIP #30
## Lead MLC₁

### 1. RHYTHM

Atrial:

Ventricular:

### 2. RATE

Atrial:

Ventricular:

### 3. P WAVE

Present:

Configuration:

Consistency:

Relation to QRS:

### 4. P-R INTERVAL

Duration:

Consistency:

### 5. QRS COMPLEX

Present:

Configuration:

Consistency:

Duration:

### 6. DATA ANALYSIS

### 7. RHYTHM INTERPRETATION

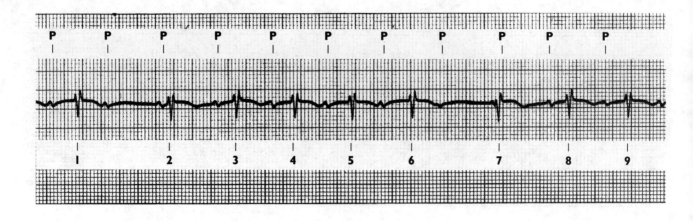

Figure 2-30B

# ECG RHYTHM STRIP #30
## Lead MLC₁

## 1. RHYTHM

Atrial: Regular

Ventricular: Irregular

## 2. RATE

Atrial: 100

Ventricular: 80

## 3. P WAVE

Present: Yes

Configuration: Normal

Consistency: Consistent

Relation to QRS: Variable

## 4. P-R INTERVAL

Duration: 0.20-0.34 seconds except in beats 2 and 7

Consistency: Inconsistent; progressively lengthens

## 5. QRS COMPLEX

Present: Yes

Configuration: Abnormal rSr'

Consistency: Consistent

Duration: 0.08 seconds

## 6. DATA ANALYSIS

The abnormal values include:
- a slower ventricular versus atrial rate
- an irregular ventricular rhythm
- a variable P to QRS relation
- a prolonged and inconsistent P-R interval
- an abnormal QRS complex (rSr')

Several nonconducted P waves account for the slower ventricular rate and the pauses in the ventricular rhythm. Since the atrial rhythm is regular, the change in the P-R interval as well as the pauses are causing the irregular ventricular rhythm. The nonconducted P waves and prolonged P-R intervals indicate AV block.

The P-R intervals are consistently long (> 0.20 seconds) except in beats 2 and 7 where the P-R intervals are too short to have conducted those QRS complexes. This makes them dissociated beats, with nonconducted P waves. The pacemaker depolarizing the ventricles must be junctional since the QRS complexes are the same as those with the conducted beats.

The P-R intervals progressively increase until a P wave is not conducted, consistent with Wenckebach.

The rSr' in MCL₁ is consistent with a right-sided intraventicular conduction defect.

## 7. RHYTHM INTERPRETATION

Sinus rhythm with second degree AV block–Mobitz I (Wenckebach), two junctional escape beats, and a right-sided intraventicular conduction defect

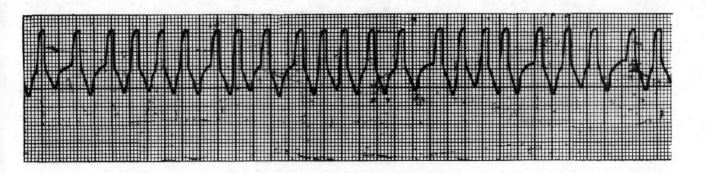

Figure 2-31A

# ECG RHYTHM STRIP #31
## Lead II

## I. RHYTHM

Atrial:

Ventricular:

## 2. RATE

Atrial:

Ventricular:

## 3. P WAVE

Present:

Configuration:

Consistency:

Relation to QRS:

## 4. P-R INTERVAL

Duration:

Consistency:

## 5. QRS COMPLEX

Present:

Configuration:

Consistency:

Duration:

## 6. DATA ANALYSIS

## 7. RHYTHM INTERPRETATION

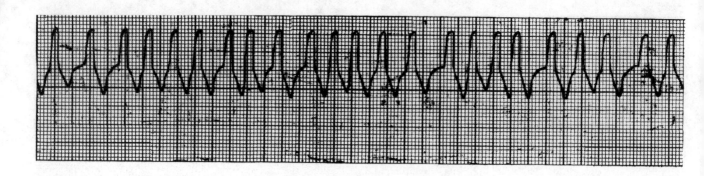

Figure 2-31B

# ECG RHYTHM STRIP #31
## Lead II

## 1. RHYTHM

Atrial: Indeterminable

Ventricular: Irregularly irregular

## 2. RATE

Atrial: Indeterminable

Ventricular: 200

## 3. P WAVE  Unidentifiable

Present: —

Configuration: —

Consistency: —

Relation to QRS: —

## 4. P-R INTERVAL  Undefined

Duration: —

Consistency: —

## 5. QRS COMPLEX

Present: Yes

Configuration: Abnormal

Consistency: Consistent

Duration: 0.12 seconds

## 6. DATA ANALYSIS

The abnormal values include:
- an unidentifiable P wave—making the atrial rate, rhythm, and P-R interval indeterminable
- a ventricular rate of 200 beats per minute
- an irregularly, irregular ventricular rhythm
- an abnormal QRS complex

Although the QRS complexes are wide, the irregularly irregular ventricular rhythm is consistent with underlying atrial fibrillation. (Ventricular tachycardia is a predominantly regular rhythm.)

The abnormal QRS complexes may be caused by a permanent or rate-related bundle branch block, aberrancy, or preexcitation syndrome (i.e., Wolff-Parkinson-White). A 12 lead ECG and/or previous ECG tracings are needed to make a differential diagnosis.

## 7. RHYTHM INTERPRETATION

Atrial fibrillation with uncontrolled ventricular response and an intraventricular conduction delay

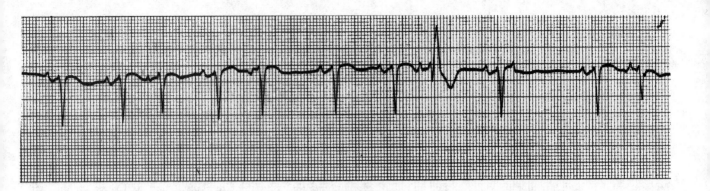

Figure 2-32A

# ECG RHYTHM STRIP #32
## Lead V₁

**1. RHYTHM**

    Atrial:

    Ventricular:

**2. RATE**

    Atrial:

    Ventricular:

**3. P WAVE**

    Present:

    Configuration:

    Consistency:

    Relation to QRS:

**4. P-R INTERVAL**

    Duration:

    Consistency:

**5. QRS COMPLEX**

    Present:

    Configuration:

    Consistency:

    Duration:

**6. DATA ANALYSIS**

**7. RHYTHM INTERPRETATION**

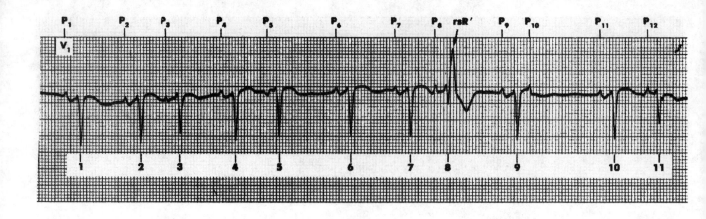

Figure 2-32B

# ECG RHYTHM STRIP #32
## Lead V₁

## I. RHYTHM

Atrial: Irregular

Ventricular: Irregular

## 2. RATE

Atrial: 100 (note P on T after $QRS_9$)

Ventricular: 90

## 3. P WAVE

Present: Yes

Configuration: Sinus—diphasic
Others—variable in configuration

Consistency: Inconsistent; varies in configuration and polarity

Relation to QRS: 1:1 except for nonconducted P wave (follows $QRS_9$)

## 4. P-R INTERVAL

Duration: 0.16 seconds, except for beat 5, which is 0.12 seconds

Consistency: Consistent except with beat 5

## 5. QRS COMPLEX

Present: Yes

Configuration: Normal, except for beat 8 (abnormal—rsR')

Consistency: Consistent except for beat 8

Duration: Normal—0.08 seconds
Abnormal—0.15 seconds

## 6. DATA ANALYSIS

The abnormal values include:
- a slower ventricular versus atrial rate (due to nonconducted P wave)
- an irregular rhythm
- an inconsistent P wave
- a shorter P-R interval with beat 5
- a wide, abnormal QRS with beat 8

Diphasic P waves are seen in beats 1, 2, 4, 6, 7, 9, and 10. These predominant P's are sinus in origin, since the underlying rhythm is regular (P-P intervals identical where consecutive P's occur, i.e., between beats 1 & 2 and 6 & 7) and the rate is normal (approximately 90). The morphology of the P waves (diphasic) could be normal for lead V₁; however, a 12 lead ECG is necessary to rule out atrial abnormality. If the first P-P interval represents the basic sinus cycle, P waves 3, 5, 8, 10, and 12 are premature. These same P waves are also different in configuration from the sinus P waves, representing premature ectopic foci.

The shorter P-R interval with beat 5, which is also associated with the only negative P wave, is probably due to a pacemaker site close to (low atrial) or in the AV junction.

The wide, abnormal QRS complex (beat 8) shows a RBBB configuration and is preceded by a P wave with a normal P-R interval. This is consistent with an aberrantly conducted PAC. A P wave not followed by a QRS complex is present in the ST segment following $QRS_9$. Due to its high degree of prematurity, it ($P_{10}$) does not conduct to the ventricles.

## 7. RHYTHM INTERPRETATION

Sinus rhythm with frequent PAC's—one aberrantly conducted and one nonconducted

278

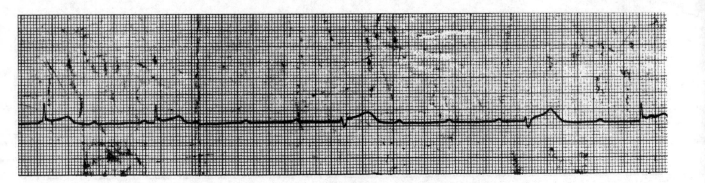

Figure 2-33A

# ECG RHYTHM STRIP #33
## Lead II

**1. RHYTHM**

    Atrial:

    Ventricular:

**2. RATE**

    Atrial:

    Ventricular:

**3. P WAVE**

    Present:

    Configuration:

    Consistency:

    Relation to QRS:

**4. P-R INTERVAL**

    Duration:

    Consistency:

**5. QRS COMPLEX**

    Present:

    Configuration:

    Consistency:

    Duration:

**6. DATA ANALYSIS**

**7. RHYTHM INTERPRETATION**

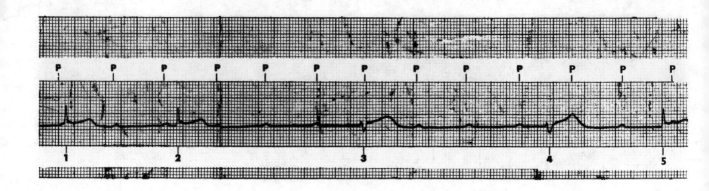

Figure 2-33B

# ECG RHYTHM STRIP #33
## Lead II

## I. RHYTHM

Atrial: Regular

Ventricular: Irregular

## 2. RATE

Atrial: 90 (P's obscure: onset $QRS_1$, in $QRS_3$, T wave of $QRS_4$)

Ventricular: 30

## 3. P WAVE

Present: Yes

Configuration: Normal

Consistency: Consistent

Relation to QRS: None; P's regular and change relation to QRS

## 4. P-R INTERVAL  Indeterminable—no relation P to QRS

Duration: —

Consistency: —

## 5. QRS COMPLEX

Present: Yes

Configuration: Normal—positive
Abnormal— negative

Consistency: Inconsistent

Duration: Beats 1, 2, & 5—0.08 seconds
Beats 3 & 4—0.11 seconds

## 6. DATA ANALYSIS

The abnormal values include:
- a ventricular rate of 30 (less than atrial rate because of nonconducted P waves)
- an irregular ventricular rhythm
- an unrelated P to QRS relation
- an inconsistent QRS complex

Since the P waves are unrelated to the QRS complex, there is AV dissociation. The atrial pacemaker is sinus—normal P's, atrial rate and rhythm. The ventricular pacemaker is initially junctional (normal QRS) at approximately 40 per minute, which subsequently fails (pause in ventricular rhythm) and is replaced by a ventricular focus (abnormal QRS) at approximately 25 per minute.

## 7. RHYTHM INTERPRETATION

Sinus rhythm with complete heart block, alternating junctional and ventricular escape rhythms

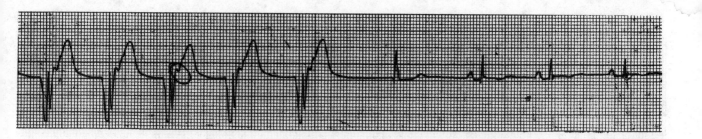

Figure 2-34A

# ECG RHYTHM STRIP #34
## Lead II

**1. RHYTHM**

Atrial:

Ventricular:

**2. RATE**

Atrial:

Ventricular:

**3. P WAVE**

Present:

Configuration:

Consistency:

Relation to QRS:

**4. P-R INTERVAL**

Duration:

Consistency:

**5. QRS COMPLEX**

Present:

Configuration:

Consistency:

Duration:

**6. DATA ANALYSIS**

**7. RHYTHM INTERPRETATION**

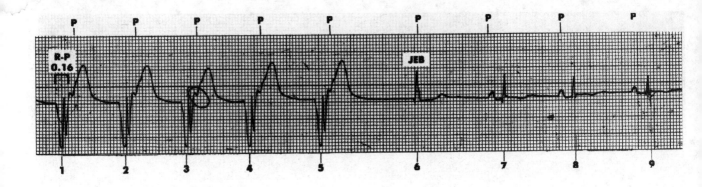

Figure 2-34B

# ECG RHYTHM STRIP #34
## Lead II

### 1. RHYTHM

Atrial: Irregular

Ventricular: Irregular

### 2. RATE

Atrial: 70 (P's hidden in ST segment of first five beats then possibly in QRS of beat 6)

Ventricular: 70

### 3. P WAVE

Present: Yes, obscure

Configuration: Normal—positive
Abnormal—negative (obscure with ST segment)

Consistency: Varies in configuration and polarity

Relation to QRS: Varies, 1 after every abnormal QRS; possibly hidden in $QRS_6$; 1:1 last 3 beats

### 4. P-R INTERVAL

Duration: 0.16 seconds with sinus conducted beats (last 3 beats)

Consistency: Consistent

R-P interval: Approximately 0.16 seconds first 5 beats, consistent

### 5. QRS COMPLEX

Present: Yes

Configuration: Abnormal—negative
Normal—positive

Consistency: Inconsistent; varies in configuration and polarity

Duration: Abnormal beats—0.16 seconds
Normal beats—0.06 seconds

### 6. DATA ANALYSIS

The abnormal values include:
- an irregular rhythm
- a variation in the P wave and relation of P to QRS
- a change in the configuration and width of the QRS complex from abnormal and wide to normal and narrow

The first 5 beats show a consistent notching in the ST segment (with identical R-P intervals) indicating retrograde conduction to the atria. The wide abnormal QRS is consistent with a ventricular origin. $QRS_6$ which follows a pause in the rhythm, resembles the sinus conducted beats—except for slurring in the downstroke of the R wave. This is most likely a distortion caused by a dissociated sinus P wave since it marches out in the sinus rhythm. $QRS_6$ is consistent with a junctional escape beat.

The irregular rhythm is due primarily to the change in the pacemaker site.

### 7. RHYTHM INTERPRETATION

Accelerated idioventricular rhythm (AIVR) with retrograde atrial conduction, junctional escape beat, sinus rhythm

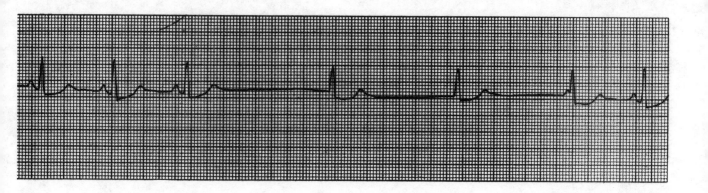

Figure 2-35A

# ECG RHYTHM STRIP #35
## Lead II

**1. RHYTHM**

Atrial:

Ventricular:

**2. RATE**

Atrial:

Ventricular:

**3. P WAVE**

Present:

Configuration:

Consistency:

Relation to QRS:

**4. P-R INTERVAL**

Duration:

Consistency:

**5. QRS COMPLEX**

Present:

Configuration:

Consistency:

Duration:

**6. DATA ANALYSIS**

**7. RHYTHM INTERPRETATION**

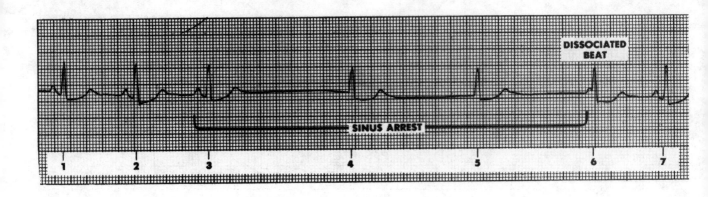

Figure 2-35B

# ECG RHYTHM STRIP #35
## Lead II

## I. RHYTHM

Atrial: Irregular

Ventricular: Irregular

## 2. RATE

Atrial: 20

Ventricular: 40

## 3. P WAVE

Present: Yes

Configuration: Normal

Consistency: Consistent

Relation to QRS: 1:1 when present except dissociated prior to $QRS_6$

## 4. P-R INTERVAL

Duration: 0.14 seconds with conducted beats

Consistency: Consistent

## 5. QRS COMPLEX

Present: Yes

Configuration: Normal

Consistency: Consistent

Duration: 0.08 seconds

## 6. DATA ANALYSIS

The abnormal values include:
- a slow atrial and ventricular rate
- an irregular rhythm
- a variable P to QRS relation

The first 3 beats and the last beat show a 1:1 P to QRS relation. There are no visible P waves associated with beats 4 and 5. The abrupt absence of atrial activity is consistent with a sinus arrest. Beat 6 has a P wave immediately preceding and distorting the initial portion of the QRS complex. This represents resumption of sinus activity. The P-R interval here (beat 6) is too short to conduct, making this a dissociated (P-QRS) beat. The QRS (beat 4) terminating the pause is identical to the normally conducted impulses and is consistent with a junctional origin. Beat 4, 5, and 6 represent a junctional escape rhythm at approximately 40 per minute.

## 7. RHYTHM INTERPRETATION

Sinus rhythm with sinus arrest and junctional escape rhythm

284

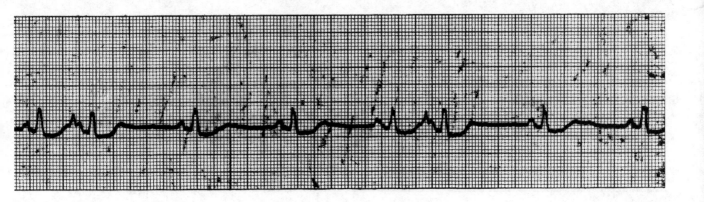

Figure 2-36A

# ECG RHYTHM STRIP #36
## Monitor Lead II

**1. RHYTHM**

    Atrial:

    Ventricular:

**2. RATE**

    Atrial:

    Ventricular:

**3. P WAVE**

    Present:

    Configuration:

    Consistency:

    Relation to QRS:

**4. P-R INTERVAL**

    Duration:

    Consistency:

**5. QRS COMPLEX**

    Present:

    Configuration:

    Consistency:

    Duration:

**6. DATA ANALYSIS**

**7. RHYTHM INTERPRETATION**

285

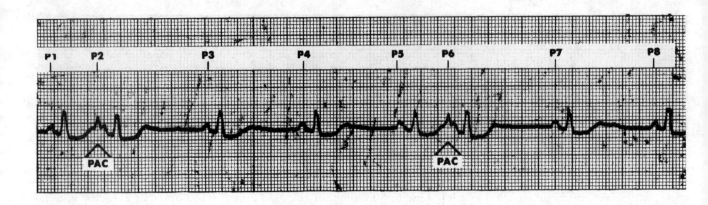

Figure 2-36B

# ECG RHYTHM STRIP #36
## Monitor Lead II

## I. RHYTHM

Atrial: Irregular

Ventricular: Irregular

## 2. RATE

Atrial: 60 (overall)

Ventricular: 60 (overall)

## 3. P WAVE

Present: Yes

Configuration: Notched, except for P's 2 and 6—peaked

Consistency: Inconsistent

Relation to QRS: 1:1

## 4. P-R INTERVAL

Duration: Beats 2 and 6—0.20 seconds
Others—0.16 seconds

Consistency: Inconsistent

## 5. QRS COMPLEX

Present: Yes

Configuration: Slightly notched

Consistency: Consistent

Duration: 0.09 seconds

## 6. DATA ANALYSIS

The abnormal values include:
- an irregular rhythm
- an inconsistent P wave
- a variable P-R interval

The underlying rhythm is represented by notched P waves (1, 3, 4, 5, 7, 8) occurring regularly (when 2 consecutive P's) at a rate of 50 beats per minute. The notching of these P waves raises the possibility of an atrial abnormality; however, a 12 lead ECG is necessary to accurately assess this.

P's 2 and 6 are different in configuration and premature in the basic sinus cycle. They conduct with longer P-R intervals (0.20 seconds) than the sinus beats due to prematurity and relative refractoriness of the AV node.

The slightly notched QRS complexes may be related to monitor lead artifact or an intraventricular conduction defect. A 12 lead ECG is needed to differentiate these possibilities.

## 7. RHYTHM INTERPRETATION

Sinus bradycardia with two PAC's

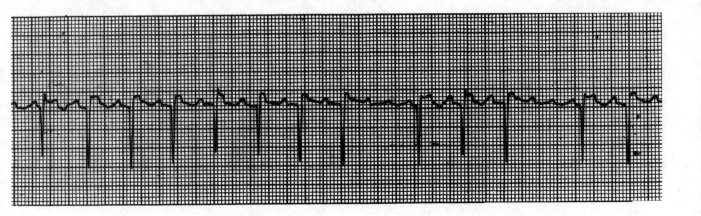

Figure 2-37A

# ECG RHYTHM STRIP #37
## Lead V₁

**I. RHYTHM**

   Atrial:

   Ventricular:

**2. RATE**

   Atrial:

   Ventricular:

**3. P WAVE**

   Present:

   Configuration:

   Consistency:

   Relation to QRS:

**4. P-R INTERVAL**

   Duration:

   Consistency:

**5. QRS COMPLEX**

   Present:

   Configuration:

   Consistency:

   Duration:

**6. DATA ANALYSIS**

**7. RHYTHM INTERPRETATION**

287

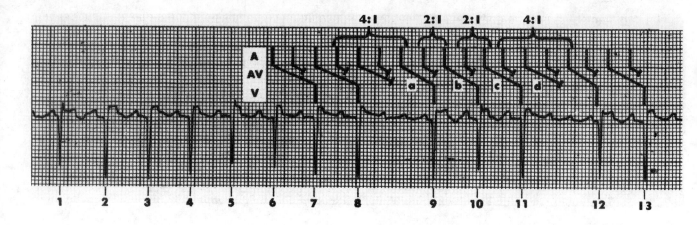

Figure 2-37B

# ECG RHYTHM STRIP #37
## Lead V₁

## 1. RHYTHM

Atrial: Regular

Ventricular: Irregular

## 2. RATE

Atrial: 250 (some P's obscure in ST-T segment)

Ventricular: 110

## 3. P WAVE

Present: Yes

Configuration: Predominantly positive

Consistency: Consistent when identifiable

Relation to QRS: Varies 2:1 to 4:1

## 4. P-R INTERVAL

Duration: Difficult to define

Consistency: Variable "P-R" (F-R)

## 5. QRS COMPLEX

Present: Yes

Configuration: Normal

Consistency: Consistent

Duration: 0.05 seconds

## 6. DATA ANALYSIS

The abnormal values include:
- an atrial rate of 250 and ventricular rate of 110
- an irregular ventricular rhythm
- an inconsistent P to QRS relation
- a variable P-R interval

The atrial rate of 250 is consistent with atrial flutter, although the morphology of the P wave is not typical of flutter. The slower ventricular rate is secondary to the nonconducted P waves.

The P-R intervals are longer than they initially appear to be. For example, the QRS complexes ending the pauses are immediately preceded by a P wave with a P-R interval of approximately 0.11 seconds. Normally, the P-R intervals with atrial flutter are greater than 0.20 seconds, due to concealed AV conduction (from the previous "P" wave). It is therefore unlikely that these P's (where P-R 0.11 seconds) are conducting the QRS's (1, 9, and 12). It is probable, then, that the preceding P is responsible for conduction with a P-R interval of 0.36 seconds. Following that pattern with a basic 2:1 conduction ratio, the P's immediately preceding each QRS are blocked and the P's in ST-T wave are conducting with progressively longer P-R intervals until an additional second P is blocked (see a, b, c, d of ladder diagram). It should be noted that the block in the upper portion of the AV node is physiologic (every other impulse is not conducted). The varying P-R intervals and AV conduction ratios (2:1 to 4:1), therefore can be explained by a Wenckebach phenomenon involving the lower portion of the AV node. Notice that the long R-R interval (of the pause) is less than two successive short R-R intervals.

## 7. RHYTHM INTERPRETATION

Atrial flutter with variable AV conduction ratios (2:1, 4:1) and Wenckebach phenomenon

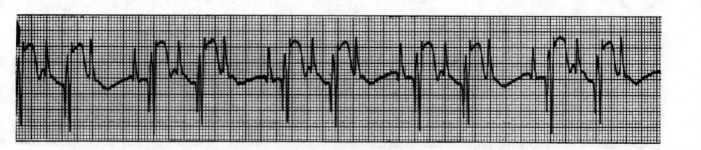

Figure 2-38A

# ECG RHYTHM STRIP #38
## Monitor Lead II

**1. RHYTHM**

    Atrial:

    Ventricular:

**2. RATE**

    Atrial:

    Ventricular:

**3. P WAVE**

    Present:

    Configuration:

    Consistency:

    Relation to QRS:

**4. P-R INTERVAL**

    Duration:

    Consistency:

**5. QRS COMPLEX**

    Present:

    Configuration:

    Consistency:

    Duration:

**6. DATA ANALYSIS**

**7. RHYTHM INTERPRETATION**

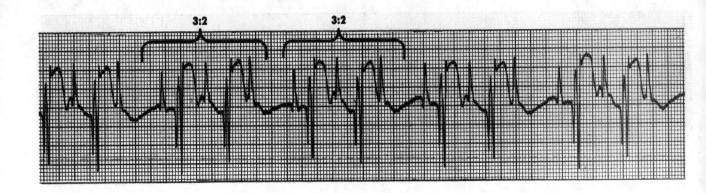

Figure 2-38B

# ECG RHYTHM STRIP #38
## Monitor Lead II

### I. RHYTHM

Atrial: Regular

Ventricular: Regularly irregular (cyclic)

### 2. RATE

Atrial: 105

Ventricular: 70

### 3. P WAVE

Present: Yes

Configuration: Tall, peaked

Consistency: Consistent

Relation to QRS: 3:2

### 4. P-R INTERVAL

Duration: 0.20 to 0.24 seconds

Consistency: Variable in repetitive pattern

### 5. QRS COMPLEX

Present: Yes

Configuration: Abnormal

Consistency: Consistent

Duration: 0.12 seconds

### 6. DATA ANALYSIS

The abnormal values include:
- a faster atrial (105) versus ventricular rate (70)
- a regularly irregular ventricular rhythm
- tall, peaked P waves with a 3:2 P to QRS relation
- a variable, and at times prolonged, P-R interval (0.20 to 0.24 seconds)
- a wide, abnormal QRS complex (0.12 seconds)

The atrial rate is slightly increased. The P wave morphology is unusual and probably is due to monitor lead placement. A 12 lead ECG would confirm the suspected mild sinus tachycardia and permit assessment for possible right atrial abnormality.

The ventricular rate is slower than the atrial rate due to the presence of AV block. Second degree AV block is identifiable by the occurrence of nonconducted sinus P waves (every third P wave). Although the ventricular rhythm is irregular, it is so in a repetitive fashion. Groups of three P waves and two QRS complexes ("group beating") are apparent. In each group the P-R interval progressively increases prior to the nonconducted sinus P wave (Wenckebach phenomenon). The QRS complexes are wide, indicating an intraventicular conduction delay. Monitor lead placement probably has distorted the QRS configuration. A 12 lead ECG is necessary to assess for the presence of a specific bundle branch block. The location of the block with Wenckebach is usually at the AV node; however, the presence of the intraventricular conduction delay raises the possibility of infranodal disease.

### 7. RHYTHM INTERPRETATION

Sinus tachycardia with Mobitz I (Wenckebach) second degree AV block and an intraventricular conduction delay

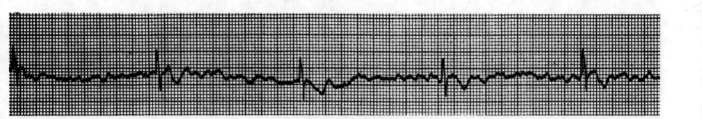

Figure 2-39A

# ECG RHYTHM STRIP #39
## Monitor Lead II

**1. RHYTHM**

    Atrial:

    Ventricular:

**2. RATE**

    Atrial:

    Ventricular:

**3. P WAVE**

    Present:

    Configuration:

    Consistency:

    Relation to QRS:

**4. P-R INTERVAL**

    Duration:

    Consistency:

**5. QRS COMPLEX**

    Present:

    Configuration:

    Consistency:

    Duration:

**6. DATA ANALYSIS**

**7. RHYTHM INTERPRETATION**

291

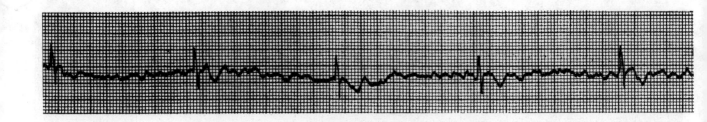

Figure 2-39B

# ECG RHYTHM STRIP #39
## Monitor Lead II

### I. RHYTHM

Atrial: Irregular

Ventricular: Regular

### 2. RATE

Atrial: Indeterminable

Ventricular: 34

### 3. P WAVE

Present: Variable atrial activity

Configuration: Abnormal, fibrillatory waves

Consistency: Inconsistent; varies in size, shape, and width

Relation to QRS: None

### 4. P-R INTERVAL  Undefined

Duration: —

Consistency: —

### 5. QRS COMPLEX

Present: Yes

Configuration: Normal

Consistency: Consistent

Duration: 0.08 seconds

### 6. DATA ANALYSIS

The abnormal values include fibrillatory waves that make the atrial rate and P-R interval indeterminable. The perfect regularity of the R-R intervals in the setting of atrial fibrillation makes the ventricular rhythm dissociated from the atrial rhythm. (An irregularly irregular ventricular rhythm characterizes the erratic conduction of fibrillatory waves to the ventricles.) Although the ventricular rate is slow at 34 beats per minute, the normal, narrow QRS is consistent with a junctional rhythm driving the ventricles during AV dissociation. This rhythm is highly suspicious for digitalis toxicity.

### 7. RHYTHM INTERPRETATION

Atrial fibrillation with complete AV dissociation and a slow junctional rhythm

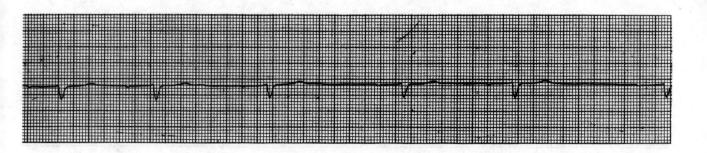

Figure 2-40A

# ECG RHYTHM STRIP #40
## Lead MCL₁

**I. RHYTHM**

Atrial:

Ventricular:

**2. RATE**

Atrial:

Ventricular:

**3. P WAVE**

Present:

Configuration:

Consistency:

Relation to QRS:

**4. P-R INTERVAL**

Duration:

Consistency:

**5. QRS COMPLEX**

Present:

Configuration:

Consistency:

Duration:

**6. DATA ANALYSIS**

**7. RHYTHM INTERPRETATION**

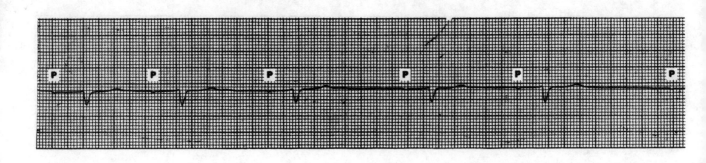

Figure 2-40B

# ECG RHYTHM STRIP #40
## Lead MCL₁

## 1. RHYTHM

Atrial: Irregular

Ventricular: Irregular

## 2. RATE

Atrial: 40

Ventricular: 40

## 3. P WAVE

Present: Yes

Configuration: Negative and flattened

Consistency: Consistent

Relation to QRS: 1:1

## 4. P-R INTERVAL

Duration: 0.36 seconds to 0.40 seconds

Consistency: Slightly variable

## 5. QRS COMPLEX

Present: Yes

Configuration: Abnormal, slurred S

Consistency: Consistent

Duration: 0.10 seconds

## 6. DATA ANALYSIS

The abnormal values include:
- a rate of 40 beats per minute
- an irregular rhythm
- a prolonged P-R interval
- a mildly abnormal QRS

The slightly negative P wave can be normal for MCL₁. A 12 lead ECG is needed to assess for the presence of a left atrial abnormality.

The first P-P interval is the shortest, making the basic rate 50 beats per minute. The rate slows due to the exaggerated sinus arrhythmia or more likely periods of sinus arrest.

The mildly abnormal QRS at 0.10 seconds is related to an intraventricular conduction defect.

## 7. RHYTHM INTERPRETATION

Marked sinus bradycardia with probable sinus arrests, variable first degree AV block, and an intraventricular conduction defect

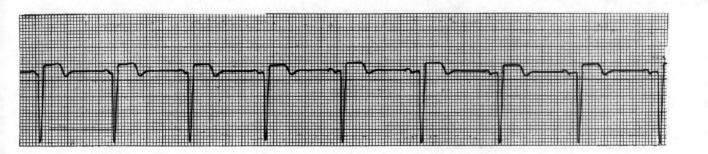

Figure 2-41A

# ECG RHYTHM STRIP #41
## Lead MCL₁

**1. RHYTHM**

    Atrial:

    Ventricular:

**2. RATE**

    Atrial:

    Ventricular:

**3. P WAVE**

    Present:

    Configuration:

    Consistency:

    Relation to QRS:

**4. P-R INTERVAL**

    Duration:

    Consistency:

**5. QRS COMPLEX**

    Present:

    Configuration:

    Consistency:

    Duration:

**6. DATA ANALYSIS**

**7. RHYTHM INTERPRETATION**

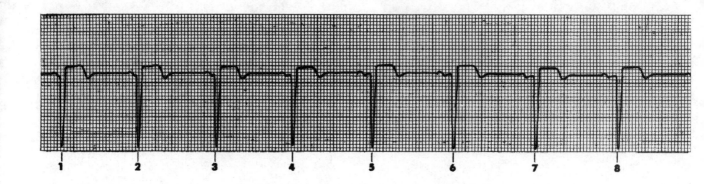

Figure 2-41B

# ECG RHYTHM STRIP #41
## Lead MCL₁

### 1. RHYTHM

Atrial: Regular

Ventricular: Slightly irregular

### 2. RATE

Atrial: 60

Ventricular: 60

### 3. P WAVE

Present: Yes

Configuration: Normal

Consistency: Consistent

Relation to QRS: Varies, none to 1:1

### 4. P-R INTERVAL

Duration: 0.11 to 0.18 seconds

Consistency: With last 4 beats only, otherwise varies

### 5. QRS COMPLEX

Present: Yes

Configuration: Normal

Consistency: Consistent

Duration: 0.08 seconds

### 6. DATA ANALYSIS

All values are normal except the the ventricular rhythm is slightly irregular, and the P to QRS relation and P-R intervals vary.

The irregular ventricular rhythm is caused by a slight slowing after beat 5. The first 5 beats represent AV dissociation since the P-R intervals vary while the atrial and ventricular rhythms remain regular. Thereafter, there is 1:1 conduction to the ventricles as the P-R intervals are consistent at 0.18 seconds. The dissociated ventricular pacemaker slowed to allow sinus conduction to the ventricles. The dissociated ventricular pacemaker is of junctional origin since the QRS complexes are identical to those of the sinus capture beats. Note that the sinus and junctional rates are nearly identical, hence the term isorhythmic AV dissociation.

### 7. RHYTHM INTERPRETATION

Junctional rhythm with isorythmic AV dissociation, sinus rhythm

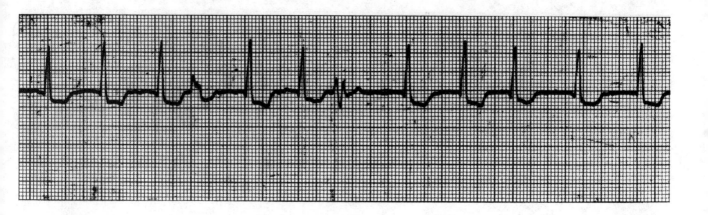

Figure 2-42A

# ECG RHYTHM STRIP #42
## Lead II

**I. RHYTHM**

Atrial:

Ventricular:

**2. RATE**

Atrial:

Ventricular:

**3. P WAVE**

Present:

Configuration:

Consistency:

Relation to QRS:

**4. P-R INTERVAL**

Duration:

Consistency:

**5. QRS COMPLEX**

Present:

Configuration:

Consistency:

Duration:

**6. DATA ANALYSIS**

**7. RHYTHM INTERPRETATION**

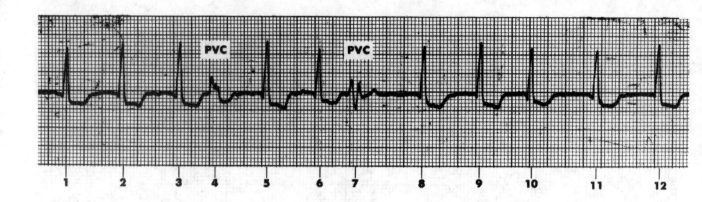

Figure 2-42B

# ECG RHYTHM STRIP #42
## Lead II

## 1. RHYTHM

Atrial: Indeterminable

Ventricular: Irregularly irregular

## 2. RATE

Atrial: Indeterminable

Ventricular: 100

## 3. P WAVE  Unidentifiable

Present: —

Configuration: —

Consistency: —

Relation to QRS: —

## 4. P-R INTERVAL  Undefined

Duration: —

Consistency: —

## 5. QRS COMPLEX

Present: Yes

Configuration: Normal—positive
2 Abnormal (bizarre)

Consistency: Inconsistent

Duration: Normal—0.08 seconds
Abnormal—0.12 seconds

## 6. DATA ANALYSIS

The abnormal values include:
- unidentifiable P waves making the atrial rate, rhythm, and P-R interval indeterminable
- an irregularly irregular ventricular rhythm
- an abnormal and wide QRS complex in beats 4 and 7

The normal QRS complexes indicate an underlying supraventricular rhythm. The irregularly irregular ventricular rhythm is due to the erratic AV conduction characteristic of atrial fibrillation.

The abnormal QRS complexes are premature—close relatively short R-R intervals. They may represent either aberrantly conducted impulses or multiform PVC's. The latter are more likely because there is a fixed coupling interval and the abnormal QRS complexes do not follow a long R-R interval. A 12 lead ECG to determine the morphology of the abnormal QRS complexes in the V leads would be helpful in making a differential diagnosis. The slight differences in the "normal" QRS complexes is probably due to respiratory variation.

## 7. RHYTHM INTERPRETATION

Atrial fibrillation with multiform PVC's

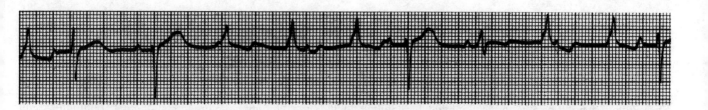

Figure 2-43A

# ECG RHYTHM STRIP #43
## Lead V₁

### 1. RHYTHM

Atrial:

Ventricular:

### 2. RATE

Atrial:

Ventricular:

### 3. P WAVE

Present:

Configuration:

Consistency:

Relation to QRS:

### 4. P-R INTERVAL

Duration:

Consistency:

### 5. QRS COMPLEX

Present:

Configuration:

Consistency:

Duration:

### 6. DATA ANALYSIS

### 7. RHYTHM INTERPRETATION

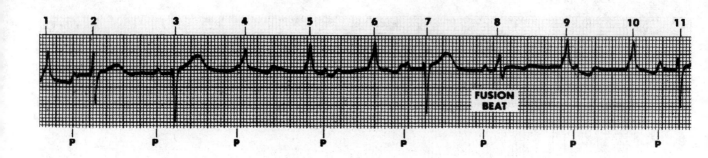

Figure 2-43B

# ECG RHYTHM STRIP #43
## Lead V₁

## I. RHYTHM

Atrial: Slightly irregular

Ventricular: Irregular

## 2. RATE

Atrial: 60 (P wave obscure at onset of QRS₄)

Ventricular: 80

## 3. P WAVE

Present: Yes

Configuration: Normal

Consistency: Consistent

Relation to QRS: Varies

## 4. P-R INTERVAL

Duration: 0.20 seconds (beats 2, 3, 7, 11) and 0.16 seconds (beat 8).

Consistency: Inconsistent

## 5. QRS COMPLEX

Present: Yes

Configuration: Normal and abnormal

Consistency: Varies in configuration and polarity

Duration: Varies 0.08 to 0.14 seconds

## 6. DATA ANALYSIS

The abnormal values include:
- an irregular rhythm
- a slower atrial versus ventricular rate
- a variable P to QRS relation
- a change in the P-R interval with beat 8
- an inconsistent QRS complex that varies from normal and narrow (beats 3 and 7) to abnormal and wide (beats 1, 5, 6, 9, and 10)

Since the configuration of the P waves is normal and consistent, the underlying atrial rhythm is sinus. The varying P-P interval is secondary to a sinus arrhythmia.

The P to QRS relationship is inconsistent. The conducted sinus beats include those with a P-R interval of 0.20 seconds (beats 2, 3, 7, and 11).

QRS complexes 3 and 7 represent normal conduction through the ventricles. The wide, abnormal QRS complexes (1, 4, 5, 6, 9, and 10) are related to an independent competing accelerated idioventricular rhythm. Note that the P waves bear no constant relationship to these impulses. Beat 8 is preceded by a sinus P, but with a shorter P-R interval (0.16 seconds). The change in the QRS complex in this beat is due to ventricular fusion.

The QRS configuration of beats 2 and 11 are more difficult to explain. Although their cycle length (QRS₁ - QRS₂, QRS₁₀ - QRS₁₁) are slightly shorter (than QRS₆ - QRS₇), raising the possibility of aberrancy, neither has a RBBB morphology (this is a lead V₁) and QRS₁₁ does **not** follow a long R-R interval—points against aberrancy. Ventricular fusion is more likely.

Although the apparent rate of the "accelerated idioventricular" focus is approximately 75 per minute (cycle length 800 milliseconds), the actual rate may be 3 times this or approximately 225 per minute (cycle length 270 milliseconds). Variable degrees of ventricular exit block from the ventricular focus could account for the apparent idioventricular rate of 75 and for the appearance of fusion beats at QRS₂ - QRS₁₁. Note that QRS₁ - QRS₂ and QRS₁₀ - QRS₁₁ have cycle lengths of 540 milliseconds (2 x 270 milliseconds), and that QRS₅, - QRS₆, and QRS₉ - QRS₁₀ have cycle lengths of approximately 800 milliseconds (3 x 270 milliseconds). Finally, because QRS₄ is slightly different than the other QRS complexes of the "accelerated idioventricular" focus and because the antecedent P-R interval is too short to permit fusion, one might hypothesize that ventricular depolarization from the ectopic ventricular focus occurred by a slightly different pathway. Alternatively one could invoke the occurrence of a second ventricular focus and fusion with the first ("accelerated idioventricular") focus.

## 7. RHYTHM INTERPRETATION

Sinus arrhythmia with accelerated idioventricular rhythm and fusion beats

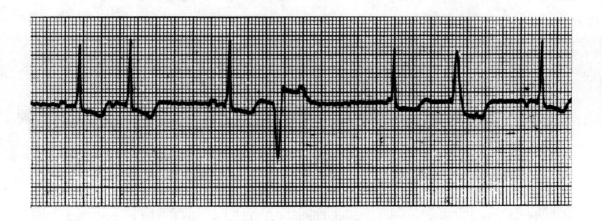

Figure 2-44A

# ECG RHYTHM STRIP #44
## Lead II

**1. RHYTHM**

    Atrial:

    Ventricular:

**2. RATE**

    Atrial:

    Ventricular:

**3. P WAVE**

    Present:

    Configuration:

    Consistency:

    Relation to QRS:

**4. P-R INTERVAL**

    Duration:

    Consistency:

**5. QRS COMPLEX**

    Present:

    Configuration:

    Consistency:

    Duration:

**6. DATA ANALYSIS**

**7. RHYTHM INTERPRETATION**

301

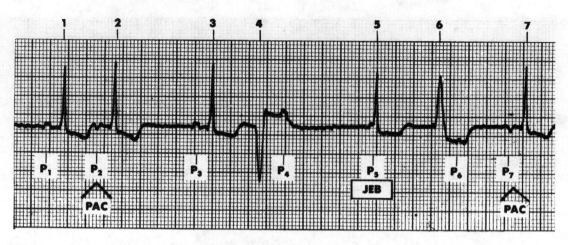

Figure 2-44B

# ECG RHYTHM STRIP #44
## Lead II

## I. RHYTHM

**Atrial:** Irregular

**Ventricular:** Irregular

## 2. RATE

**Atrial:** 70 (obscure P's-onset of QRS 5; ST of beat 6)

**Ventricular:** 70

## 3. P WAVE

**Present:** Yes

**Configuration:** Predominantly positive—slightly notched; two negative (preceding beats 2 and 7)

**Consistency:** Inconsistent

**Relation to QRS:** Varies

## 4. P-R INTERVAL

**Duration:** 0.18 seconds with conducted beats

**Consistency:** Inconsistent

## 5. QRS COMPLEX

**Present:** Yes

**Configuration:** Normal and abnormal

**Consistency:** Inconsistent

**Duration:** Normal—0.08 seconds
Abnormal—0.12 seconds

## 6. DATA ANALYSIS

The abnormal values include:
- an irregular rhythm
- inconsistent P waves
- a variable P to QRS relation
- two wide, abnormal, and inconsistent QRS complexes

The clearly visible P waves that are similar include the P's preceding QRS complexes 1 and 3 and following QRS complex 4. Beginning with the P wave preceding beat 3, the P waves march out regularly through $QRS_6$. It distorts the onset of the QRS in beat 5 and appears as a notch in the ST segment of beat 6. These P waves are probably sinus in origin, although a 12 lead ECG is necessary to rule out atrial abnormality, since the P waves are slightly notched. Only 2 of the "sinus" P waves conduct to the ventricles (the first and third). The others (P waves 4, 5, and 6) are dissociated (not conducted) because of their relationship to the QRS complexes. The pause following $QRS_4$ is terminated by a QRS of identical morphology to the "normally" conducted impulse, consistent with a junctional origin.

P's 2 and 7 are different in configuration and are both premature in the **sinus** cycle. The reason the last beat does not appear premature in the rhythm is because the preceding sinus P wave (in ST segment of beat 6) did not conduct to the ventricles (due to physiologic AV refractoriness) and therefore is not followed by a QRS complex.

The wide, abnormal QRS complexes (4 and 6) vary in configuration and are premature in the basic rhythm representing ventricular ectopy.

## 7. RHYTHM INTERPRETATION

Sinus rhythm with two PAC's; two multiform PVC's; and one junctional escape beat

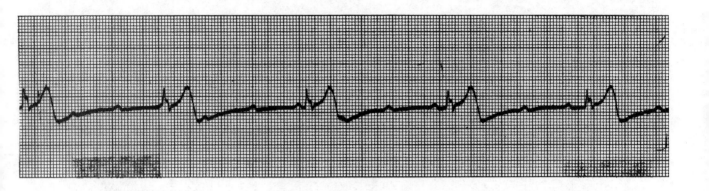

Figure 2-45A

# ECG RHYTHM STRIP #45
## Lead II

**I. RHYTHM**

Atrial:

Ventricular:

**2. RATE**

Atrial:

Ventricular:

**3. P WAVE**

Present:

Configuration:

Consistency:

Relation to QRS:

**4. P-R INTERVAL**

Duration:

Consistency:

**5. QRS COMPLEX**

Present:

Configuration:

Consistency:

Duration:

**6. DATA ANALYSIS**

**7. RHYTHM INTERPRETATION**

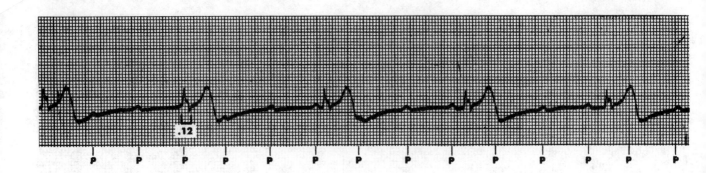

Figure 2-45B

# ECG RHYTHM STRIP #45
## Lead II

## I. RHYTHM

Atrial: Regular

Ventricular: Regular

## 2. RATE

Atrial: 110 (many P's obscure in QRS-T sequence)

Ventricular: 30

## 3. P WAVE

Present: Yes

Configuration: Normal

Consistency: Consistent

Relation to QRS: None; P-R intervals vary without change in ventricular rhythm

## 4. P-R INTERVAL Indeterminable since P's unrelated to QRS

Duration: —

Consistency: —

## 5. QRS COMPLEX

Present: Yes

Configuration: Abnormal—notched

Consistency: Consistent

Duration: 0.12 seconds

## 6. DATA ANALYSIS

The abnormal values include:
- an atrial rate of 110 and a ventricular rate of 30
- an unrelated P to QRS relation
- an abnormal, wide QRS complex (0.12 seconds)

The ventricular rate is slower than the atrial rate due to nonconducted P waves. There is AV dissociation: P's are unrelated to QRS complexes with regular (independent) atrial and ventricular rhythms.

A wide, abnormal QRS characterizes the independent escape rhythm. It may be caused by a slow junctional rhythm with an intraventricular conduction delay or a ventricular ectopic pacemaker. A 12 lead ECG may help differentiate between the two, particularly if previous ECG tracings are available for comparison.

## 7. RHYTHM INTERPRETATION

Sinus tachycardia with complete heart block and an idioventricular rhythm (versus junctional with intraventricular conduction delay)

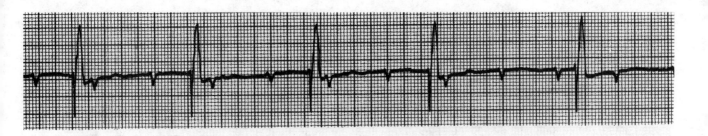

Figure 2-46A

# ECG RHYTHM STRIP #46
## Lead V₁

**1. RHYTHM**

    Atrial:

    Ventricular:

**2. RATE**

    Atrial:

    Ventricular:

**3. P WAVE**

    Present:

    Configuration:

    Consistency:

    Relation to QRS:

**4. P-R INTERVAL**

    Duration:

    Consistency:

**5. QRS COMPLEX**

    Present:

    Configuration:

    Consistency:

    Duration:

**6. DATA ANALYSIS**

**7. RHYTHM INTERPRETATION**

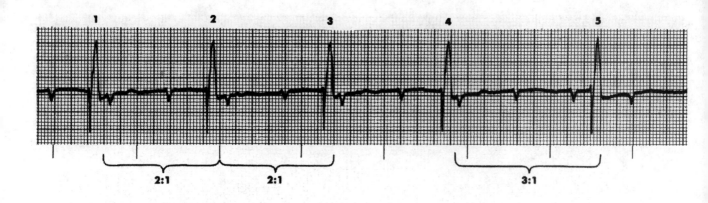

Figure 2-46B

# ECG RHYTHM STRIP #46
## Lead V₁

## 1. RHYTHM

Atrial: Regular

Ventricular: Irregular

## 2. RATE

Atrial: 80

Ventricular: 40

## 3. P WAVE

Present: Yes

Configuration: Diphasic with large terminal negative deflection

Consistency: Consistent

Relation to QRS: Predominantly 2:1; 3:1 prior to last QRS

## 4. P-R INTERVAL

Duration: 1st 4 beats; 0.50 seconds; Beat 5: 0.24 seconds

Consistency: Variable due to change with beat 5

## 5. QRS COMPLEX

Present: Yes

Configuration: Abnormal rSR'

Consistency: Consistent

Duration: 0.14 seconds

## 6. DATA ANALYSIS

The abnormal values include:
- a ventricular rate of 40
- an irregular ventricular rhythm
- a variable P to QRS relation (2:1 and 3:1)
- a prolonged and variable P-R interval
- an abnormal and wide (0.14 seconds) QRS complex

The atrial rate and rhythm are consistent with underlying sinus rhythm. The configuration of the P wave in V₁ (diphasic with large terminal negative deflection) raises the possibility of a left atrial abnormality; however, a 12 lead ECG is needed to accurately assess this.

The ventricular rate is slower than the atrial rate due to the presence of an AV block. Initially every other P wave is **not** conducted to the ventricles (2:1 conduction ratios). The P waves that are conducted prior to the 1st 4 beats are conducted with an identical marked prolongation of the P-R interval. The ventricular rhythm then becomes irregular due to a "worsening" in the conduction ratios (3:1 prior to the 5th QRS). The P-R interval prior to QRS₅ is "shorter" because the AV conduction tissues had more time to "rest." The wide QRS with an rSR' in V₁ indicates right bundle branch block. The presence of the RBBB implies the level of the block is infranodal (Mobitz II).

## 7. RHYTHM INTERPRETATION

Sinus rhythm with high grade AV block (Mobitz Type II) and RBBB

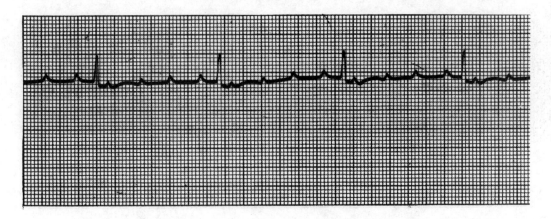

Figure 2-47A

# ECG RHYTHM STRIP #47
## Lead II

**I. RHYTHM**

    Atrial:

    Ventricular:

**2. RATE**

    Atrial:

    Ventricular:

**3. P WAVE**

    Present:

    Configuration:

    Consistency:

    Relation to QRS:

**4. P-R INTERVAL**

    Duration:

    Consistency:

**5. QRS COMPLEX**

    Present:

    Configuration:

    Consistency:

    Duration:

**6. DATA ANALYSIS**

**7. RHYTHM INTERPRETATION**

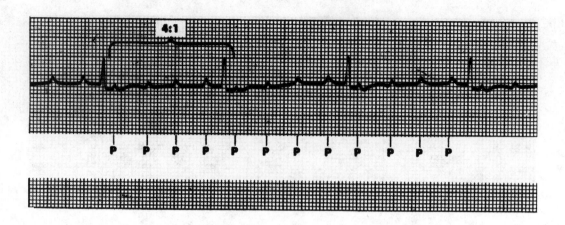

Figure 2-47B

# ECG RHYTHM STRIP #47
## Lead II

## 1. RHYTHM

Atrial: Regular

Ventricular: Regular

## 2. RATE

Atrial: 190

Ventricular: 45

## 3. P WAVE

Present: Yes

Configuration: Peaked

Consistency: Consistent

Relation to QRS: 4:1

## 4. P-R INTERVAL

Duration: 0.22 seconds

Consistency: Consistent

## 5. QRS COMPLEX

Present: Yes

Configuration: Normal

Consistency: Consistent

Duration: 0.04 seconds

## 6. DATA ANALYSIS

The abnormal values include:
- an atrial rate of 190 and ventricular rate of 45
- a 4:1 P to QRS relation
- a prolonged P-R interval at 0.22 seconds

The atrial rate is consistent with atrial tachy-cardia (rate 150 to 210). Quinidine-like drug effect, however, could slow the atrial rate of atrial flutter (rate 250 to 350) to this level.

The nonconducted P waves (4:1 P to QRS relation) and prolonged P-R interval are indicative of AV block. Physiologic AV refractoriness could account for nonconduction of the P wave immediately following the QRS complexes but not the 2nd and 3rd P waves following each QRS.

## 7. RHYTHM INTERPRETATION

Atrial tachycardia with block (rule out atrial flutter with slow atrial rate)

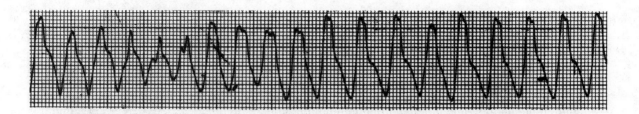

Figure 2-48A

# ECG RHYTHM STRIP #48
## Lead II

**1. RHYTHM**

   Atrial:

   Ventricular:

**2. RATE**

   Atrial:

   Ventricular:

**3. P WAVE**

   Present:

   Configuration:

   Consistency:

   Relation to QRS:

**4. P-R INTERVAL**

   Duration:

   Consistency:

**5. QRS COMPLEX**

   Present:

   Configuration:

   Consistency:

   Duration:

**6. DATA ANALYSIS**

**7. RHYTHM INTERPRETATION**

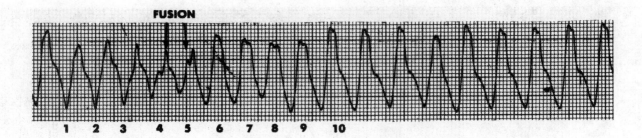

FUSION

1  2  3  4  5  6  7  8  9  10

Figure 2-48B

## ECG RHYTHM STRIP #48
### Lead II

### 1. RHYTHM

Atrial: Indeterminable

Ventricular: Slightly irregular

### 2. RATE

Atrial: Indeterminable

Ventricular: 170

### 3. P WAVE

Present: None identified

Configuration: —

Consistency: —

Relation to QRS: —

### 4. P-R INTERVAL Indeterminable

Duration: —

Consistency: —

### 5. QRS COMPLEX

Present: Yes

Configuration: Abnormal

Consistency: Inconsistent; varies in configuration and polarity

Duration: > 0.14 seconds

### 6. DATA ANALYSIS

The abnormal values include:
- unidentifiable P waves (therefore atrial rate, rhythm, and P-R interval indeterminable)
- a ventricular rate of 170
- an abnormal, wide, and inconsistent QRS complex

The wide, abnormal QRS complexes (without identifiable P waves) are consistent with a ventricular origin.

The QRS complexes appear to change polarity—the initial three beats being negative and similar in configuration and the 6th through last beats being positive and similar in configuration. QRS complexes 4 and 5 are probably fusion beats as the two ventricular pacemaker sites compete for control. Alternatively one might call the rhythm "Toursade of Pointes"—a peculiar form of ventricular tachycardia characterized by progressive changes in the amplitude and polarity of the QRS complexes such that the QRS complexes appear to be twisting around an isoelectric baseline.

### 7. RHYTHM INTERPRETATION

Multiform ventricular tachycardia

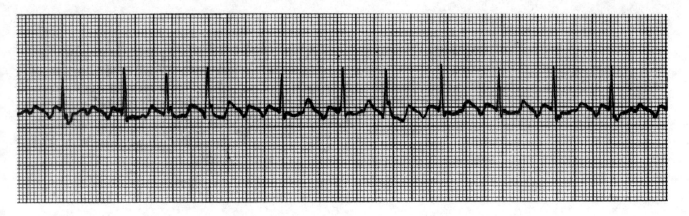

Figure 2-49A

## ECG RHYTHM STRIP #49
### Lead II

**1. RHYTHM**

    Atrial:

    Ventricular:

**2. RATE**

    Atrial:

    Ventricular:

**3. P WAVE**

    Present:

    Configuration:

    Consistency:

    Relation to QRS:

**4. P-R INTERVAL**

    Duration:

    Consistency:

**5. QRS COMPLEX**

    Present:

    Configuration:

    Consistency:

    Duration:

**6. DATA ANALYSIS**

**7. RHYTHM INTERPRETATION**

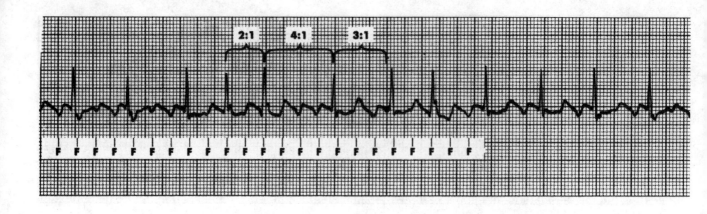

Figure 2-49B

## ECG RHYTHM STRIP #49
### Lead II

### 1. RHYTHM

Atrial: Regular (march out)

Ventricular: Irregular

### 2. RATE

Atrial: 300 (P's obscure in QRS-T sequence of every beat)

Ventricular: 100

### 3. P WAVE

Present: Yes, multiple

Configuration: Abnormal, saw-toothed

Consistency: Consistent when clearly identifiable

Relation to QRS: Varies: 2:1, 3:1, 4:1

### 4. P-R INTERVAL  Indeterminable

Duration: —

Consistency: —

### 5. QRS COMPLEX

Present: Yes

Configuration: Normal

Consistency: Consistent except when distorted by P waves

Duration: 0.06 seconds

### 6. DATA ANALYSIS

The abnormal values include:
- an atrial rate of 300 and a ventricular rate of 100 (slower due to nonconducted P waves)
- an irregular ventricular rhythm
- multiple, abnormal P waves that are partly obscure in the QRS-T sequence
- a variable P to QRS relation

The atrial rate of 300, regular atrial rhythm, and morphology of the P waves are consistent with atrial flutter. The ventricular rhythm is irregular due to variable AV conduction ratios.

### 7. RHYTHM INTERPRETATION

Atrial flutter with variable AV conduction ratios

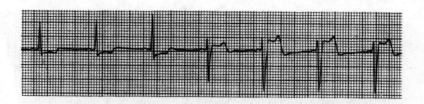

Figure 2-50A

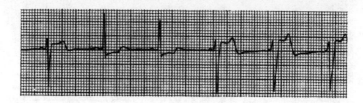

Figure 2-50B

# ECG RHYTHM STRIP #50 (Continuous Strip)
## Lead II

**1. RHYTHM**

    Atrial:

    Ventricular:

**2. RATE**

    Atrial:

    Ventricular:

**3. P WAVE**

    Present:

    Configuration:

    Consistency:

    Relation to QRS:

**4. P-R INTERVAL**

    Duration:

    Consistency:

**5. QRS COMPLEX**

    Present:

    Configuration:

    Consistency:

    Duration:

**6. DATA ANALYSIS**

**7. RHYTHM INTERPRETATION**

313

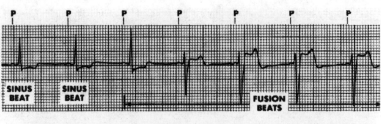

Figure 2-50C

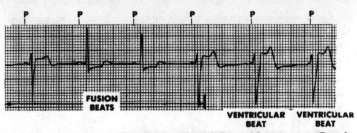

Figure 2-50D

# ECG RHYTHM STRIP #50 (Continuous Strip)
## Lead II

## I. RHYTHM

Atrial: Regular

Ventricular: Regular

## 2. RATE

Atrial: 75

Ventricular: 75

## 3. P WAVE

Present: Yes

Configuration: Normal

Consistency: Consistent

Relation to QRS: 1 before each QRS: some conduct, some dissociated (P-R's too short)

## 4. P-R INTERVAL

Duration: 0.06 to 0.14 seconds

Consistency: Inconsistent

## 5. QRS COMPLEX

Present: Yes

Configuration: Normal—positive
Abnormal—negative

Consistency: Inconsistent; varies in configuration and polarity

Duration: 0.06 to 0.12 seconds

## 6. DATA ANALYSIS

The abnormal values include:
- a variable P to QRS relation
- an inconsistent and sometimes short P-R interval
- a change in the QRS complex from normal and narrow to abnormal and wide

The atrial activity is characterized by a normal, regular P wave at a rate of 75 indicating an underlying sinus rhythm.

Although a sinus P wave can be seen preceding each QRS, the relationship to the subsequent QRS varies as the P-R interval changes. At the same time, the QRS complex varies in configuration becoming wider and more abnormal as the P-R interval becomes shorter. The change in the QRS complex can be explained by various degrees of fusion, since there is no change in cycle length. There is, therefore, an independent (competing) ventricular rhythm at the same rate as the sinus rhythm (i.e., periods of isorhythmic AV dissociation). Most of the beats in this strip are fusion since the P-R intervals and QRS complexes are so inconsistent—even if only slightly. The "pure" sinus beats are probably 1 and 2, and the "pure" ventricular beats are probably the last 2—widest QRS and shortest P-R intervals.

## 7. RHYTHM INTERPRETATION

Sinus rhythm with incomplete isorhythmic AV dissociation, accelerated idioventricular rhythm, and various degrees of ventricular fusion beats

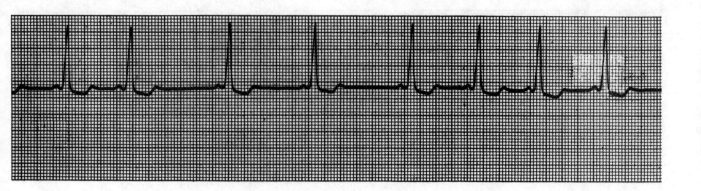

Figure 2-51A

## ECG RHYTHM STRIP #51
### Lead II

**1. RHYTHM**

    Atrial:

    Ventricular:

**2. RATE**

    Atrial:

    Ventricular:

**3. P WAVE**

    Present:

    Configuration:

    Consistency:

    Relation to QRS:

**4. P-R INTERVAL**

    Duration:

    Consistency:

**5. QRS COMPLEX**

    Present:

    Configuration:

    Consistency:

    Duration:

**6. DATA ANALYSIS**

**7. RHYTHM INTERPRETATION**

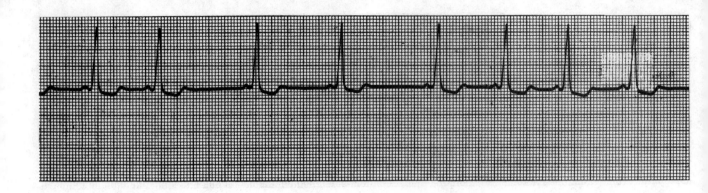

Figure 2-51B

# ECG RHYTHM STRIP #51
## Lead II

## 1. RHYTHM

Atrial: Irregular

Ventricular: Irregular

## 2. RATE

Atrial: 60

Ventricular: 60

## 3. P WAVE

Present: Yes

Configuration: Normal

Consistency: Consistent

Relation to QRS: 1:1

## 4. P-R INTERVAL

Duration: 0.10 to 0.11 seconds

Consistency: Consistent

## 5. QRS COMPLEX

Present: Yes

Configuration: Abnormal—slight slurring of
initial upstoke

Consistency: Consistent

Duration: 0.12 seconds

## 6. DATA ANALYSIS

All values are normal except that:
- the rhythm is irregular
- the P-R interval is shortened at 0.10 to 0.11 seconds
- the QRS complex is wide and abnormal

The rhythm is irregular due to a variation in the P-P interval. Since the P waves appear identical, sinus arrhythmia and/or sinus arrests may account for the variability in the P-P interval.

The short P-R interval and wide, abnormal QRS complex suggest the possibility of pre-excitation as in the WPW syndrome. A 12 lead ECG is needed to confirm this diagnosis.

## 7. RHYTHM INTERPRETATION

Sinus arrhythmia with possible sinus arrest. Short P-R interval, intraventricular conduction delay (rule out WPW syndrome)

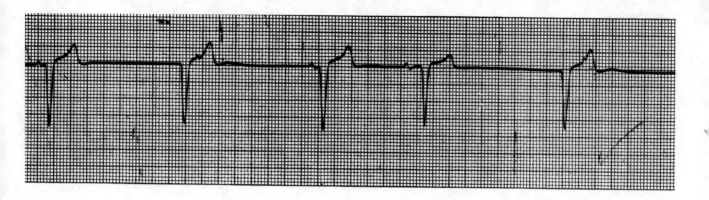

Figure 2-52A

# ECG RHYTHM STRIP #52
## Lead V₁

**I. RHYTHM**

Atrial:

Ventricular:

**2. RATE**

Atrial:

Ventricular:

**3. P WAVE**

Present:

Configuration:

Consistency:

Relation to QRS:

**4. P-R INTERVAL**

Duration:

Consistency:

**5. QRS COMPLEX**

Present:

Configuration:

Consistency:

Duration:

**6. DATA ANALYSIS**

**7. RHYTHM INTERPRETATION**

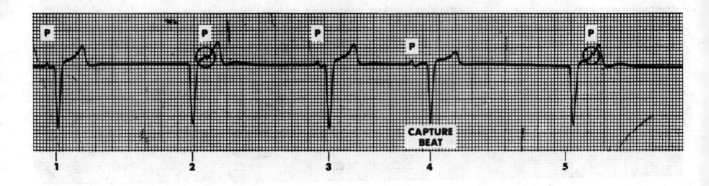

Figure 2-52B

# ECG RHYTHM STRIP #52
## Lead V₁

## 1. RHYTHM

Atrial: Irregular

Ventricular: Irregular

## 2. RATE

Atrial: 40 (P's present in ST of beats 2 and 5)

Ventricular: 40 (overall)

## 3. P WAVE

Present: Yes

Configuration: Normal

Consistency: Consistent

Relation to QRS: Varies

## 4. P-R INTERVAL

Duration: Beats 1 and 3—0.12 seconds
Beat 4—0.20 seconds

Consistency: Inconsistent

## 5. QRS COMPLEX

Present: Yes

Configuration: Beat 4: normal
Others: slight slurring on
upstroke of QS wave

Consistency: Consistent except beat 4

Duration: 0.11 seconds
0.10 seconds in beat 4

## 6. DATA ANALYSIS

The abnormal values include:
- a rate of 40 beats per minute
- an irregular rhythm
- a variable P to QRS relation
- an inconsistent P-R interval when measurable
- a slight inconsistency in the QRS complex

The atrial rhythm is characterized by normal, consistent P waves at a slow rate and varying cycle lengths (long pauses). This probably reflects a combination of sinus arrhythmia and periods of sinus arrest. The P to QRS relation varies—some P's precede the QRS while others follow. Beat 4 represents the only normally conducted beat (capture beat)—the P-R interval is long enough to permit conduction of the sinus impulse to the ventricles, and the QRS is "premature" when compared to the 1st three QRS complexes.

The remaining four beats must be dissociated since the remaining ventricular rhythm is basically regular, the P to QRS relation varies, and the pseudo P-R interval with beats 1 and 3 is shorter (0.10 to 0.12 seconds). During (the) AV dissociation, the ventricular rate is 35 per minute and the QRS complex is wide and slightly slurred. The QRS complexes (beats 1, 2, 3, and 5) are probably of ventricular origin although a slow junctional rhythm with LBBB aberration cannot be excluded.

## 7. RHYTHM INTERPRETATION

Sinus bradycardia and arrhythmia with periods of sinus arrest and incomplete AV dissociation with probable ventricular rhythm (versus slow junctional rhythm and intraventricular conduction defect)

318

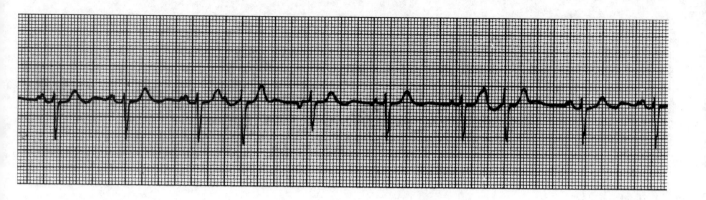

Figure 2-53A

# ECG RHYTHM STRIP #53
## Monitor Lead II

**1. RHYTHM**

   Atrial:

   Ventricular:

**2. RATE**

   Atrial:

   Ventricular:

**3. P WAVE**

   Present:

   Configuration:

   Consistency:

   Relation to QRS:

**4. P-R INTERVAL**

   Duration:

   Consistency:

**5. QRS COMPLEX**

   Present:

   Configuration:

   Consistency:

   Duration:

**6. DATA ANALYSIS**

**7. RHYTHM INTERPRETATION**

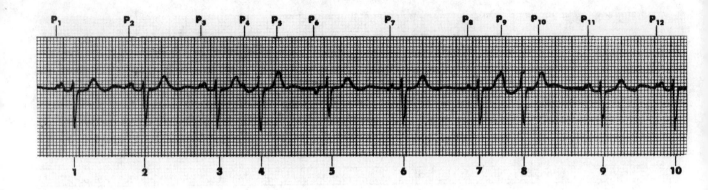

Figure 2-53B

# ECG RHYTHM STRIP #53
## Monitor Lead II

## I. RHYTHM

Atrial: Irregular

Ventricular: Irregular

## 2. RATE

Atrial: 90

Ventricular: 80

## 3. P WAVE

Present: Yes

Configuration: Sinus—notched; others variable
in configuraiton

Consistency: Inconsistent

Relation to QRS: Predominantly 1:1 with 2 not
followed by QRS complexes
($P_5$ and $P_{10}$)

## 4. P-R INTERVAL

Duration: 0.14 to 0.24 seconds

Consistency: Inconsistent

## 5. QRS COMPLEX

Present: Yes

Configuration: Normal

Consistency: Slight variation

Duration: 0.08 seconds

## 6. DATA ANALYSIS

The abnormal values include:
- a slower ventricular versus atrial rate
- an irregular rhythm
- a variable P wave configuration (sometimes notched) and P to QRS relation (usually 1:1)
- an inconsistent and sometimes prolonged P-R interval

The first three and last two P waves are identical and establish a basic sinus rhythm at 70 per minute. The notching of these P waves raises the possibility of an atrial abnormality; however, a 12 lead ECG is necessary to accurately assess this. $P_4$ through $P_{10}$ show variable morphology. Some are premature when compared to the sinus cycle, others are not. The latter suggests periods of wandering atrial pacemaker (WAP), but the prematurity of the other P waves is atypical of WAP. The T waves following QRS complexes 4 and 8 are distorted (P on T) and are not followed by QRS complexes. These findings are consistent with nonconducted PAC's.

The slight variability of the QRS configuration may relate in part to respiratory variation. In addition, QRS complexes 4 and 8 may be conducted with slight aberrancy.

## 7. RHYTHM INTERPRETATION

Sinus rhythm with frequent multifocal ectopic atrial beats (WAP with PAC's); some conducted with first degree AV block, others nonconducted

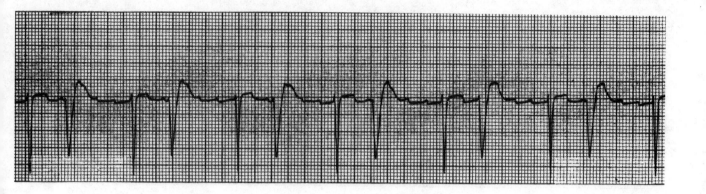

Figure 2-54A

# ECG RHYTHM STRIP #54
## Lead MCL₁

**1. RHYTHM**

    Atrial:

    Ventricular:

**2. RATE**

    Atrial:

    Ventricular:

**3. P WAVE**

    Present:

    Configuration:

    Consistency:

    Relation to QRS:

**4. P-R INTERVAL**

    Duration:

    Consistency:

**5. QRS COMPLEX**

    Present:

    Configuration:

    Consistency:

    Duration:

**6. DATA ANALYSIS**

**7. RHYTHM INTERPRETATION**

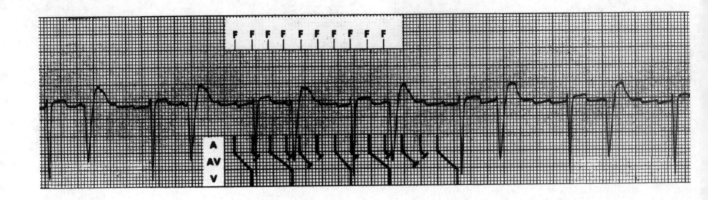

Figure 2-54B

# ECG RHYTHM STRIP #54
## Lead MCL₁

### 1. RHYTHM

Atrial: Regular

Ventricular: Irregular (regularly irregular or cyclic)

### 2. RATE

Atrial: 275

Ventricular: 100

### 3. P WAVE

Present: Yes

Configuration: Diphasic

Consistency: Consistent

Relation to QRS: Varies

### 4. P-R INTERVAL

Duration: 0.22 seconds (F-R) with normal QRS

Consistency: Consistent

### 5. QRS COMPLEX

Present: Yes

Configuration: Alternates between normal and abnormal

Consistency: Inconsistent

Duration: Normal—0.08 seconds
Abnormal—0.14 seconds

### 6. DATA ANALYSIS

The abnormal values include:
- an atrial rate of 275 beats per minutes
- a regularly irregular ventricular rhythm
- a variable P to QRS relation
- alternating wide QRS complexes

The atrial rate is consistent with atrial flutter, though the P wave morphology shows an atypical flutter wave.

Every other QRS complex is wide and abnormal, ending a short cycle that was preceded by a longer cycle. This raises the possibility of aberrancy. Alternatively, the wide QRS complexes may be due to ventricular ectopy. If aberrancy were the case, one could then demonstrate a Wenckebach phenomenon (see ladder diagram). Physiologically every other atrial impulse would be blocked in the upper portion of the AV node. The flutter wave immediately preceding the wide QRS would not be able to conduct to the ventricles (P-R too short). One could then invoke a progressive increase in the P-R interval. In addition, the R-R intervals. This discussion is all for naught if the wide QRS complexes represents ventricular ectopy.

The P to QRS relationship varies, accounting for the irregular ventricular rhythm.

### 7. RHYTHM INTERPRETATION

Atrial flutter with ventricular bigeminy (rule out aberrantly conducted flutter waves)

322

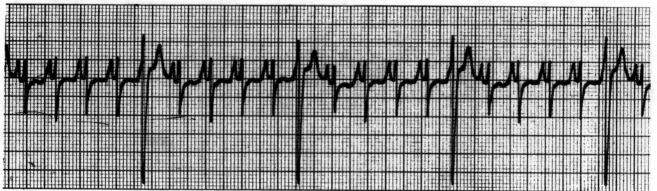

Figure 2-55A

# ECG RHYTHM STRIP #55
## Monitor Lead II

**I. RHYTHM**

    Atrial:

    Ventricular:

**2. RATE**

    Atrial:

    Ventricular:

**3. P WAVE**

    Present:

    Configuration:

    Consistency:

    Relation to QRS:

**4. P-R INTERVAL**

    Duration:

    Consistency:

**5. QRS COMPLEX**

    Present:

    Configuration:

    Consistency:

    Duration:

**6. DATA ANALYSIS**

**7. RHYTHM INTERPRETATION**

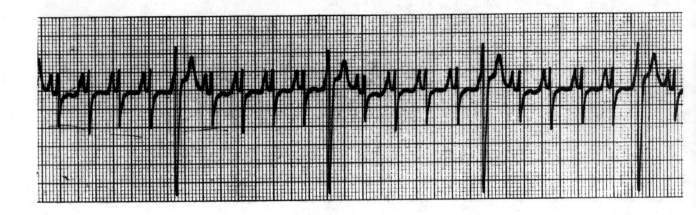

Figure 2-55B

# ECG RHYTHM STRIP #55
## Monitor Lead II

## I. RHYTHM

Atrial: Regular

Ventricular: Irregular (regularly irregular or cyclic)

## 2. RATE

Atrial: 175 (P's obscure in abnormal QRS's)

Ventricular: 175

## 3. P WAVE

Present: Yes

Configuration: Tall, peaked

Consistency: Consistent

Relation to QRS: 1:1 except with abnormal beats where P's hidden in QRS

## 4. P-R INTERVAL

Duration: 0.10 seconds

Consistency: Consistent

## 5. QRS COMPLEX

Present: Yes

Configuration: Normal and abnormal

Consistency: Inconsistent

Duration: Normal—0.06 seconds
Abnormal—0.11 seconds

## 6. DATA ANALYSIS

The abnormal values include:
- a rate of 175 beats per minute
- an irregular ventricular rhythm
- a variable P to QRS relation
- a P-R interval of 0.10 seconds
- an inconsistent QRS complex

The P waves march out regularly in the atrial rhythm, some of which are hidden in the abnormal QRS complexes. The abnormal QRS complexes are premature in the basic rhythm and occur regularly with every 5th beat—making the ventricular rhythm cyclic. Since the P waves hidden in these abnormal beats are part of the basic rhythm, they are dissociated from the QRS complexes.

The tachycardia is of supraventricular origin since the QRS complexes in question are narrow. The short P-R interval as well as the rate (175 per minute) suggests that this is not sinus tachycardia unless this strip was taken from an infant or during exercise.

The short P-R interval may be a normal variation but raises the possibility of an ectopic pacemaker site (i.e., close to the AV junction) or preexcitation. Clinical information and a 12 lead ECG would be helpful in making the differential diagnosis. If this is sinus tachycardia, a 12 lead ECG will also assist in assessing the presence of a right atrial abnormality (tall, peaked P waves inferiorly).

## 7. RHYTHM INTERPRETATION

Supraventricular tachycardia with frequent unifocal PVC's

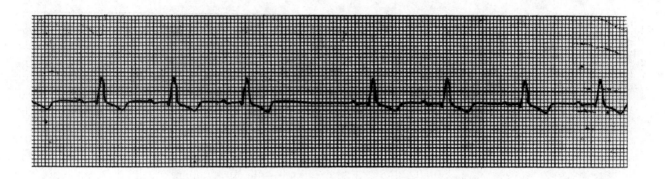

Figure 2-56A

# ECG RHYTHM STRIP #56
## Monitor Lead II

**1. RHYTHM**

   Atrial:

   Ventricular:

**2. RATE**

   Atrial:

   Ventricular:

**3. P WAVE**

   Present:

   Configuration:

   Consistency:

   Relation to QRS:

**4. P-R INTERVAL**

   Duration:

   Consistency:

**5. QRS COMPLEX**

   Present:

   Configuration:

   Consistency:

   Duration:

**6. DATA ANALYSIS**

**7. RHYTHM INTERPRETATION**

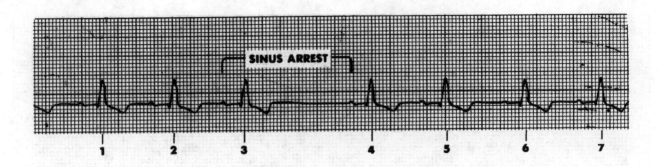

Figure 2-56B

# ECG RHYTHM STRIP #56
## Monitor Lead II

### I. RHYTHM

Atrial: Irregular

Ventricular: Irregular

### 2. RATE

Atrial: 70

Ventricular: 70

### 3. P WAVE

Present: Yes

Configuration: Normal

Consistency: Consistent

Relation to QRS: 1:1

### 4. P-R INTERVAL

Duration: 0.22 seconds
0.18 seconds beat 4 only

Consistency: Consistent except with beat 4

### 5. QRS COMPLEX

Present: Yes

Configuration: Slight notching

Consistency: Consistent

Duration: 0.11 seconds

### 6. DATA ANALYSIS

All values are normal except that:
- the rhythm is irregular
- the P-R interval is prolonged at 0.22 seconds (varies with beat 4)
- the QRS complex is prolonged

There is a pause in the rhythm following beat 3. This, along with a slight slowing in the basic rhythm following beat 5, accounts for the irregular rhythm.

The P-R intervals are prolonged at 0.22 seconds except with beat 4. This is probably related to the preceding pause in the rhythm allowing the AV node time to "rest." A P wave is not found in the "pause" and the P-P interval of the "pause" is not a precise multiple of the basic sinus cycle. These findings are consistent with the occurrence of a sinus arrest.

The prolonged (0.11 seconds) and slightly notched QRS complex is related to an intraventricular conduction defect.

### 7. RHYTHM INTERPRETATION

Sinus arrhythmia with sinus arrest, first degree AV block and an intraventricular conduction defect

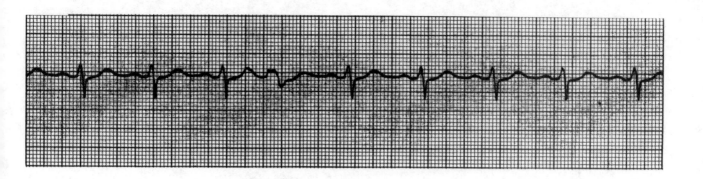

Figure 2-57A

## ECG RHYTHM STRIP #57
### Monitor Lead II

**1. RHYTHM**

    Atrial:

    Ventricular:

**2. RATE**

    Atrial:

    Ventricular:

**3. P WAVE**

    Present:

    Configuration:

    Consistency:

    Relation to QRS:

**4. P-R INTERVAL**

    Duration:

    Consistency:

**5. QRS COMPLEX**

    Present:

    Configuration:

    Consistency:

    Duration:

**6. DATA ANALYSIS**

**7. RHYTHM INTERPRETATION**

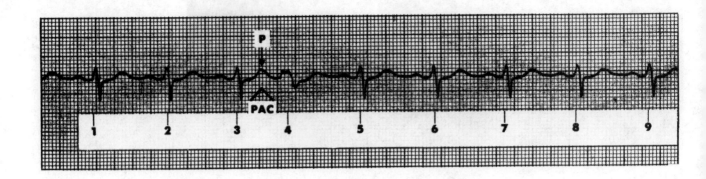

Figure 2-57B

# ECG RHYTHM STRIP #57
## Monitor Lead II

## I. RHYTHM

Atrial: Irregular

Ventricular: Irregular

## 2. RATE

Atrial: 75 (one P wave obscure on T wave after QRS$_3$)

Ventricular: 75

## 3. P WAVE

Present: Yes

Configuration: Widened

Consistency: Consistent when visible

Relation to QRS: 1:1

## 4. P-R INTERVAL

Duration: 0.21 seconds

Consistency: Consistent

## 5. QRS COMPLEX

Present: Yes

Configuration: Normal, 1 abnormal

Consistency: Consistent except for QRS$_4$

Duration: 0.11 seconds
0.20 seconds in QRS$_4$

## 6. DATA ANALYSIS

The abnormal values include:
- an irregular rhythm (due to 4th premature P-QRS-T sequence)
- a prolonged P-R interval at 0.21 seconds
- a slightly prolonged QRS complex
- a change in the QRS complex is beat 4—bizarre and wide (0.20 seconds)

The T wave following beat 3 is different than the others—raising the possibility of an obscure, premature P wave. Since the bizarre, wide QRS complex appears to be preceded by a P wave, its abnormality is caused by aberrant conduction rather than a ventricular ectopic pacemaker. The absence of a compensatory pause further supports this diagnosis.

The prolonged P-R intervals may be partly related to an intra-atrial conduction delay, since the P waves appear widened. A 12 lead ECG is necessary to assess for left atrial abnormality. The QRS complexes are slightly prolonged in duration indicating an intraventricular conduction defect.

## 7. RHYTHM INTERPRETATION

Sinus rhythm with first degree AV block, one aberrantly conducted PAC, and an intraventricular conduction defect

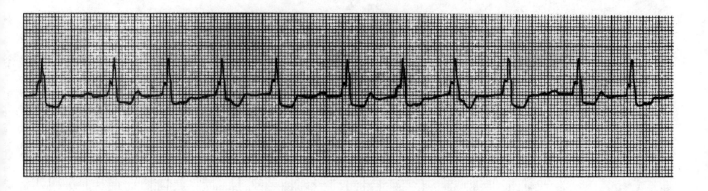

Figure 2-58A

# ECG RHYTHM STRIP #58
## Monitor Lead II

**1. RHYTHM**

    Atrial:

    Ventricular:

**2. RATE**

    Atrial:

    Ventricular:

**3. P WAVE**

    Present:

    Configuration:

    Consistency:

    Relation to QRS:

**4. P-R INTERVAL**

    Duration:

    Consistency:

**5. QRS COMPLEX**

    Present:

    Configuration:

    Consistency:

    Duration:

**6. DATA ANALYSIS**

**7. RHYTHM INTERPRETATION**

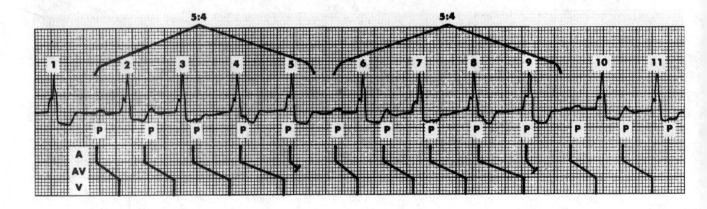

Figure 2-58B

# ECG RHYTHM STRIP #58
## Monitor Lead II

## 1. RHYTHM

Atrial: Regular

Ventricular: Irregular (regularly irregular or cyclic)

## 2. RATE

Atrial: 100 (P's obscure in QRS-T sequence except in beat following pauses)

Ventricular: 80

## 3. P WAVE

Present: Yes

Configuration: Normal

Consistency: Consistent when visible

Relation to QRS: 5:4

## 4. P-R INTERVAL

Duration: 0.30 to 0.54 seconds

Consistency: Inconsistent, progressively lengthens

## 5. QRS COMPLEX

Present: Yes

Configuration: Abnormal—notched

Consistency: Consistent

Duration: 0.12 seconds

## 6. DATA ANALYSIS

The abnormal values include:
- a slower ventricular versus atrial rate
- an irregular ventricular rhythm
- a 5:4 P to QRS relation
- a prolonged and inconsistent P-R interval
- abnormal, wide QRS complexes (0.12 seconds)

Although it is difficult to detect P waves, the P-P interval is regular. The pauses are due to non-conduction of sinus P waves (hidden in QRS complexes 1, 5, and 9) from the atria to the ventricles consistent with second degree AV block. The P-R intervals progressively increase until a P wave is not conducted, indicating a Wenckebach mechanism. The second degree AV block accounts for the irregular ventricular rhythm and an intraventricular conduction delay accounts for the wide, abnormal QRS.

## 7. RHYTHM INTERPRETATION

Sinus rhythm with second degree AV block–Mobitz 1 (Wenckebach) and an intraventricular conduction delay

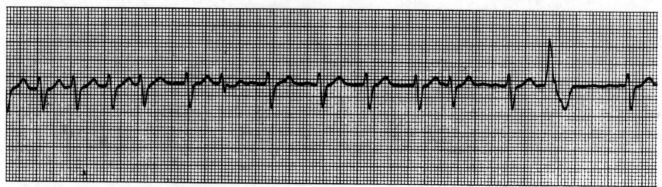

Figure 2-59A

# ECG RHYTHM STRIP #59
## Lead II

**1. RHYTHM**

    Atrial:

    Ventricular:

**2. RATE**

    Atrial:

    Ventricular:

**3. P WAVE**

    Present:

    Configuration:

    Consistency:

    Relation to QRS:

**4. P-R INTERVAL**

    Duration:

    Consistency:

**5. QRS COMPLEX**

    Present:

    Configuration:

    Consistency:

    Duration:

**6. DATA ANALYSIS**

**7. RHYTHM INTERPRETATION**

331

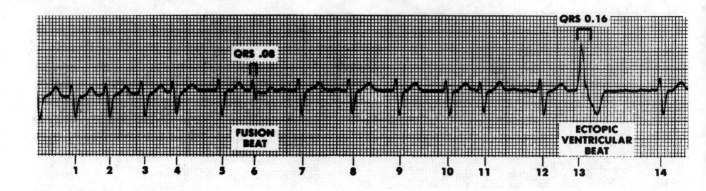

Figure 2-59B

# ECG RHYTHM STRIP #59
## Lead II

## I. RHYTHM

Atrial: Irregular

Ventricular: Irregularly irregular

## 2. RATE

Atrial: Indeterminable

Ventricular: 120

## 3. P WAVE

Present: No (discrete P waves not present)

Configuration: Flattened

Consistency: Varies in size, shape, and width when seen

Relation to QRS: Indeterminable

## 4. P-R INTERVAL   Undefined

Duration: —

Consistency: —

## 5. QRS COMPLEX

Present: Yes

Configuration: Normal and abnormal

Consistency: Varies slightly

Duration: Beat 6—0.08 seconds
Beat 13—0.16 seconds
Others—0.12

## 6. DATA ANALYSIS

Most of the values are abnormal. With the exception of two beats, the QRS complexes are normal and occur at a rate greater than 100, indicating a supraventricular tachycardia. The identification of a fine fibrillatory baseline—irregular flattened and variable atrial activity—and an irregularly irregular ventricular rhythm are the keys to interpretation and point to atrial fibrillation.

$QRS_{13}$ is wide and bizarre, consistent with an ectopic ventricular beat. Although the R-R interval preceding this beat is slightly prolonged (raising the possibility of aberrancy), the QRS does not show RBBB configuration (which is usually seen with aberrancy). Furthermore, $QRS_6$ is narrower than the "normal" QRS complexes and is consistent with a ventricular fusion beat. This is further evidence that $QRS_{13}$ is of ventricular origin. The remaining QRS complexes are slightly prolonged in duration, consistent with an intraventricular conduction delay.

## 7. RHYTHM INTERPRETATION

Atrial fibrillation with one ectopic ventricular beat, one ventricular fusion beat, and an intraventricular conduction delay

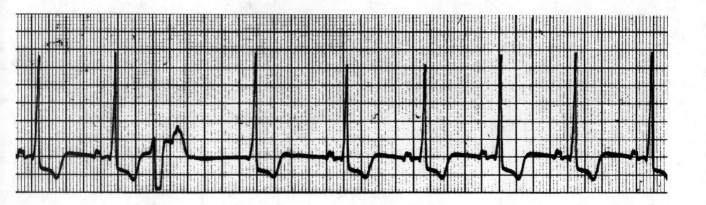

Figure 2-60A

# ECG RHYTHM STRIP #60
## Monitor Lead II

**I. RHYTHM**

Atrial:

Ventricular:

**2. RATE**

Atrial:

Ventricular:

**3. P WAVE**

Present:

Configuration:

Consistency:

Relation to QRS:

**4. P-R INTERVAL**

Duration:

Consistency:

**5. QRS COMPLEX**

Present:

Configuration:

Consistency:

Duration:

**6. DATA ANALYSIS**

**7. RHYTHM INTERPRETATION**

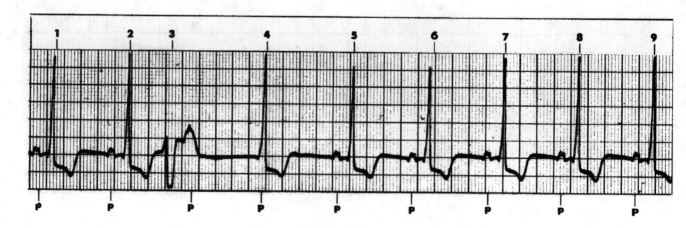

Figure 2-60B

# ECG RHYTHM STRIP #60
## Monitor Lead II

## I. RHYTHM

Atrial: Regular (marches out)

Ventricular: Irregular

## 2. RATE

Atrial: 70 (P hidden in 3rd T wave and $QRS_4$)

Ventricular: 70

## 3. P WAVE

Present: Yes

Configuration: Predominantly positive—
notched

Consistency: Consistent when seen

Relation to QRS: 1:1 except in beats 3 and 4

## 4. P-R INTERVAL

Duration: 0.18 seconds

Consistency: Consistent

## 5. QRS COMPLEX

Present: Yes

Configuration: Normal, increased amplitude;
one abnormal

Consistency: Consistent except for beat 3

Duration: Normal QRS—0.09 seconds
Abnormal QRS—0.14 seconds

## 6. DATA ANALYSIS

The abnormal values include:
- an irregular ventricular rhythm
- a change in the P to QRS relation in beats 3 and 4
- a wide (0.14 seconds), abnormal QRS in beat 3

The atrial rate is consistent with sinus rhythm. The notching of these P waves raises the possibility of atrial abnormality, however, a 12 lead ECG is necessary to accurately assess this.

The P waves measure out regularly, although obscure in beats 3 and 4. This makes them dissociated sinus P's with an independent pacemaker depolarizing the ventricles.

$QRS_3$ is wide and bizarre, consistent with an ectopic ventricular focus. $QRS_4$ appears slightly wide due to distortion by the sinus P wave. It is, however, identical to the "normal" QRS complexes and terminates a "pause" following the PVC. It is a junctional escape beat.

## 7. RHYTHM INTERPRETATION

Sinus rhythm with one PVC and a junction escape beat

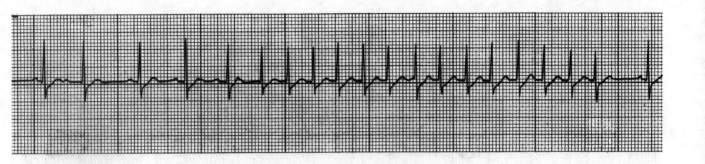

Figure 2-61A

# ECG RHYTHM STRIP #61
## Lead II

**1. RHYTHM**

· Atrial:

Ventricular:

**2. RATE**

Atrial:

Ventricular:

**3. P WAVE**

Present:

Configuration:

Consistency:

Relation to QRS:

**4. P-R INTERVAL**

Duration:

Consistency:

**5. QRS COMPLEX**

Present:

Configuration:

Consistency:

Duration:

**6. DATA ANALYSIS**

**7. RHYTHM INTERPRETATION**

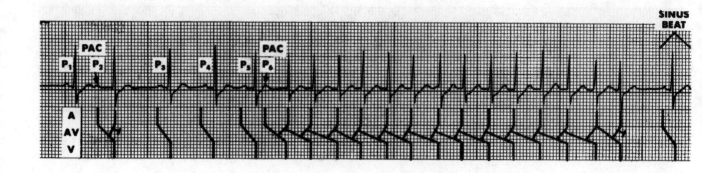

SINUS BEAT

Figure 2-61B

# ECG RHYTHM STRIP #61
## Lead II

## I. RHYTHM

**Atrial:** Irregular

**Ventricular:** Irregular

## 2. RATE

**Atrial:** Average 160 (assuming P wave is buried in QRS-T sequence with run of tachycardia)

**Ventricular:** Average 160 (varies 110 to 200)

## 3. P WAVE

**Present:** Yes

**Configuration:** Normal and positive when seen

**Consistency:** Slight variation

**Relation to QRS:** 1:1 beats 1 to 6 then suspect retrograde conduction

## 4. P-R INTERVAL

**Duration:** 0.12 to 0.26 seconds

**Consistency:** Varies when measurable; increases with premature beats

## 5. QRS COMPLEX

**Present:** Yes

**Configuration:** Normal

**Consistency:** Consistent

**Duration:** 0.06 seconds

## 6. DATA ANALYSIS

The abnormal values include:
- an overall rate of 160 beats per minute
- an irregular rhythm
- a slight variation in the configuration of the P waves
- an inconsistent P-R interval

P waves 1, 3, 4, 5, and last appear similar and are probably sinus in origin. If the 4th to 5th P-P interval represents the basic sinus cycle, P waves 2 and 6 (on T wave after $QRS_5$) are premature—conducting with long P-R intervals. This is related to the premature arrival of the ectopic pacemaker in the AV node and physiologic refractoriness.

The pause following the 1st PAC (2nd P wave) may be due to an atrial echo beat falling within the second QRS (see ladder diagram). The PAC is conducted with a prolonged P-R interval, which permits differential pathway AV nodal conduction and ultimately retrograde conduction back to the atria.

The ventricular rate abruptly increases following beat 5. The paroxysmal tachycardia is initiated by a PAC (P on T wave of $QRS_5$). As with the first PAC this one is also conducted with a prolonged P-R interval permitting differential pathway AV nodal conduction. Retrograde conduction to the atria again occurs, but this time conduction also returns to the ventricles (see ladder diagram). A re-entrant (reciprocating) tachycardia has been established. It spontaneously terminates and the last beat is sinus.

## 7. RHYTHM INTERPRETATION

Sinus tachycardia, PAC's, and paroxysmal AV nodal reentrant tachycardia

336

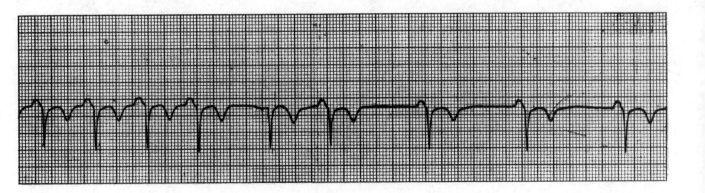

Figure 2-62A

# ECG RHYTHM STRIP #62
## Lead MCL₁

**1. RHYTHM**

    Atrial:

    Ventricular:

**2. RATE**

    Atrial:

    Ventricular:

**3. P WAVE**

    Present:

    Configuration:

    Consistency:

    Relation to QRS:

**4. P-R INTERVAL**

    Duration:

    Consistency:

**5. QRS COMPLEX**

    Present:

    Configuration:

    Consistency:

    Duration:

**6. DATA ANALYSIS**

**7. RHYTHM INTERPRETATION**

337

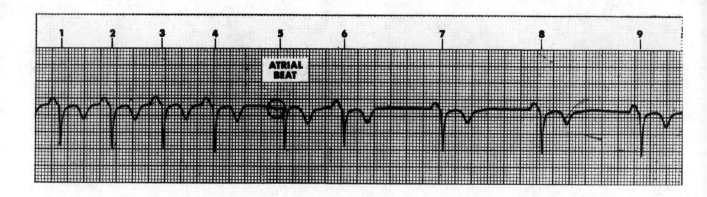

ATRIAL BEAT

Figure 2-62B

# ECG RHYTHM STRIP #62
## Lead MCL₁

## I. RHYTHM

Atrial: Irregular

Ventricular: Irregular

## 2. RATE

Atrial: Average 70, varies from 100 to 50

Ventricular: Same as atrial

## 3. P WAVE

Present: Yes

Configuration: Positive and prolonged;
        5th beat—negative

Consistency: Consistent except with beat 5

Relation to QRS: 1:1

## 4. P-R INTERVAL

Duration: 0.12 seconds

Consistency: Consistent

## 5. QRS COMPLEX

Present: Yes

Configuration: Normal

Consistency: Consistent

Duration: 0.06 seconds

## 6. DATA ANALYSIS

The abnormal values include:
- an abrupt change in rate (last 4 beats approximately half the rate of first 4 beats)
- an irregular rhythm
- a variable P wave (in beat 5 only)

The P waves of the dominant rhythm are probably sinus. A 12 lead ECG would be needed to rule out left atrial abnormality (prolonged P wave duration) and to confirm a sinus origin, as an ectopic atrial rhythm cannot be entirely excluded. The 5th P wave, which is different and follows a pause in the initial rhythm, represents an ectopic atrial escape beat.

The sinus P-P intervals in the latter portion of the strip are approximately twice the initial P-P intervals (rate from 100 to 50) consistent with SA exit block with 2:1 conduction. In addition, the initial P-P intervals (1st 4 beats) are precisely the same. The overall findings indicate a Mobitz Type II SA exit block.

## 7. RHYTHM INTERPRETATION

Probable sinus rhythm with Mobitz II SA exit block and one atrial escape beat

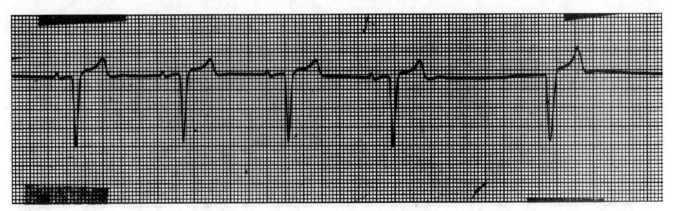

Figure 2-63A

# ECG RHYTHM STRIP #63
## Lead V₁

**1. RHYTHM**

    Atrial:

    Ventricular:

**2. RATE**

    Atrial:

    Ventricular:

**3. P WAVE**

    Present:

    Configuration:

    Consistency:

    Relation to QRS:

**4. P-R INTERVAL**

    Duration:

    Consistency:

**5. QRS COMPLEX**

    Present:

    Configuration:

    Consistency:

    Duration:

**6. DATA ANALYSIS**

**7. RHYTHM INTERPRETATION**

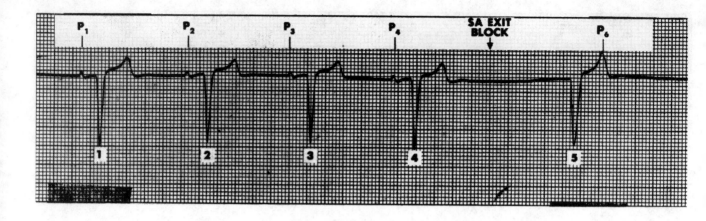

Figure 2-63B

# ECG RHYTHM STRIP #63
## Lead V₁

## 1. RHYTHM

Atrial: Irregular

Ventricular: Irregular

## 2. RATE

Atrial: 40 (P on T after $QRS_5$)

Ventricular: 40

## 3. P WAVE

Present: Yes

Configuration: Normal

Consistency: Consistent

Relation to QRS: 1:1 except with beat 5

## 4. P-R INTERVAL

Duration: 0.20 seconds

Consistency: Consistent

## 5. QRS COMPLEX

Present: Yes

Configuration: Normal except last beat is slurred

Consistency: Consistent except beat 5

Duration: 0.10 seconds
0.12 seconds in $QRS_5$

## 6. DATA ANALYSIS

The abnormal values include:
- a rate of 40 beats per minute
- an irregular rhythm
- the absence of a P wave preceding the last beat
- a change in the configuration and width of the last QRS from normal and narrow to slurred and wide

The T wave following $QRS_5$ is unusually pointed, suggesting a superimposed P wave. Further supporting this is the fact that the P-P interval from the P wave before $QRS_4$ to the proposed P wave following $QRS_5$ is equal to two sinus cycle lengths. This finding is consistent with SA exit block, although the $P_2$-$P_3$ interval is slightly less than the $P_1$-$P_2$ interval. There is no further decrease in the P-P intervals ($P_2$-$P_3$=$P_3$-$P_4$).

The wide QRS terminating the sinus pause is of probable ventricular origin although a junctional beat with LBBB aberrancy cannot be excluded.

## 7. RHYTHM INTERPRETATION

Sinus bradycardia with SA exit block (probably Mobitz II), and probable ventricular escape beat

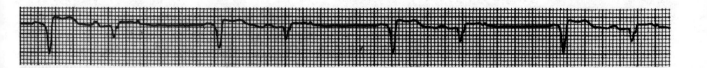

Figure 2-64A

# ECG RHYTHM STRIP #64
## Lead II

**1. RHYTHM**

    Atrial:

    Ventricular:

**2. RATE**

    Atrial:

    Ventricular:

**3. P WAVE**

    Present:

    Configuration:

    Consistency:

    Relation to QRS:

**4. P-R INTERVAL**

    Duration:

    Consistency:

**5. QRS COMPLEX**

    Present:

    Configuration:

    Consistency:

    Duration:

**6. DATA ANALYSIS**

**7. RHYTHM INTERPRETATION**

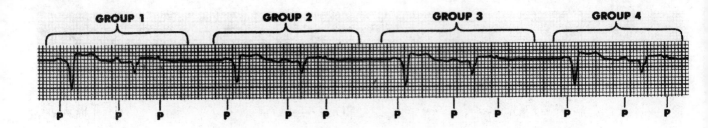

Figure 2-64B

# ECG RHYTHM STRIP #64
## Lead II

## 1. RHYTHM

Atrial: Regularly irregular

Ventricular: Regularly irregular

## 2. RATE

Atrial: 90

Ventricular: 60

## 3. P WAVE

Present: Yes

Configuration: Normal—first two P
waves in each group
Abnormal—third P wave
in each group

Consistency: Variable

Relation to QRS: Variable

## 4. P-R INTERVAL

Duration: Second P-R interval of each
group 0.24 seconds

Consistency: Second P-R interval of each
group—yes (conducted beats);
First P-R interval of each
group—slight variability

## 5. QRS COMPLEX

Present: Yes

Configuration: Abnormal—varies from
slurred to notched QS

Consistency: Inconsistent

Duration: 1st QRS—0.11 seconds
2nd QRS—0.10 seconds

## 6. DATA ANALYSIS

The abnormal values include:
- a slower ventricular versus atrial rate
- a regularly irregular rhythm
- an inconsistent P wave configuration and a variable P to
  QRS relation
- a prolonged (0.24 seconds) P-R interval with conducted beats
- an inconsistent, abnormal QRS complex

Careful scrutiny of the baseline reveals that groups of three P waves
(atrial trigeminy) are present. The first P wave in each group is partially distorted (by the first QRS in each group) but is essentially
identical to the second P wave in each group and establishes a basic
sinus rhythm at 90 per minute. The third P wave in each group is
different in morphology, premature in the basic sinus cycle, and is
not followed by a QRS. These represent nonconducted PAC's. The
second P wave in each group is conducted to the ventricles with
first degree AV block. The first P wave in each group shows a significantly shorter and slightly variable "P-R interval" and is
not conducted to the ventricles. The nonconducted PAC's
account for the ventricular rate being slower than the atrial rate.

The QRS complexes occur in groups of two (ventricular bigeminy).
Overall, then, each group consists of three P waves and two
QRS complexes. The second QRS in each group represents
ventricular depolarization from the descending sinus impulse.
The slight QRS prolongation and notching indicate an intraventricular conduction defect. The first QRS complexes in
each group are different in duration and configuration than
the intrinsically conducted impulses (second QRS complexes)
and follow P-R intervals that are too short to conduct in this
patient. These ventricular ectopic beats terminate periods of
ventricular asystole, in part produced by the nonconducted
PAC's, and are escape beats. The rate of the ventricular escape
beats (equivalent to a rate of 50 per minute) is slightly faster than
an intrinsic idioventricular pacemaker rate (15 to 40 per minute).

## 7. RHYTHM INTERPRETATION

Sinus rhythm with first degree AV block, nonconducted PAC's,
intraventricular conduction defect, and accelerated ventricular
escape beats

342

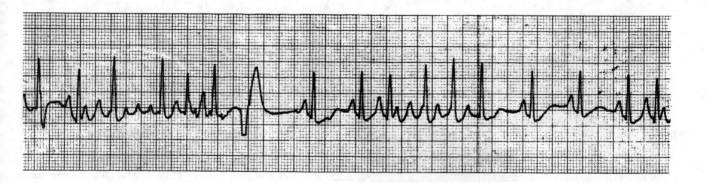

Figure 2-65A

# ECG RHYTHM STRIP #65
## Monitor Lead II

**I. RHYTHM**

Atrial:

Ventricular:

**2. RATE**

Atrial:

Ventricular:

**3. P WAVE**

Present:

Configuration:

Consistency:

Relation to QRS:

**4. P-R INTERVAL**

Duration:

Consistency:

**5. QRS COMPLEX**

Present:

Configuration:

Consistency:

Duration:

**6. DATA ANALYSIS**

**7. RHYTHM INTERPRETATION**

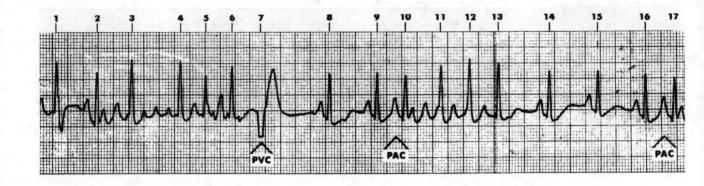

Figure 2-65B

# ECG RHYTHM STRIP #65
## Monitor Lead II

## I. RHYTHM

Atrial:  Irregular

Ventricular:  Irregular

## 2. RATE

Atrial:  Variable; sinus 90, "flutter" 370

Ventricular:  Variable; sinus 90, "flutter" 90 to 160

## 3. P WAVE

Present:  Yes

Configuration:  Varies from "normal" to peaked to coarse flutter-fibrillatory waves

Consistency:  Variable

Relation to QRS:  Variable

## 4. P-R INTERVAL

Duration:  0.14 seconds with sinus beats

Consistency:  Variable

## 5. QRS COMPLEX

Present:  Yes

Configuration:  Predominantly normal; $QRS_7$ is abnormal, wide, and bizarre

Consistency:  Slightly variability with normal QRS complexes

Duration:  Normal—0.08 seconds
Abnormal—0.12 seconds

## 6. DATA ANALYSIS

Most of the values are abnormal. The P waves before QRS complexes 2, 8, 9, 14, 15, and 16 are identical and establish a basic sinus rhythm at 90 per minute. These P waves are somewhat peaked. A 12 lead ECG would be necessary to ascertain whether a right atrial abnormality exists. The P wave preceding QRS complexes 10 and 17 fall premature in the basic sinus cycle, are more peaked than the sinus P waves, and are PAC's. Following QRS complexes 2 and 10 there are bursts of atrial activity with some variation in morphology at a rate of 370 per minute. The fluctuating atrial morphology is consistent with coarse atrial fibrillation but the regularity of the atrial rate is consistent with atrial flutter.

Some of the atrial activity distorts QRS complexes 3, 5, 11, and 12. There is variable conduction of the atrial activity to the ventricles accounting for the varying ventricular rate. $QRS_7$ is wide, bizarre, and "premature" when compared to the basic sinus cycle and is a PVC. The positive portion of $QRS_1$ resembles the other QRS complexes such that its "negative" defection may be artifactual or distortion from a P wave. The variability in amplitude of the QRS complexes may relate to respiratory variation.

## 7. RHYTHM INTERPRETATION

Sinus rhythm with PAC's, one PVC, and paroxysmal atrial flutter-fibrillation

344

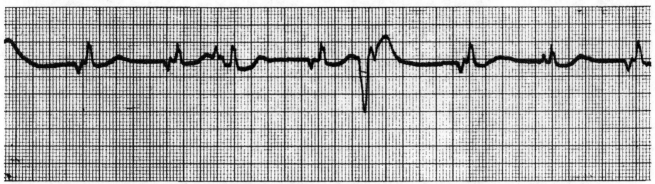

Figure 2-66A

# ECG RHYTHM STRIP #66
## Lead II

**I. RHYTHM**

　　Atrial:

　　Ventricular:

**2. RATE**

　　Atrial:

　　Ventricular:

**3. P WAVE**

　　Present:

　　Configuration:

　　Consistency:

　　Relation to QRS:

**4. P-R INTERVAL**

　　Duration:

　　Consistency:

**5. QRS COMPLEX**

　　Present:

　　Configuration:

　　Consistency:

　　Duration:

**6. DATA ANALYSIS**

**7. RHYTHM INTERPRETATION**

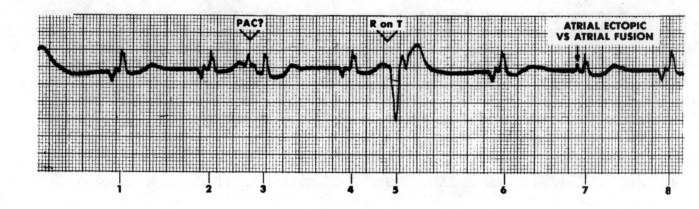

Figure 2-66B

# ECG RHYTHM STRIP #66
## Lead II

## I. RHYTHM

Atrial: Irregular

Ventricular: Irregular

## 2. RATE

Atrial: 60

Ventricular: 60

## 3. P WAVE

Present: Yes

Configuration: Abnormal—most negative; 2 positive

Consistency: Varies in polarity

Relation to QRS: 1:1 except with beat 5 (P follows QRS)

## 4. P-R INTERVAL

Duration: 0.12 seconds
0.20 seconds in beat 3

Consistency: Inconsistent

## 5. QRS COMPLEX

Present: Yes

Configuration: Most positive with slight notching: one negative, wide

Consistency: Changes in configuration and polarity in beat 5

Duration: Positive QRS—0.09 seconds
Negative QRS—0.12 seconds

## 6. DATA ANALYSIS

The abnormal values include:
- an irregular rhythm
- an inconsistent P wave
- a change in the P to QRS relation with beat 5 (P follows QRS)
- a variable P-R interval
- an inconsistent QRS complex.

The basic rhythm is characterized by negative P waves (beats 1, 2, 4, 6, 8) which in lead 2 represent retrograde conduction through the atria. This, in turn, indicates a low atrial or junctional rhythm (difficult to differentiate considering borderline P-R interval).

$P_3$ is different and premature in the basic rhythm and is therefore of different origin (ectopic atrial or sinus?).

Beat 5 is initiated by an abnormal, wide and different QRS complex and is premature in the basic rhythm—falls on downslope of preceding T wave. It is followed by a retrograde P wave which is related to it since the P is also premature in the basic rhythm.

The origin of $P_7$ is difficult to determine. The P wave itself appears diphasic with an initial flat negative component followed by a sharp positive wave deflection. Since it is not premature, it may represent a wandering atrial pacemaker or some type of atrial fusion beat.

## 7. RHYTHM INTERPRETATION

Ectopic supraventricular rhythm (junctional versus atrial) with PVC (R on T) and probable PAC

346

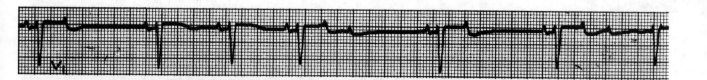

Figure 2-67A

# ECG RHYTHM STRIP #67
## Lead V₁

### I. RHYTHM

Atrial:

Ventricular:

### 2. RATE

Atrial:

Ventricular:

### 3. P WAVE

Present:

Configuration:

Consistency:

Relation to QRS:

### 4. P-R INTERVAL

Duration:

Consistency:

### 5. QRS COMPLEX

Present:

Configuration:

Consistency:

Duration:

### 6. DATA ANALYSIS

### 7. RHYTHM INTERPRETATION

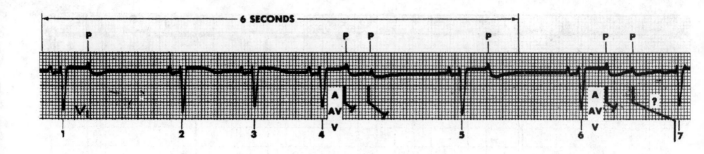

Figure 2-67B

# ECG RHYTHM STRIP #67
## Lead V₁

## I. RHYTHM

Atrial: Irregular

Ventricular: Irregular

## 2. RATE

Atrial: 90

Ventricular: 50

## 3. P WAVE

Present: Yes

Configuration: Sinus P waves—diphasic
Ectopic P waves—positive

Consistency: Inconsistent

Relation to QRS: Variable

## 4. P-R INTERVAL

Duration: 0.14 seconds

Consistency: Consistent when P followed
by QRS

## 5. QRS COMPLEX

Present: Yes

Configuration: Normal

Consistency: Consistent

Duration: 0.09 seconds

## 6. DATA ANALYSIS

The abnormal values include:
- a ventricular rate of 50 (less than atrial rate)
- an irregular rhythm
- an inconsistent P wave configuration
- a variable P to QRS relation

The P waves prior to QRS complexes 2, 3, and 4 are identical in configuration and establish a basic sinus rhythm at 65 per minute. The diphasic morphology could be normal for lead $V_1$, but a 12 lead ECG is needed to rule out atrial abnormality.

The single P waves following QRS complexes 1 and 5 and the two P waves following QRS complexes 4 and 6 are premature when compared to the basic sinus cycle; are different in configuration when compared to the sinus P waves; and are not followed by QRS complexes. These represent nonconducted PAC's. The second PAC in each couplet may not be conducted to the ventricles due to concealed conduction to the AV node by the first PAC (see ladder diagram).

$QRS_7$ is not immediately preceded by a P wave, and since it is identical to the other QRS complexes, it raises the possibility of a junctional beat. However, since the P-P interval of the second set of back to back PAC's is *slightly* longer than the P-P interval of the first set, it is possible that the second PAC of the second couplet finds the AV conducting tissues partially refractory and conducts to the ventricles (QRS) with marked first degree AV block (see ladder diagram). Favoring this hypothesis and against $QRS_7$ being a junctional "escape" beat is the fact that $QRS_6$-$QRS_7$ does not represent the longest R-R interval, as would be expected with an "escape" beat.

## 7. RHYTHM INTERPRETATION

Sinus rhythm with PAC's (most nonconducted).

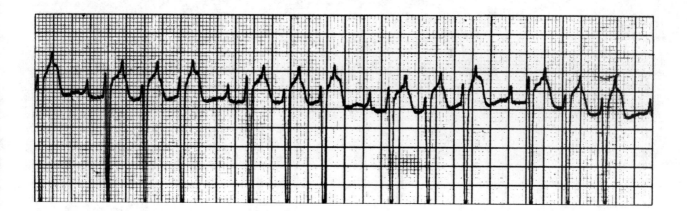

Figure 2-68A

# ECG RHYTHM STRIP #68
## Lead V₁

**1. RHYTHM**

   Atrial:

   Ventricular:

**2. RATE**

   Atrial:

   Ventricular:

**3. P WAVE**

   Present:

   Configuration:

   Consistency:

   Relation to QRS:

**4. P-R INTERVAL**

   Duration:

   Consistency:

**5. QRS COMPLEX**

   Present:

   Configuration:

   Consistency:

   Duration:

**6. DATA ANALYSIS**

**7. RHYTHM INTERPRETATION**

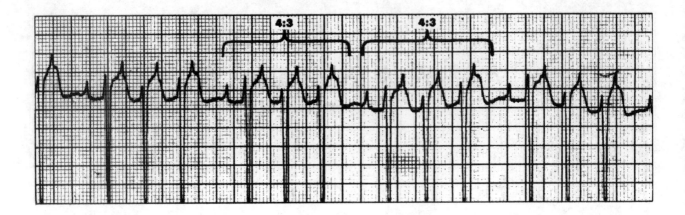

Figure 2-68B

# ECG RHYTHM STRIP #68
## Lead V₁

### 1. RHYTHM

Atrial: Regular

Ventricular: Regularly irregular

### 2. RATE

Atrial: 160

Ventricular: 120

### 3. P WAVE

Present: Yes

Configuration: Tall, peaked

Consistency: Consistent

Relation to QRS: 4:3

### 4. P-R INTERVAL

Duration: 0.24 to 0.27 seconds

Consistency: Variable in repetitive fashion

### 5. QRS COMPLEX

Present: Yes

Configuration: Normal

Consistency: Consistent

Duration: 0.08 seconds

### 6. DATA ANALYSIS

The abnormal values include:
- an atrial rate of 160 and a slower ventricular rate of 120
- a regularly irregular ventricular rhythm
- tall, peaked P waves with a 4:3 P to QRS relation
- a prolonged and variable P-R interval

The unusual P wave morphology in V₁ and fast rate (160 per minute) suggest that this rhythm is not sinus tachycardia but rather an ectopic atrial tachycardia. A 12 lead ECG is needed to accurately assess the origin of the atrial activity.

The ventricular rate is slower than the atrial rate due to the presence of second degree AV block. Characteristic of the Wenckebach phenomenon, group beating (four P waves, three QRS complexes) is apparent, the nonconducted P waves are preceded by a progressive increase in the P-R intervals, and the R-R interval encompassing the nonconducted P wave is shorter than two consecutive R-R cycles. If the underlying rhythm is atrial tachycardia, digitalis excess is a strong consideration.

### 7. RHYTHM INTERPRETATION

Supraventricular tachycardia (sinus versus ectopic atrial) with Mobitz I (Wenckebach) second degree AV block

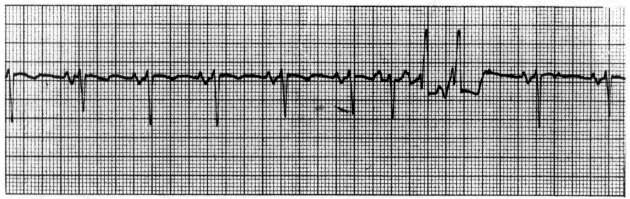

Figure 2-69A

# ECG RHYTHM STRIP #69
## Lead V₁

**1. RHYTHM**

Atrial:

Ventricular:

**2. RATE**

Atrial:

Ventricular:

**3. P WAVE**

Presence:

Appearance:

Consistency:

Relation to QRS:

**4. P-R INTERVAL**

Duration:

Consistency:

**5. QRS COMPLEX**

Presence:

Appearance:

Consistency:

Duration:

**6. DATA ANALYSIS**

**7. INTERPRETATION**

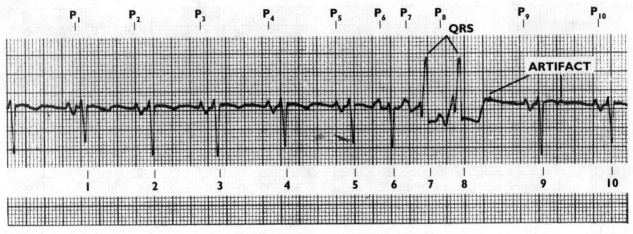

Figure 2-69B

# ECG RHYTHM STRIP #69

## I. RHYTHM

Atrial: Irregular

Ventricular: Irregular

## 2. RATE

Atrial: 90

Ventricular: 90

## 3. P WAVE

Presence: Yes

Appearance: Sinus—diphasic
Others—positive and notched

Consistency: Inconsistent; varies in configuration
and polarity

Relation to QRS: 1:1

## 4. P-R INTERVAL

Duration: 0.16 seconds, except for beats 7 and
8 (0.18 seconds)

Consistency: Consistent except with beats 7
and 8

## 5. QRS COMPLEX

Presence: Yes

Appearance: Normal, except for beats 7 and 8
(abnormal—rSR[1])

Consistency: Consistent except for beats 7 and 8

Duration: Normal—0.07 seconds
Abnormal—0.11 seconds

## 6. DATA ANALYSIS

The abnormal values include:
- an irregular rhythm
- an inconsistent P wave
- a longer P-R interval with beats 7 and 8
- a wide, abnormal QRS with beats 7 and 8

Diphasic P waves are seen in beats 1 through 5,
9, and 10. These predominant P's are sinus in
origin, since the underlying rhythm is regular
and the rate is normal (approximately 80). The
morphology of the P waves (diphasic) could be
normal for $V_1$, however, a 12 lead ECG is necessary to rule out atrial abnormality. P waves 6, 7,
and 8 are premature and different in configuration from the sinus P waves, representing premature atrial ectopic foci.

The longer P-R intervals with beats 7 and 8 are
related to the prematurity of the ectopic atrial
beats and relative refractoriness of the AV node.

The wide, abnormal QRS complexes (beats 7
and 8) show a RBBB configuration and are preceded by ectopic P waves. This is consistent with
aberrantly conducted PACs.

Careful inspection of the ST-T wave following
QRS 8 and 9 reveal a deformity that is most
likely artifact, since the timing of the sinus node
is not interrupted.

## 7. INTERPRETATION

Sinus rhythm with two aberrantly conducted
PACs.

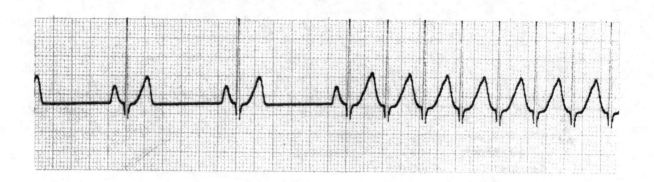

Figure 2-70A

# ECG RHYTHM STRIP #70
## Monitor Lead II

### 1. RHYTHM

Atrial:

Ventricular:

### 2. RATE

Atrial:

Ventricular:

### 3. P WAVE

Presence:

Appearance:

Consistency:

Relation to QRS:

### 4. P-R INTERVAL

Duration:

Consistency:

### 5. QRS COMPLEX

Presence:

Appearance:

Consistency:

Duration:

### 6. DATA ANALYSIS

### 7. INTERPRETATION

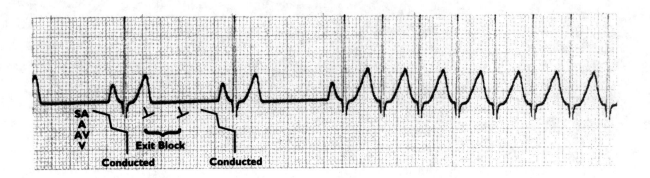

Figure 2-70B

# ECG RHYTHM STRIP #70
## Monitor Lead II

## 1. RHYTHM

Atrial: Irregular

Ventricular: Irregular

## 2. RATE

Atrial: Varies from 50 to 150

Ventricular: Same as atrial

## 3. P WAVE

Presence: Yes

Appearance: Normal peaked, then superimposed on T wave

Consistency: Inconsistent

Relation to QRS: 1:1

## 4. P-R INTERVAL

Duration: 0.14 seconds, then undeterminable

Consistency: Consistent when measurable

## 5. QRS COMPLEX

Presence: Yes

Appearance: Normal

Consistency: Consistent

Duration: 0.06 seconds

## 6. DATA ANALYSIS

The first 3 beats probably represent sinus activity
at a slow rate. Since the P wave is peaked and
prolonged in duration, a 12 lead ECG is needed
to rule out right atrial abnormality.

The rate changes from 50 to 150 abruptly following the third beat. The QRS of normal duration
indicates that this tachycardia originates above the
ventricles. The T waves with the tachycardia are
taller and more peaked, indicating a superimposed
P wave when compared to the first two T waves. A
12 lead ECG would be helpful in determining the
exact origin of the supraventricular tachycardia.

**Note:** Sinus tachycardia with SA exit block
Mobitz II with 3:1 conduction (first 3 beats) is
also a possibility, since the atrial rate exactly triples
with the supraventricular tachycardia (see diagram).

## 7. INTERPRETATION

Sinus bradycardia and (paroxysmal) supraventricular tachycardia

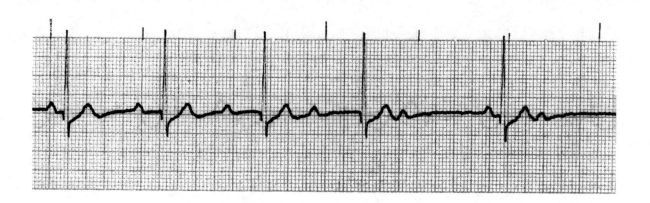

Figure 2-71A

## ECG RHYTHM STRIP #71
### Lead II

**1. RHYTHM**

Atrial:

Ventricular:

**2. RATE**

Atrial:

Ventricular:

**3. P WAVE**

Presence:

Appearance:

Consistency:

Relation to QRS:

**4. P-R INTERVAL**

Duration:

Consistency:

**5. QRS COMPLEX**

Presence:

Appearance:

Consistency:

Duration:

**6. DATA ANALYSIS**

**7. INTERPRETATION**

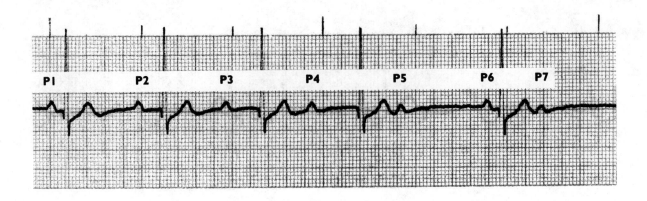

P1    P2    P3    P4    P5    P6    P7

Figure 2-71B

# ECG RHYTHM STRIP #71
## Lead II

## 1. RHYTHM

Atrial:  Regular, except for 1 premature cycle

Ventricular:  Irregular

## 2. RATE

Atrial:  70

Ventricular:  50

## 3. P WAVE

Presence:  Yes

Appearance:  Normal

Consistency:  Consistent, except for the 7th
P wave (flatter)

Relation to QRS:  Varies 1:1 and 2:1

## 4. P-R INTERVAL

Duration:  0.18 to 0.54 seconds

Consistency:  Progressively increases until QRS
dropped

## 5. QRS COMPLEX

Presence:  Yes

Appearance:  Normal

Consistency:  Consistent

Duration:  0.07 seconds

## 6. DATA ANALYSIS

The abnormal values include:
- one premature P wave
- an irregular ventricular rhythm
- a slower ventricular vs atrial rate
- a slight change in the P wave configuration
  with the 7th P wave
- a variable P to QRS relation
- a prolonged and inconsistent P-R interval

Except for the 7th P wave, the atrial rate and
rhythm are consistent with sinus origin. The 7th
P wave is premature when compared to the sinus
cycle with a slightly different configuration. It is
not followed by a QRS complex. This finding is
consistent with a nonconducted PAC.

In addition to the nonconducted PAC, the 5th
sinus P wave is not conducted. Both nonconducted P waves account for the slower ventricular
rate and the pauses in the ventricular rhythm.

The P-R intervals progressively increase until the
5th P wave is not conducted, consistent with
second degree AV block (Wenckebach).

## 7. INTERPRETATION

Sinus rhythm with second degree AV block
Mobitz 1 (Wenckebach) and one nonconducted
PAC

# • Part III •

## Pacemaker Rhythm Strips

# PACEMAKER ECG RHYTHM STRIP ANALYSIS GUIDE

Interpretation of ECG rhythm strips of patients with mechanical pacemakers is often difficult. If one has an understanding of the basic types and modes of operation of commonly used pacemakers and employs a systematic approach to analysis, accurate interpretation will more easily be accomplished.

Pacemakers are either *single chamber,* with a lead implanted only in the right atrium (A) or right ventricle (V), or *dual chamber,* with leads implanted in both (D) the right atrium and right ventricle. Dual chamber pacemakers may be programmed to function as single chamber pacemakers.

In 1974, the Intersociety Commission for Heart Disease (ICHD) introduced a pacing modality identification code to facilitate understanding pacemaker function. A comprehensive knowledge of this code is essential for analyzing and interpreting pacemaker strips.

| The *first* letter stands for the *chamber paced* | The *second* letter stands for the *chamber sensed* | The *third* letter stands for the *mode of response* to the sensed event |
|---|---|---|
| A = Atrium<br>V = Ventricle<br>D = Atrium and ventricle<br>O = None | A = Atrium<br>V = Ventricle<br>D = Atrium and ventricle<br>O = None | I = Inhibited<br>T = Triggered<br>D = Inhibited and triggered<br>O = None |

This three letter pacemaker code is sufficient for interpretation of most pacemaker ECG rhythm strips.

## SINGLE CHAMBER PACEMAKERS

| Code | Chamber paced | Chamber sensed | Mode of response | Method of operation |
|---|---|---|---|---|
| VVI | Ventricle | Ventricle | Inhibition | Ventricular demand |
| VOO | Ventricle | None | None | Ventricular fixed rate |
| AAI | Atrium | Atrium | Inhibition | Atrial demand |
| AOO | Atrium | None | None | Atrial fixed rate |

## DUAL CHAMBER PACEMAKERS

| Code | Chamber paced | Chamber sensed | Mode of response | Method of operation |
|---|---|---|---|---|
| DDD | Atrium and ventricle | Atrium and ventricle | Inhibition and triggered | Fully automatic |
| VAT | Ventricle | Atrium | Atrial triggered | Atrial synchronous |
| VDD | Ventricle | Atrium and ventricle | Atrial triggered ventricular inhibited | Atrial synchronous |
| DOO | Atrium and ventricle | None | None | A-V sequential fixed rate |
| DVI | Atrium and Ventricle | Ventricle | Inhibition | A-V sequential |

The most common type of *single chamber* pacemaker is the *ventricular demand* pacemaker. The chamber paced is the ventricle (V), the chamber sensed is the ventricle (V), and the mode of response to a sensed QRS complex is inhibition (I); hence the designation VVI. If a magnet is placed over the pulse generator of a VVI pacemaker, it loses its ability to sense (O) and there is no mode of response (O). Under this circumstance the pacemaker functions in the fixed rate mode (VOO). Less commonly implanted but still useful when AV block is not a concern is the single chamber atrial demand pacemaker (AAI).

Most *dual chamber* pacemakers implanted today have the capability of functioning in the fully automatic mode (DDD). At any given point in time the pacemaker may be functioning in the atrial demand (AAI), ventricular demand (VVI), atrial synchronous (VAT, VDD), or A-V (atrial-ventricular) sequential (DVI) mode. When functioning in the atrial synchronous mode (VAT), the *sensing* of a P wave by the atrial lead *triggers* discharge of the ventricular pacing component after a predetermined AV (atrioventricular) delay. This is the most common "triggered" mode of response. Pacemaker "triggering" or "firing" *into* sensed P waves (AAT) or sensed QRS complexes (VVT) is a modality present in older single chamber pacemakers that is infrequently used today.

The pacemaker analysis worksheet for steps 1 through 5 maintains the same format as the basic and complex rhythm strip analysis but applys only to the *intrinsic* (nonmechanical pacemaker induced) rhythm, complexes, and conduction. Steps 6 through 12 pertain to mechanical pacemaker activity and assist in recognition of its presence, type, and function. The analysis process is detailed below:

## 6. Mechanical Pacemaker Spikes

Determine whether mechanical pacemaker spikes are present and their relationship to P waves and QRS complexes. If pacer spikes are:

a. immediately followed by P waves, atrial pacing is present.
b. immediately followed by wide QRS complexes, ventricular pacing is present.
c. consistently preceded by P waves with a constant AV delay, dual chamber atrial synchronous pacing is present.

## 7. Mechanical Pacemaker Rate

Calculate the mechanical pacemaker rate.

Measure the interval between two successive pacer spikes and divide into 60.

### Remember:

• One "large" box = 0.20 seconds, one "small" box = 0.04 seconds.

## 8. AV Delay

Calculate the AV delay.

In pacemaker terminology, the AV delay is measured from the onset of a paced or sensed atrial depolarization (P wave) to the onset of a paced ventricular depolarization (QRS complex) as seen in dual chamber pacemakers functioning in the A-V sequential (atrial pacer spike–ventricular pacer spike) or atrial synchronous (intrinsic P wave–ventricular pacer spike) modes. For analysis purposes the AV delay in this workbook also includes the interval from the onset of a paced atrial depolarization to an intrinsic QRS complex (atrial pacer spike–intrinsic QRS) as seen in single chamber atrial pacemakers or dual chamber pacemakers functioning in the AAI mode.

### Remember:

• The absolute AV delay is less important than its constancy.

For example, with a single chamber VVI pacemaker it may appear that pacer spikes are consistently preceded by P waves (implying atrial synchronism), but careful measurement reveals the AV delay is variable (confirming the presence of AV dissociation at least some of the time). In contrast, the presence of a constant intrinsic P wave–ventricular pacer spike interval (AV delay) implies the presence of a dual chamber pacemaker functioning in the atrial synchronous mode.

## 9. Fusion/pseudofusion Beats

Are fusion or pseudofusion beats present?

The presence of multiform QRS complexes in patients with mechanical ventricular pacing is common. Ventricular depolarizations (QRS complexes) may be due to intrinsic conduction of supraventricular impulses (with or without intraventricular conduction defects or delays), ventricular ectopy, pacemaker discharge, or fusion. *Fusion beats* are common and are usually the result of ventricular depolarization that is due in part to a descending supraventricular impulse and in part to mechanical pacemaker discharge.

At times pacemaker spikes may occur at the beginning of, or "within," QRS complexes, often distorting them but not contributing to ventricular depolarization. That is, the QRS complex results entirely from intrinsic depolarization with no contribution from the pacemaker discharge. These complexes are *pseudofusion beats* in that they only simulate fusion. Pseudofusion beats may be explainable based on normal pacemaker function but at times indicate pacemaker sensing malfunction.

## 10. Unexpected Pauses

Are there any unexpected pauses?

After the mechanical pacemaker rate (atrial and/or ventricular) is calculated, the finding of a prolonged pause (period of atrial and/or ventricular asystole) or prolonged pacer spike–pacer spike interval raises the possibility of pacemaker malfunction *(failure to discharge)*.

## 11. Sensing Function

Assess sensing function.

Once the mechanical pacemaker rate (atrial and/or ventricular) is calculated and depending on the type and mode of the pacemaker, the finding of an unexpectedly *short* interval between an intrinsic P wave and atrial pacer spike or between an intrinsic QRS complex and ventricular pacer spike raises the possibility of pacemaker *sensing malfunction.*

### Remember:

- Many pacemaker ECG rhythm strips do not show intrinsic atrial or ventricular activity so sensing function cannot be assessed.

## 12. Capture Function

Assess capture function.

Are there any atrial and/or ventricular pacer spikes that occur outside of the intrinsic atrial and/or ventricular refractory period that are not immediately followed by a P wave or QRS complex? Such findings suggest pacemaker *capture malfunction.*

### Remember:

- If an ECG rhythm strip shows a dual chamber pacemaker functioning only in the atrial synchronous mode, atrial capture function cannot be assessed. Also, if the underlying atrial mechanism is atrial fibrillation, atrial pacemaker capture would not be expected, and therefore capture function cannot be assessed.

## 13. Data Analysis

Analyze the data collected:

a. Identify the underlying intrinsic (nonmechanical pacemaker induced) rhythm and existing intrinsic abnormalities.
b. Review the evidence that indicates what type of pacemaker is present and its mode of operation
c. Explain any unusual beats or pauses.
d. Review any evidence suggestive of pacemaker malfunction.

### Remember:

- Always consider whether or not apparent "pacemaker malfunction" *may* be explainable!

## 14. Interpretation

Interpret the rhythm strip.

Your interpretation should summarize the data analysis. Identify the underlying rhythm, type of pacemaker and mode of operation, and any abnormalities present.

*After completing the worksheet, compare your findings with the appropriate corresponding analysis.*

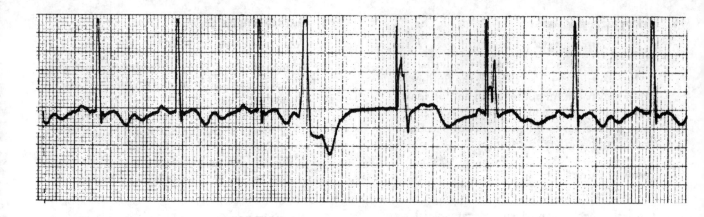

Figure 3-1A

## ECG PACEMAKER STRIP #1

### INTRINSIC

#### 1. RHYTHM

Atrial:

Ventricular:

#### 2. RATE

Atrial:

Ventricular:

#### 3. P WAVE

Present:

Configuration:

Consistency:

Relation to QRS:

#### 4. P-R INTERVAL

Duration:

Consistency:

#### 5. QRS COMPLEX

Present:

Configuration:

Consistency:

Duration:

### MECHANICAL PACEMAKER

#### 6. MECHANICAL PACEMAKER SPIKES

Present:

Immediately Followed by P Wave:

Immediately Followed by QRS:

Consistently Preceded by P Wave:

#### 7. MECHANICAL PACEMAKER RATE

Atrial:

Ventricular:

## 8. AV DELAY

Intrinsic P Wave – Ventricular Pacemaker:

Atrial Pacer – Ventricular Pacer:

Atrial Pacer – Intrinsic QRS:

## 9. FUSION/PSEUDOFUSION BEATS

Present:

## 10. UNEXPECTED PAUSES

Present:

## 11. SENSING FUNCTION

Atrial:

Ventricular:

## 12. CAPTURE FUNCTION

Atrial:

Ventricular:

## 13. DATA ANALYSIS

## 14. INTERPRETATION

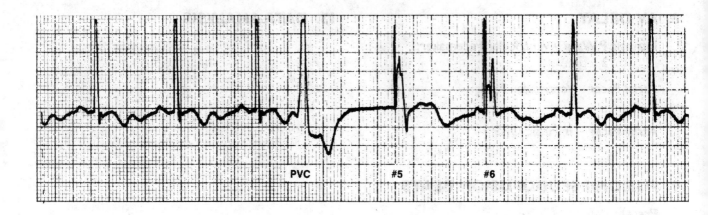

Figure 3-1B

# ECG PACEMAKER STRIP #1

## INTRINSIC

### 1. RHYTHM

Atrial: Regular

Ventricular: Regular except for one premature beat

### 2. RATE

Atrial: 68

Ventricular: 68

### 3. P WAVE

Present: Yes

Configuration: Normal

Consistency: Yes

Relation to QRS: 1:1 except follows QRS #4 (premature beat) and "buried" in QRS #5

### 4. P-R INTERVAL

Duration: 0.20 seconds

Consistency: Yes

### 5. QRS COMPLEX

Present: Yes

Configuration: Normal except QRS #4

Consistency: Yes, except QRS #4

Duration: 0.08 seconds, except QRS #4 (0.13 seconds)

## MECHANICAL PACEMAKER

### 6. MECHANICAL PACEMAKER SPIKES

Present: Yes

Immediately Followed by P Wave: No

Immediately Followed by QRS: Yes

Consistently Preceded by P Wave: No

### 7. MECHANICAL PACEMAKER RATE

Atrial: —

Ventricular: 60

364

## 8. AV DELAY

Intrinsic P Wave – Ventricular Pacemaker:
0.12 seconds (Beat #6)

Atrial Pacer – Ventricular Pacer: —

Atrial Pacer – Intrinsic QRS: —

## 9. FUSION/PSEUDOFUSION BEATS

Present: Yes, QRS #6 (fusion)

## 10. UNEXPECTED PAUSES

Present: No

## 11. SENSING FUNCTION

Atrial: —

Ventricular: Normal

## 12. CAPTURE FUNCTION

Atrial: —

Ventricular: Normal

## 13. DATA ANALYSIS

The underlying atrial mechanism is sinus at 68 per minute. The 4th P wave occurs on the ST segment of the premature beat and the 5th P wave is "buried" in QRS #5. The 4th QRS is premature, wide, and of different configuration than the normal QRS complexes, consistent with a PVC. The expected compensatory pause following the PVC is interrupted by the occurrence of a mechanical pacemaker spike. The spike is immediately followed by a wide QRS complex consistent with a mechanical ventricular pacemaker. A second pacer spike occurs at a rate equivalent to 60 per minute. A P wave occurs prior to this pacer spike but with a shorter "P-R" interval than the other complexes. The QRS (#6) configuration following this pacer spike is different from QRS #5 and represents a fusion beat, as ventricular depolarization results in part from the descending sinus impulse and in part from the ventricular pacemaker discharge. Ventricular sensing and capture function are normal.

## 14. INTERPRETATION

Sinus rhythm with one PVC, VVI pacemaker, and one fusion beat

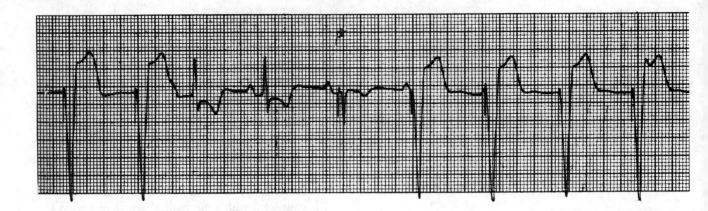

Figure 3-2A

# ECG PACEMAKER STRIP #2

## INTRINSIC

### I. RHYTHM

Atrial:

Ventricular:

### 2. RATE

Atrial:

Ventricular:

### 3. P WAVE

Present:

Configuration:

Consistency:

Relation to QRS:

### 4. P-R INTERVAL

Duration:

Consistency:

### 5. QRS COMPLEX

Present:

Configuration:

Consistency:

Duration:

## MECHANICAL PACEMAKER

### 6. MECHANICAL PACEMAKER SPIKES

Present:

Immediately Followed by P Wave:

Immediately Followed by QRS:

Consistently Preceded by P Wave:

### 7. MECHANICAL PACEMAKER RATE

Atrial:

Ventricular:

## 8. AV DELAY

Intrinsic P Wave – Ventricular Pacemaker:

Atrial Pacer – Ventricular Pacer:

Atrial Pacer – Intrinsic QRS:

## 9. FUSION/PSEUDOFUSION BEATS

Present:

## 10. UNEXPECTED PAUSES

Present:

## 11. SENSING FUNCTION

Atrial:

Ventricular:

## 12. CAPTURE FUNCTION

Atrial:

Ventricular:

## 13. DATA ANALYSIS

## 14. INTERPRETATION

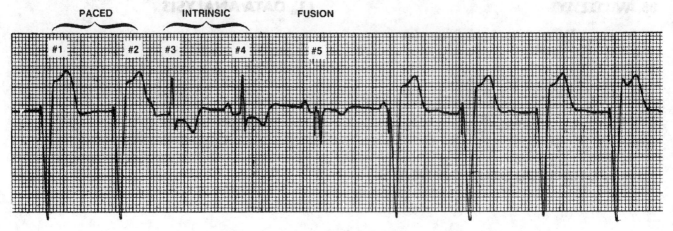

Figure 3-2B

## ECG PACEMAKER STRIP #2

## INTRINSIC

### 1. RHYTHM

Atrial: Regular

Ventricular: Regular (QRS #3, #4, #5)

### 2. RATE

Atrial: 65

Ventricular: 72 (QRS #3, #4, #5)

### 3. P WAVE

Present: Yes, but often buried in QRS-ST complex

Configuration: Normal

Consistency: Yes

Relation to QRS: 1:1 with intrinsic QRS complexes

### 4. P-R INTERVAL

Duration: Beat #3 0.28 seconds, beat #4 0.20 seconds

Consistency: Variable

### 5. QRS COMPLEX

Present: Yes

Configuration: QRS #3, #4 normal, QRS #5 abnormal (fusion)

Consistency: No

Duration: 0.08 seconds

## MECHANICAL PACEMAKER

### 6. MECHANICAL PACEMAKER SPIKES

Present: Yes

Immediately Followed by P Wave: No

Immediately Followed by QRS: Yes

Consistently Preceded by P Wave: No

### 7. MECHANICAL PACEMAKER RATE

Atrial: —

Ventricular: 70

## 8. AV DELAY

Intrinsic P Wave – Ventricular Pacemaker:
    0.16 seconds (beat #5),
    0.12 seconds (beat #6)

Atrial Pacer – Ventricular Pacer: —

Atrial Pacer – Intrinsic QRS: —

## 9. FUSION/PSEUDOFUSION BEATS

Present: Yes, QRS #5 (fusion)

## 10. UNEXPECTED PAUSES

Present: No

## 11. SENSING FUNCTION

Atrial: —

Ventricular: Normal

## 12. CAPTURE FUNCTION

Atrial: —

Ventricular: Normal

## 13. DATA ANALYSIS

The underlying atrial mechanism is sinus at a rate of 65 per minute. Many of the P waves are buried in the QRS-ST complexes. Only three P waves are conducted to the ventricles (P-QRS complexes #3, #4, #5). The P-R interval of complex #3 is prolonged probably secondary to concealed AV conduction from the previous beat. Mechanical pacemaker spikes are present and are immediately followed by wide QRS complexes, consistent with a ventricular pacemaker. QRS #5 represents a fusion beat in that ventricular depolarization results in part from the descending sinus impulse and in part from the ventricular pacemaker discharge. Ventricular sensing and capture function are normal.

## 14. INTERPRETATION

Sinus rhythm with concealed AV conduction, VVI pacemaker, and one fusion beat

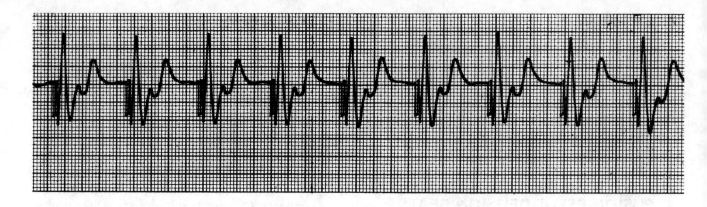

Figure 3-3A

# ECG PACEMAKER STRIP #3

## INTRINSIC

### 1. RHYTHM

Atrial:

Ventricular:

### 2. RATE

Atrial:

Ventricular:

### 3. P WAVE

Present:

Configuration:

Consistency:

Relation to QRS

### 4. P-R INTERVAL

Duration:

Consistency:

### 5. QRS COMPLEX

Present:

Configuration:

Consistency:

Duration:

## MECHANICAL PACEMAKER

### 6. MECHANICAL PACEMAKER SPIKES

Present:

Immediately Followed by P Wave:

Immediately Followed by QRS:

Consistently Preceded by P Wave:

### 7. MECHANICAL PACEMAKER RATE

Atrial:

Ventricular:

## 8. AV DELAY

Intrinsic P Wave – Ventricular Pacemaker:

Atrial Pacer – Ventricular Pacer:

Atrial Pacer – Intrinsic QRS:

## 9. FUSION/PSEUDOFUSION BEATS

Present:

## 10. UNEXPECTED PAUSES

Present:

## 11. SENSING FUNCTION

Atrial:

Ventricular:

## 12. CAPTURE FUNCTION

Atrial:

Ventricular:

## 13. DATA ANALYSIS

## 14. INTERPRETATION

371

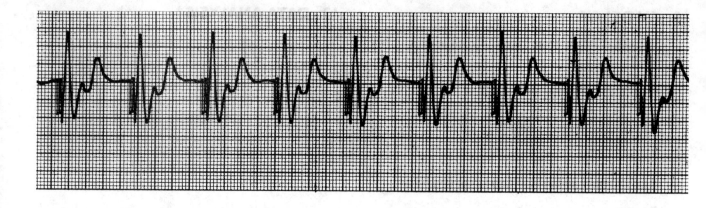

Figure 3-3B

## ECG PACEMAKER STRIP #3

### INTRINSIC

#### I. RHYTHM

Atrial: Regular

Ventricular: No intrinsic QRS complexes

#### 2. RATE

Atrial: 72

Ventricular: No intrinsic rhythm

#### 3. P WAVE

Present: Yes, distorting ST segment

Configuration: Negative depolarization

Consistency: Yes

Relation to QRS: Follows QRS 1:1

#### 4. P-R INTERVAL: No intrinsic P-R interval

Duration:

Consistency:

#### 5. QRS COMPLEX: No intrinsic QRS complexes

Present:

Configuration:

Consistency:

Duration:

### MECHANICAL PACEMAKER

#### 6. MECHANICAL PACEMAKER SPIKES

Present: Yes

Immediately Followed by P Wave: No

Immediately Followed by QRS: Yes

Consistently Preceded by P Wave: No

#### 7. MECHANICAL PACEMAKER RATE

Atrial: —

Ventricular: 72

## 8. AV DELAY

Intrinsic P Wave – Ventricular Pacemaker: —

Atrial Pace – Ventricular Pacer: —

Atrial Pacer – Intrinsic QRS: —

## 9. FUSION/PSEUDOFUSION BEATS

Present: No

## 10. UNEXPECTED PAUSES

Present: No

## 11. SENSING FUNCTION

Atrial: —

Ventricular: Indeterminable (no ventricular sensing)

## 12. CAPTURE FUNCTION

Atrial: —

Ventricular: Normal

## 13. DATA ANALYSIS

Although intrinsic P waves are present, they consistently follow the QRS complexes distorting the ST segments and have a negative polarity consistent with retrograde atrial depolarization. Mechanical pacemaker spikes are present and are immediately followed by QRS complexes, consistent with a mechanical ventricular pacemaker (presumably VVI). Ventricular sensing function cannot be assessed from this rhythm strip.

## 14. INTERPRETATION

Mechanical ventricular pacemaker (presumably VVI) with retrograde atrial capture

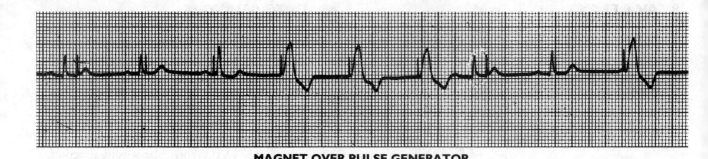

**MAGNET OVER PULSE GENERATOR**

Figure 3-4A

# ECG PACEMAKER STRIP #4

## INTRINSIC

### 1. RHYTHM

Atrial:

Ventricular:

### 2. RATE

Atrial:

Ventricular:

### 3. P WAVE

Present:

Configuration:

Consistency:

Relation to QRS:

### 4. P-R INTERVAL

Duration:

Consistency:

### 5. QRS COMPLEX

Present:

Configuration:

Consistency:

Duration:

## MECHANICAL PACEMAKER

### 6. MECHANICAL PACEMAKER SPIKES

Present:

Immediately Followed by P Wave:

Immediately Followed by QRS:

Consistently Preceded by P Wave:

### 7. MECHANICAL PACEMAKER RATE

Atrial:

Ventricular:

## 8. AV DELAY

Intrinsic P Wave – Ventricular Pacemaker:

Atrial Pacer – Ventricular Pacer:

Atrial Pacer – Intrinsic QRS:

## 9. FUSION/PSEUDOFUSION BEATS

Present:

## 10. UNEXPECTED PAUSES

Present:

## 11. SENSING FUNCTION

Atrial:

Ventricular:

## 12. CAPTURE FUNCTION

Atrial:

Ventricular:

## 13. DATA ANALYSIS

## 14. INTERPRETATION

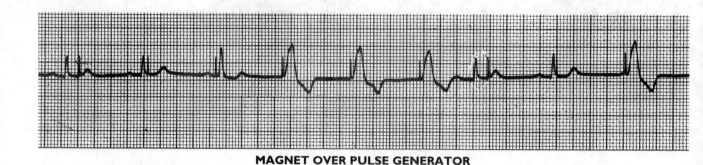

Figure 3-4B

# ECG PACEMAKER STRIP #4

## INTRINSIC

### I. RHYTHM

Atrial: Slightly irregular

Ventricular: Regular (QRS #1-2, QRS #7-8)

### 2. RATE

Atrial: 62

Ventricular: 64

### 3. P WAVE

Present: Yes except buried in QRST #4, 5, 9

Configuration: Normal

Consistency: Yes

Relation to QRS: 1:1 with intrinsic QRS
complexes

### 4. P-R INTERVAL

Duration: 0.19 seconds except 0.24 seconds
complex #7

Consistency: Yes except complex #7

### 5. QRS COMPLEX

Present: Yes

Configuration: Normal

Consistency: Yes except QRS #3

Duration: 0.06 seconds

## MECHANICAL PACEMAKER

### 6. MECHANICAL PACEMAKER SPIKES

Present: Yes

Immediately Followed by P Wave: No

Immediately Followed by QRS: Some complexes

Consistently Preceded by P Wave: No

### 7. MECHANICAL PACEMAKER RATE

Atrial: —

Ventricular: 73

## 8. AV DELAY

Intrinsic P Wave – Ventricular Pacer: —

Atrial Pacer – Ventricular Pacer: —

Atrial Pacer – Intrinsic QRS: —

## 9. FUSION/PSEUDOFUSION BEATS

Present: Yes, QRS #3 (fusion)

## 10. UNEXPECTED PAUSES

Present: No

## 11. SENSING FUNCTION

Atrial: —

Ventricular: Indeterminable (no ventricular sensing)

## 12. CAPTURE FUNCTION

Atrial: —

Ventricular: Normal

## 13. DATA ANALYSIS

Although all visible P waves are of similar configuration, there is a slight variability to the P-P interval consistent with underlying sinus arrhythmia. P waves #4, 5, and 9 are buried in the QRST complexes. The P-R intervals of the intrinsic complexes are normal with the exception of complex #7, which is prolonged. This is most likely due to concealed conduction to the AV node from the preceding ventricular depolarization. Mechanical pacemaker spikes occurring at a regular rate of 62 per minute are apparent. Clinical information indicates that a magnet has been placed over the pulse generator, which converts the pacemaker to a fixed rate mode. When the pacemaker spikes occur outside of the refractory period of the intrinsic QRS complexes, they are followed immediately by a wide QRS consistent with ventricular pacing. QRS #3 is a fusion beat, as ventricular depolarization is in part due to the descending sinus impulse and in part from the mechanical pacemaker discharge. Since the pacemaker is in the fixed rate mode (VOO), sensing function cannot be assessed. Capture function is normal.

## 14. INTERPRETATION

Sinus arrhythmia with concealed AV conduction, mechanical ventricular pacemaker (presumably VVI) functioning in the VOO mode, and one fusion beat

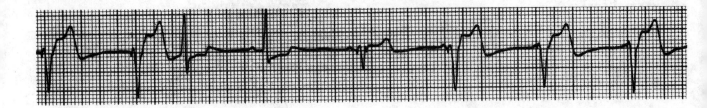

Figure 3-5A

# ECG PACEMAKER STRIP #5

## INTRINSIC

### 1. RHYTHM

Atrial:

Ventricular:

### 2. RATE

Atrial:

Ventricular:

### 3. P WAVE

Present:

Configuration:

Consistency:

Relation to QRS:

### 4. P-R INTERVAL

Duration:

Consistency:

### 5. QRS COMPLEX

Present:

Configuration:

Consistency:

Duration:

## MECHANICAL PACEMAKER

### 6. MECHANICAL PACEMAKER SPIKES

Present:

Immediately Followed by P Wave:

Immediately Followed by QRS:

Consistently Preceded by P Wave:

### 7. MECHANICAL PACEMAKER RATE

Atrial:

Ventricular:

## 8. AV DELAY

Intrinsic P Wave – Ventricular Pacemaker:

Atrial Pacer – Ventricular Pacer:

Atrial Pacer – Intrinsic QRS:

## 9. FUSION/PSEUDOFUSION BEATS

Present:

## 10. UNEXPECTED PAUSES

Present:

## 11. SENSING FUNCTION

Atrial:

Ventricular:

## 12. CAPTURE FUNCTION

Atrial:

Ventricular:

## 13. DATA ANALYSIS

## 14. INTERPRETATION

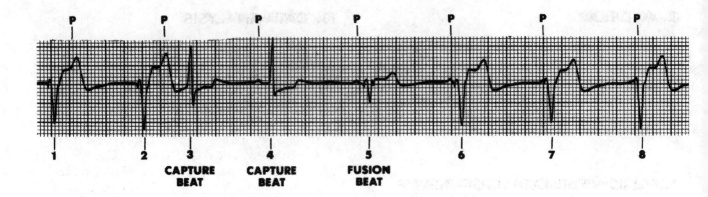

P P P P P P P

1  2  3  4  5  6  7  8

**CAPTURE BEAT** (beat 3)   **CAPTURE BEAT** (beat 4)   **FUSION BEAT** (beat 5)

Figure 3-5B

# ECG PACEMAKER STRIP #5

## INTRINSIC

### 1. RHYTHM

Atrial: Regular

Ventricular: Indeterminable (only two intrinsic QRS complexes)

### 2. RATE

Atrial: 56

Ventricular: Indeterminable

### 3. P WAVE

Present: Yes, concealed in ST-T wave of QRS #1 and #2 and the beginning of #7 and #8

Configuration: Normal

Consistency: Yes

Relation to QRS: Variable

### 4. P-R INTERVAL

Duration: Beat #3 > 0.20 seconds, beat #4 0.16 seconds

Consistency: Variable

### 5. QRS COMPLEX

Present: Yes

Configuration: #3 abnormal, #4 normal

Consistency: Variable

Duration: QRS #3: 0.10 seconds, QRS #4: 0.08 seconds

## MECHANICAL PACEMAKER

### 6. MECHANICAL PACEMAKER SPIKES

Present: Yes

Immediately Followed by P Wave: No

Immediately Followed by QRS: Yes

Consistently Preceded by P Wave: No

### 7. MECHANICAL PACEMAKER RATE

Atrial: —

Ventricular: 60

## 8. AV DELAY

Intrinsic P Wave – Ventricular Pacer: —

Atrial Pacer – Ventricular Pacer: —

Atrial Pacer – Intrinsic QRS: —

## 9. FUSION/PSEUDOFUSION BEATS

Present: Yes, #5 (fusion)

## 10. UNEXPECTED PAUSES

Present: No

## 11. SENSING FUNCTION

Atrial: —

Ventricular: Normal

## 12. CAPTURE FUNCTION

Atrial: —

Ventricular: Normal

## 13. DATA ANALYSIS

The underlying atrial mechanism is sinus brady-cardia at 56 per minute. Using the established P-P interval, it is apparent that the first two P waves are concealed in the T waves following QRS #1 and #2 and that the initial portion of the last two P waves can be seen just prior to QRS #7 and #8. The 4th QRS cycle is the only normal intrinsic P-QRS complex. The P wave hidden in the T wave prior to QRS #3 is con-ducted with a first degree AV block because of concealed conduction to the AV node by the 2nd ventricular depolarization. Furthermore, QRS #3 is wider than QRS #4 because it is conducted with slight aberrancy, since it ends a short cycle preceded by a longer cycle. Mechanical pacemak-er spikes occurring at a rate of 60 per minute are apparent. Wide QRS complexes immediately fol-low the pacer spikes, consistent with ventricular pacing, and no pacer spikes occur in the vicinity of QRS complexes #3 and #4, consistent with the demand mode (VVI). All ventricular depolar-izations are mechanical pacemaker induced except QRS complexes #3 and #4. The latter are sinus capture beats. QRS #5 is a fusion beat since ventricular depolarization results in part from the descending sinus impulse and in part from the mechanical pacemaker discharge. Pacemaker sensing and capture function are normal.

## 14. INTERPRETATION

Sinus bradycardia with concealed AV conduction, VVI pacemaker, and one fusion beat

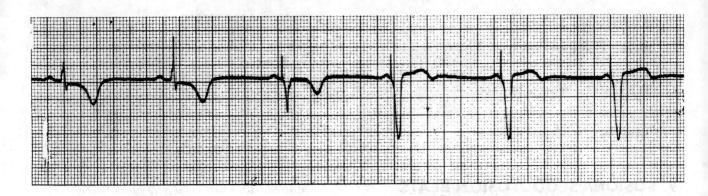

Figure 3-6A

# ECG PACEMAKER STRIP #6

## INTRINSIC

### I. RHYTHM

Atrial:

Ventricular:

### 2. RATE

Atrial:

Ventricular:

### 3. P WAVE

Present:

Configuration:

Consistency:

Relation to QRS:

### 4. P-R INTERVAL

Duration:

Consistency:

### 5. QRS COMPLEX

Present:

Configuration:

Consistency:

Duration:

## MECHANICAL PACEMAKER

### 6. MECHANICAL PACEMAKER SPIKES

Present:

Immediately Followed by P Wave:

Immediately Followed by QRS:

Consistently Preceded by P Wave:

### 7. MECHANICAL PACEMAKER RATE

Atrial:

Ventricular:

## 8. AV DELAY

Intrinsic P Wave – Ventricular Pacemaker:

Atrial Pacer – Ventricular Pacer:

Atrial Pacer – Intrinsic QRS:

## 9. FUSION/PSEUDOFUSION BEATS

Present:

## 10. UNEXPECTED PAUSES

Present:

## 11. SENSING FUNCTION

Atrial:

Ventricular:

## 12. CAPTURE FUNCTION

Atrial:

Ventricular:

## 13. DATA ANALYSIS

## 14. INTERPRETATION

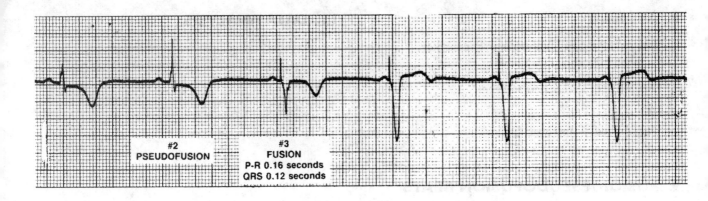

Figure 3-6B

# ECG PACEMAKER STRIP #6

## INTRINSIC

### I. RHYTHM

Atrial: Regular

Ventricular: Regular (QRS #1, #2, #3)

### 2. RATE

Atrial: 45

Ventricular: 45 (QRS #1, #2, #3)

### 3. P WAVE

Present: Yes

Configuration: Normal

Consistency: Yes

Relation to QRS: 1:1 (QRS #1, #2, #3)

### 4. P-R INTERVAL

Duration: 0.20 seconds (QRS #1, #2)
0.16 seconds (QRS #3)

Consistency: Variable

### 5. QRS COMPLEX

Present: Yes

Configuration: QRS #1, #2 normal
QRS #3, #4 abnormal (fusion)

Consistency: No

Duration: QRS #1, #2: 0.08 seconds
QRS #3: 0.12 seconds

## MECHANICAL PACEMAKER

### 6. MECHANICAL PACEMAKER SPIKES

Present: Yes

Immediately Followed by P Wave: No

Immediately Followed by QRS: Yes

Consistently Preceded by P Wave: Yes, but
variable P-R

### 7. MECHANICAL PACEMAKER RATE

Atrial: —

Ventricular: 45

## 8. AV DELAY

Intrinsic P Wave – Ventricular Pacer:
  0.11-0.22 seconds

Atrial Pacer – Ventricular Pacer: —

Atrial Pacer – Intrinsic QRS: —

## 9. FUSION/PSEUDOFUSION BEATS

Present: Yes, QRS #3 (fusion)
  QRS #1, #2 (pseudofusion)

## 10. UNEXPECTED PAUSES

Present: No

## 11. SENSING FUNCTION

Atrial: —

Ventricular: Indeterminable (ventricular sensing
  not present)

## 12. CAPTURE FUNCTION

Atrial: —

Ventricular: Normal

## 13. DATA ANALYSIS

The underlying atrial mechanism is sinus bradycardia at 45 per minute. The 1st three P waves are
conducted to ventricles. Pacemaker spikes at a
rate of 45 per minute are seen immediately prior
to QRS complexes #3, #4, #5 and #6, consistent
with a mechanical ventricular pacemaker.
Although P waves do precede each of the pacing
spikes (including P-QRS complexes #1 and #2),
the "P-R" intervals (AV delay) are variable, indicating atrial tracking is *not* present. QRS complexes #4, #5, and #6 result from ventricular
depolarization caused by the mechanical ventricular pacemaker discharge. QRS #3 is a fusion
beat in that ventricular depolarization results in
part from the descending sinus impulse and in
part from the ventricular pacemaker discharge.
QRS complexes #1 and #2 are pseudofusion
beats because both are distorted by the occurrence of a pacing spike shortly after the onset of
the QRS. Ventricular depolarization, however, is
a result only of intrinsic conduction of the
descending sinus impulse. The occurrence of pacing spikes *shortly* after the onset of intrinsic QRS
complexes #1 and #2 does *not* imply a sensing
problem. Depending on where the pacemaker is
located in the ventricle and where ventricular
depolarization starts, this finding may be normal.
Ventricular capture function is normal.

## 14. INTERPRETATION

Sinus bradycardia, mechanical ventricular pacemaker (presumably VVI) with fusion and pseudofusion beats

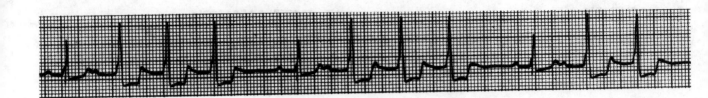

Figure 3-7A

# ECG PACEMAKER STRIP #7

## INTRINSIC

### 1. RHYTHM

Atrial:

Ventricular:

### 2. RATE

Atrial:

Ventricular:

### 3. P WAVE

Present:

Configuration:

Consistency:

Relation to QRS:

### 4. P-R INTERVAL

Duration:

Consistency:

### 5. QRS COMPLEX

Present:

Configuration:

Consistency:

Duration:

## MECHANICAL PACEMAKER

### 6. MECHANICAL PACEMAKER SPIKES

Present:

Immediately Followed by P Wave:

Immediately Followed by QRS:

Consistently Preceded by P Wave:

### 7. MECHANICAL PACEMAKER RATE

Atrial:

Ventricular:

## 8. AV DELAY

Intrinsic P Wave – Ventricular Pacemaker:

Atrial Pacer – Ventricular Pacer:

Atrial Pacer – Intrinsic QRS:

## 9. FUSION/PSEUDOFUSION BEATS

Present:

## 10. UNEXPECTED PAUSES

Present:

## 11. SENSING FUNCTION

Atrial:

Ventricular:

## 12. CAPTURE FUNCTION

Atrial:

Ventricular:

## 13. DATA ANALYSIS

## 14. INTERPRETATION

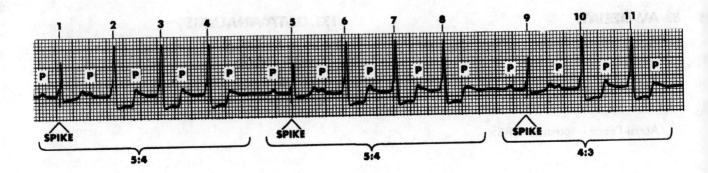

Figure 3-7B

# ECG PACEMAKER STRIP #7

## INTRINSIC

### 1. RHYTHM

Atrial: Regular

Ventricular: Irregular

### 2. RATE

Atrial: 110

Ventricular: 90

### 3. P WAVE

Present: Yes (many P waves obscured in ST-T waves)

Configuration: Normal

Consistency: Yes, when visible

Relation to QRS: 5:4 and 4:3

### 4. P-R INTERVAL

Duration: 0.20 to 0.30 seconds

Consistency: No, progressively lengthens before pause

### 5. QRS COMPLEX

Present: Yes

Configuration: Pacemaker spike distorts beats #1, #5 and #9; remaining have slurred upstroke

Consistency: No, varies in width and amplitude

Duration: Beats #1, #5, and #9: 0.08 seconds
Others: 0.09 seconds

## MECHANICAL PACEMAKER

### 6. MECHANICAL PACEMAKER SPIKES

Present: Yes

Immediately Followed by P Wave: No

Immediately Followed by QRS: Yes

Consistently Preceded by P Wave: Yes

### 7. MECHANICAL PACEMAKER RATE

Atrial: —

Ventricular: 60

388

## 8. AV DELAY

Intrinsic P Wave – Ventricular Pacer:
0.25 seconds

Atrial Pacer – Ventricular Pacer: —

Atrial Pacer – Intrinsic QRS: —

## 9. FUSION/PSEUDOFUSION BEATS

Present: Yes, QRS #1, #5, #9 (fusion)

## 10. UNEXPECTED PAUSES

Present: No

## 11. SENSING FUNCTION

Atrial: —

Ventricular: Normal

## 12. CAPTURE FUNCTION

Atrial: —

Ventricular: Normal

## 13. DATA ANALYSIS

The underlying atrial mechanism is sinus tachycardia at 110 per minute. The P-P interval is consistent and the P waves can be seen to distort the ST-T waves following the taller QRS complexes. The P-R intervals progressively increase until a P wave is not conducted. The ventricular rhythm is characterized by group beating (groups of 4 and 3) and shortening of the R-R intervals before the pauses. The pauses are less than twice the shortest R-R interval. The findings are consistent with Mobitz I (Wenckebach) second degree AV block. QRS complexes #1, #5, and #9 are different in configuration and bear a relationship to a mechanical pacemaker spike. These represent fusion beats since ventricular depolarization is in part due to the descending sinus impulse and in part from the mechanical pacemaker discharge. Although the three pacemaker spikes "follow" P waves after an "AV delay" of 0.25 seconds (raising the possibility of atrial synchrony and a dual chamber pacemaker), the absence of pacemaker spikes when the P-R interval exceeds 0.25 seconds is consistent with the presence of a ventricular pacemaker. The pacemaker is functioning in the demand mode (VVI) since it discharges only after the pauses at a rate equivalent to 60 per minute. Capture and sensing function are normal. The slurred upstroke of the QRS complexes may be related to monitor lead artifact or an intraventricular conduction defect. A 12 lead ECG is needed to differentiate these.

## 14. INTERPRETATION

Sinus tachycardia with Mobitz I (Wenckebach) second degree AV block, VVI pacemaker, and fusion beats

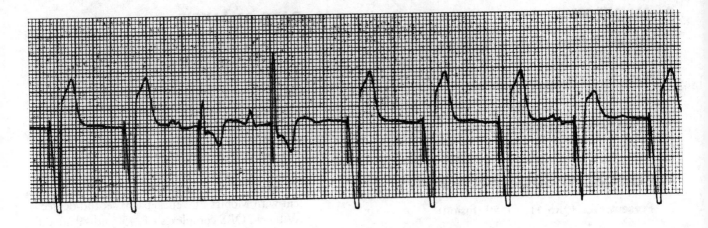

Figure 3-8A

## ECG PACEMAKER STRIP #8

| | |
|---|---|
| **INTRINSIC** | **MECHANICAL PACEMAKER** |

### INTRINSIC

**1. RHYTHM**

Atrial:

Ventricular:

**2. RATE**

Atrial:

Ventricular:

**3. P WAVE**

Present:

Configuration:

Consistency:

Relation to QRS:

**4. P-R INTERVAL**

Duration:

Consistency:

**5. QRS COMPLEX**

Present:

Configuration:

Consistency:

Duration:

### MECHANICAL PACEMAKER

**6. MECHANICAL PACEMAKER SPIKES**

Present:

Immediately Followed by P Wave:

Immediately Followed by QRS:

Consistently Preceded by P Wave:

**7. MECHANICAL PACEMAKER RATE**

Atrial:

Ventricular:

## 8. AV DELAY

Intrinsic P Wave – Ventricular Pacemaker:

Atrial Pacer – Ventricular Pacer:

Atrial Pacer – Intrinsic QRS:

## 9. FUSION/PSEUDOFUSION BEATS

Present:

## 10. UNEXPECTED PAUSES

Present:

## 11. SENSING FUNCTION

Atrial:

Ventricular:

## 12. CAPTURE FUNCTION

Atrial:

Ventricular:

## 13. DATA ANALYSIS

## 14. INTERPRETATION

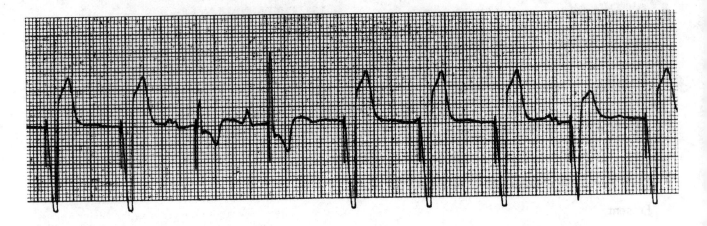

Figure 3-8B

# ECG PACEMAKER STRIP #8

## INTRINSIC

### I. RHYTHM

Atrial: Irregular

Ventricular: Indeterminable

### 2. RATE

Atrial: Overall bradycardic (only three P waves present)

Ventricular: 72 (QRS #3 and #4)

### 3. P WAVE

Present: Yes (only 3)

Configuration: Abnormal

Consistency: Variable

Relation to QRS: 1st two P waves conducted
3rd is not conducted

### 4. P-R INTERVAL

Duration: 0.35 seconds (#1), 0.30 seconds (#2)

Consistency: Variable

### 5. QRS COMPLEX

Present: QRS #3 and #4

Configuration: QRS #3 abnormal (fusion), #4 normal

Consistency: Variable

Duration: 0.11 seconds

## MECHANICAL PACEMAKER

### 6. MECHANICAL PACEMAKER SPIKES

Present: Yes

Immediately Followed by P Wave: No

Immediately Followed by QRS: Yes

Consistently Preceded by P Wave: No

### 7. MECHANICAL PACEMAKER RATE

Atrial: —

Ventricular: 72

## 8. AV DELAY

Intrinsic P Wave – Ventricular Pacemaker:
0.35, 0.30 seconds

Atrial Pacer – Ventricular Pacer: —

Atrial Pacer – Intrinsic QRS: —

## 9. FUSION/PSEUDOFUSION BEATS

Present: Yes, QRS #3 (fusion), QRS #4
(pseduofusion)

## 10. UNEXPECTED PAUSES

Present: No

## 11. SENSING FUNCTION

Atrial: —

Ventricular: Indeterminable (no ventricular
sensing)

## 12. CAPTURE FUNCTION

Atrial: —

Ventricular: Normal

## 13. DATA ANALYSIS

The underlying supraventricular rhythm is consistent with wandering atrial pacemaker since the three P waves have a different configuration. The overall bradycardic atrial rate may be secondary to sinus and/or atrial arrests. P waves #1 and #2 are conducted with first degree AV block. QRS complexes immediately follow the mechanical pacemaker spikes, consistent with a mechanical ventricular pacemaker (presumably ventricular "demand" or VVI). Pacing spikes #3 and #4 are on time and appropriate for the pacing rate of 72 per minute. Although atrial activity occurs prior to pacing spikes #3 and #4, the "AV delay" is variable, ruling out atrial synchrony and a dual chamber pacemaker. QRS #3 is a fusion beat since ventricular depolarization results in part from the descending supraventricular impulse (P wave #1) and in part from the ventricular pacemaker discharge (pacing spike #3). QRS #4 appears to result entirely from the descending supraventricular impulse. The occurrence of the "on time" pacing spike #4 immediately prior to the intrinsic QRS (#4) gives the "appearance of fusion" (pseudofusion).

## 14. INTERPRETATION

Wandering atrial pacemaker with sinus and/or atrial arrests, variable first degree AV block, mechanical ventricular pacemaker (presumably VVI) with fusion and pseudofusion beats

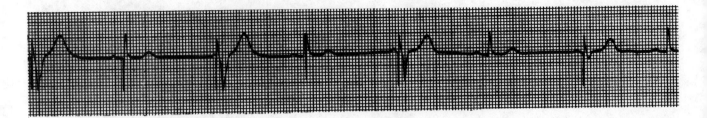

Figure 3-9A

# ECG PACEMAKER STRIP #9

## INTRINSIC

### 1. RHYTHM

Atrial:

Ventricular:

### 2. RATE

Atrial:

Ventricular:

### 3. P WAVE

Present:

Configuration:

Consistency:

Relation to QRS:

### 4. P-R INTERVAL

Duration:

Consistency:

### 5. QRS COMPLEX

Present:

Configuration:

Consistency:

Duration:

## MECHANICAL PACEMAKER

### 6. MECHANICAL PACEMAKER SPIKES

Present:

Immediately Followed by P Wave:

Immediately Followed by QRS:

Consistently Preceded by P Wave:

### 7. MECHANICAL PACEMAKER RATE

Atrial:

Ventricular:

## 8. AV DELAY

Intrinsic P Wave – Ventricular Pacemaker:

Atrial Pacer – Ventricular Pacer:

Atrial Pacer – Intrinsic QRS:

## 9. FUSION/PSEUDOFUSION BEATS

Present:

## 10. UNEXPECTED PAUSES

Present:

## 11. SENSING FUNCTION

Atrial:

Ventricular:

## 12. CAPTURE FUNCTION

Atrial:

Ventricular:

## 13. DATA ANALYSIS

## 14. INTERPRETATION

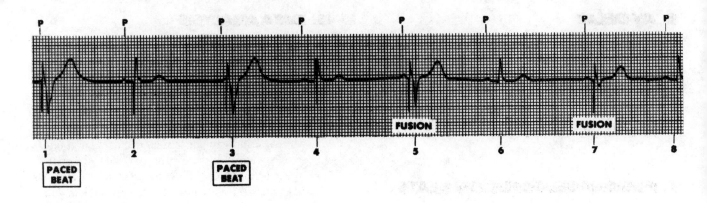

Figure 3-9B

# ECG PACEMAKER STRIP #9

## INTRINSIC

### I. RHYTHM

Atrial: Slightly irregular

Ventricular: Slightly irregular

### 2. RATE

Atrial: 50

Ventricular: 50

### 3. P WAVE

Present: Yes, hidden in 1st QRS, distorted by 3rd QRS

Configuration: Normal

Consistency: Yes

Relation to QRS: Variable

### 4. P-R INTERVAL

Duration: 0.16 seconds (beats #2, #4, #6)

Consistency: Yes (with intrinsic beats)

### 5. QRS COMPLEX

Present: Yes

Configuration: Normal (intrinsic complexes)

Consistency: Yes (intrinsic complexes)

Duration: 0.08 seconds (intrinsic complexes)

## MECHANICAL PACEMAKER

### 6. MECHANICAL PACEMAKER SPIKES

Present: Yes

Immediately Followed by P Wave: No

Immediately Followed by QRS: Yes

Consistently Preceded by P Wave: No

### 7. MECHANICAL PACEMAKER RATE

Atrial: —

Ventricular: 50

## 8. AV DELAY

Intrinsic P Wave – Ventricular Pacer: —

Atrial Pacer – Ventricular Pacer: —

Atrial Pacer – Intrinsic QRS: —

## 9. FUSION/PSEUDOFUSION BEATS

Present: Yes, QRS #4 (pseudofusion), #5, #7 (fusion)

## 10. UNEXPECTED PAUSES

Present: No

## 11. SENSING FUNCTION

Atrial: —

Ventricular: ? Normal

## 12. CAPTURE FUNCTION

Atrial: —

Ventricular: Normal

## 13. DATA ANALYSIS

The underlying atrial mechanism is sinus arrhythmia and bradycardia since the P wave configuration is similar, the P-P intervals vary, and the overall rate is approximately 50 per minute. The 1st QRS complex conceals the P wave and the 3rd partially conceals the P wave. Mechanical pacemaker spikes occurring at a rate of 50 per minute are apparent. Wide QRS complexes immediately follow pacer spikes #1 and #3, consistent with a ventricular pacemaker, and no pacer spike occurs in the vicinity of QRS #6, consistent with the demand mode (VVI). The sinus P wave is conducted normally to the ventricles in beats #2, #4, #6, and #8 and represent capture beats. QRS complexes #5 and #7 represent fusion beats since ventricular depolarization is due in part from the descending sinus impulse and in part from the mechanical pacemaker discharge. A pacemaker artifact occurs at the onset of QRS #2. The QRS is totally normal because the sinus impulse fully penetrates the ventricles causing normal depolarization. The discharge of the pacemaker was appropriate since no ventricular activity occurred during the pacing rate of 50 per minute. A pacemaker spike "falls within" QRS #4, 0.04 seconds after its onset. Although this finding raises the possibility of pacemaker sensing malfunction, depending on where in the ventricles the pacemaker is located, this still may be physiologic or "normal." Pacemaker capture function is normal.

## 14. INTERPRETATION

Sinus bradycardia and arrhythmia, VVI pacemaker with possible sensing malfunction, and fusion beats

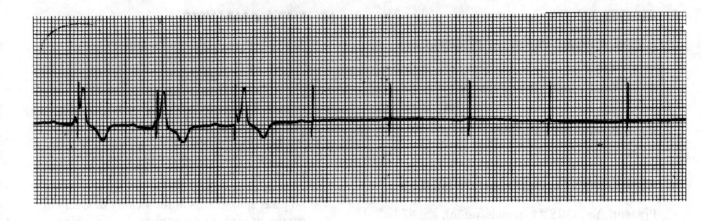

Figure 3-10A

# ECG PACEMAKER STRIP #10

## INTRINSIC

### 1. RHYTHM

Atrial:

Ventricular:

### 2. RATE

Atrial:

Ventricular:

### 3. P WAVE

Present:

Configuration:

Consistency:

Relation to QRS:

### 4. P-R INTERVAL

Duration:

Consistency:

### 5. QRS COMPLEX

Present:

Configuration:

Consistency:

Duration:

## MECHANICAL PACEMAKER

### 6. MECHANICAL PACEMAKER SPIKES

Present:

Immediately Followed by P Wave:

Immediately Followed by QRS:

Consistently Preceded by P Wave:

### 7. MECHANICAL PACEMAKER RATE

Atrial:

Ventricular:

## 8. AV DELAY

Intrinsic P Wave – Ventricular Pacemaker:

Atrial Pacer – Ventricular Pacer:

Atrial Pacer – Intrinsic QRS:

## 9. FUSION/PSEUDOFUSION BEATS

Present:

## 10. UNEXPECTED PAUSES

Present:

## 11. SENSING FUNCTION

Atrial:

Ventricular:

## 12. CAPTURE FUNCTION

Atrial:

Ventricular:

## 13. DATA ANALYSIS

## 14. INTERPRETATION

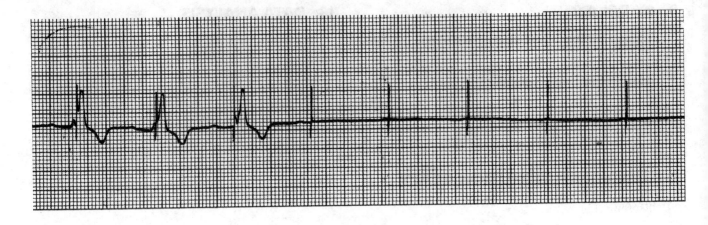

Figure 3-10B

# ECG PACEMAKER STRIP #10

## INTRINSIC

### 1. RHYTHM

Atrial:  Regular

Ventricular:  No intrinsic QRS complexes

### 2. RATE

Atrial:  68

Ventricular:  No intrinsic QRS complexes

### 3. P WAVE

Present:  Yes, some buried in pacer spike

Configuration:  Low amplitude

Consistency:  Yes

Relation to QRS:  1:1

### 4. P-R INTERVAL  No intrinsic P-R interval

Duration:

Consistency:

### 5. QRS COMPLEX  No intrinsic QRS complexes

Present:

Configuration:

Consistency:

Duration:

## MECHANICAL PACEMAKER

### 6. MECHANICAL PACEMAKER SPIKES

Present:  Yes

Immediately Followed by P Wave:  No

Immediately Followed by QRS:  Yes

Consistently Preceded by P Wave:  No

### 7. MECHANICAL PACEMAKER RATE

Atrial:  —

Ventricular:  68

## 8. AV DELAY

Intrinsic P Wave – Ventricular Pacer: Variable

Atrial Pacer – Ventricular Pacer: —

Atrial Pacer – Intrinsic QRS: —

## 9. FUSION/PSEUDOFUSION BEATS

Present: No

## 10. UNEXPECTED PAUSES

Present: Yes

## 11. SENSING FUNCTION

Atrial: —

Ventricular: Indeterminable (no ventricular sensing)

## 12. CAPTURE FUNCTION

Atrial: —

Ventricular: Abnormal, no capture after spikes #4 to #9.

## 13. DATA ANALYSIS

The underlying atrial mechanism appears to be sinus at 68 per minute. The P waves are of low amplitude, and some are obscured by mechanical pacemaker spikes, which also occur at a rate of 68 per minute. The 1st three pacing spikes are immediately followed by QRS complexes, consistent with a ventricular pacemaker. The 1st three pacing spikes are also preceded by a sinus P wave with a relatively constant AV delay (0.28 seconds), raising the possibility of atrial tracking and therefore a dual chamber pacemaker. However, the P waves "march through" subsequent pacing spikes, indicating atrial tracking is *not* present. Furthermore, if a dual chamber pacemaker were present and sudden failure of atrial sensing occurred (of P wave #4), one would expect the appearance of two pacing spikes (atrial and ventricular) with the 4th and subsequent "cycles." Ventricular capture fails with the 4th and subsequent ventricular pacer discharges. Ventricular sensing function cannot be assessed from this rhythm strip.

## 14. INTERPRETATION

Sinus rhythm, mechanical ventricular pacemaker (presumably VVI) with capture malfunction

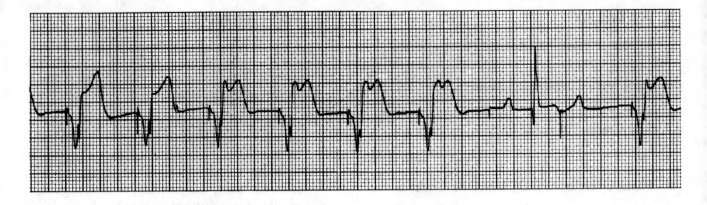

Figure 3-11A

## ECG PACEMAKER STRIP #11

### INTRINSIC

**1. RHYTHM**

Atrial:

Ventricular:

**2. RATE**

Atrial:

Ventricular:

**3. P WAVE**

Present:

Configuration:

Consistency:

Relation to QRS:

**4. P-R INTERVAL**

Duration:

Consistency:

**5. QRS COMPLEX**

Present:

Configuration:

Consistency:

Duration:

### MECHANICAL PACEMAKER

**6. MECHANICAL PACEMAKER SPIKES**

Present:

Immediately Followed by P Wave:

Immediately Followed by QRS:

Consistently Preceded by P Wave:

**7. MECHANICAL PACEMAKER RATE**

Atrial:

Ventricular:

## 8. AV DELAY

Intrinsic P Wave – Ventricular Pacemaker:

Atrial Pacer – Ventricular Pacer:

Atrial Pacer – Intrinsic QRS:

## 9. FUSION/PSEUDOFUSION BEATS

Present:

## 10. UNEXPECTED PAUSES

Present:

## 11. SENSING FUNCTION

Atrial:
Ventricular:

## 12. CAPTURE FUNCTION

Atrial:
Ventricular:

## 13. DATA ANALYSIS

## 14. INTERPRETATION

403

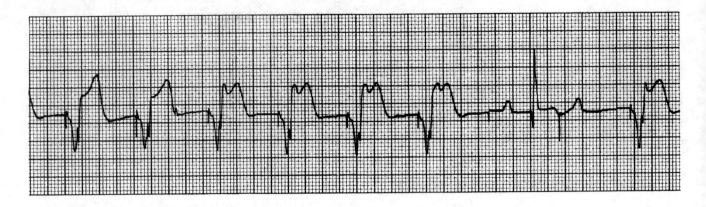

Figure 3-11B

## ECG PACEMAKER STRIP # 11

### INTRINSIC

#### 1. RHYTHM

Atrial: Regular

Ventricular: Indeterminable (only one intrinsic QRS)

#### 2. RATE

Atrial: 75

Ventricular: Indeterminable (only one intrinsic QRS)

#### 3. P WAVE

Present: Yes, but often buried in QRS-ST complex

Configuration: Normal

Consistency: Yes, when visible

Relation to QRS: 2:1 (prior to QRS #7)

#### 4. P-R INTERVAL

Duration: 0.32 seconds

Consistency: Indeterminable (only one intrinsic QRS)

#### 5. QRS COMPLEX

Present: QRS #7 (only intrinsic)

Configuration: Normal

Consistency: Indeterminable

Duration: 0.10 seconds

### MECHANICAL PACEMAKER

#### 6. MECHANICAL PACEMAKER SPIKES

Present: Yes

Immediately Followed by P Wave: No

Immediately Followed by QRS: Yes

Consistently Preceded by P Wave: No

#### 7. MECHANICAL PACEMAKER RATE

Atrial: —

Ventricular: 70

## 8. AV DELAY

Intrinsic P Wave – Ventricular Pacer: —

Atrial Pacer – Ventricular Pacer: —

Atrial Pacer – Intrinsic QRS: —

## 9. FUSION/PSEUDOFUSION BEATS

Present: No

## 10. UNEXPECTED PAUSES

Present: Yes, between QRS #6 and #7, and #7 and #8

## 11. SENSING FUNCTION

Atrial: —

Ventricular: Abnormal, QRS #7 should have been sensed

## 12. CAPTURE FUNCTION

Atrial: —

Ventricular: Abnormal, pacing spike #7 (and possibly #8) should have captured ventricles

## 13. DATA ANALYSIS

The underlying atrial mechanism is sinus. Most of the sinus impulses are buried in the QRS-ST complexes. There is only one intrinsic QRS complex (#7). The P wave immediately preceding this QRS is conducted with first degree AV block. In addition, the P wave prior to the conducted P wave and the P wave following QRS #7 are not conducted and constitute second degree AV block. Since two consecutive P waves are not conducted, one cannot determine whether this represents Mobitz I or Mobitz II. QRS complexes immediately follow the mechanical pacemaker spikes, consistent with a mechanical ventricular pacemaker (presumably ventricular "demand" or VVI). The unexpected pause between QRS #6 and #7 occurs because pacing spike #7 does not capture the ventricles. The unexpected pause between QRS #7 and QRS #8 occurs because QRS #7 was not sensed by the pacemaker.

## 14. INTERPRETATION

Sinus rhythm with first and second degree AV block, VVI pacemaker with sensing and capture malfunction

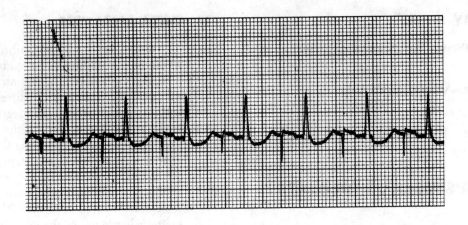

Figure 3-12A

## ECG PACEMAKER STRIP #12

### INTRINSIC

**I. RHYTHM**

    Atrial:

    Ventricular:

**2. RATE**

    Atrial:

    Ventricular:

**3. P WAVE**

    Present:

    Configuration:

    Consistency:

    Relation to QRS:

**4. P-R INTERVAL**

    Duration:

    Consistency:

**5. QRS COMPLEX**

    Present:

    Configuration:

    Consistency:

    Duration:

### MECHANICAL PACEMAKER

**6. MECHANICAL PACEMAKER SPIKES**

    Present:

    Immediately Followed by P Wave:

    Immediately Followed by QRS:

    Consistently Preceded by P Wave:

**7. MECHANICAL PACEMAKER RATE**

    Atrial:

    Ventricular:

## 8. AV DELAY

Intrinsic P Wave – Ventricular Pacemaker:

Atrial Pacer – Ventricular Pacer:

Atrial Pacer – Intrinsic QRS:

## 9. FUSION/PSEUDOFUSION BEATS

Present:

## 10. UNEXPECTED PAUSES

Present:

## 11. SENSING FUNCTION

Atrial:

Ventricular:

## 12. CAPTURE FUNCTION

Atrial:

Ventricular:

## 13. DATA ANALYSIS

## 14. INTERPRETATION

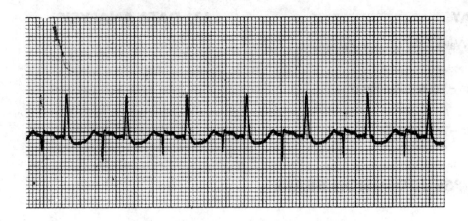

Figure 3-12B

# ECG PACEMAKER STRIP #12

## INTRINSIC

### 1. RHYTHM

Atrial: No intrinsic atrial rhythm

Ventricular: Regular

### 2. RATE

Atrial: No intrinsic atrial rhythm

Ventricular: 92

### 3. P WAVE: No intrinsic P waves

Present:

Configuration:

Consistency:

Relation to QRS:

### 4. P-R INTERVAL: No intrinsic P-R interval

Duration:

Consistency:

### 5. QRS COMPLEX

Present: Yes

Configuration: Normal

Consistency: Yes

Duration: 0.08 seconds

## MECHANICAL PACEMAKER

### 6. MECHANICAL PACEMAKER SPIKES

Present: Yes

Immediately Followed by P Wave: Yes

Immediately Followed by QRS: No

Consistently Preceded by P Wave: No

### 7. MECHANICAL PACEMAKER RATE

Atrial: 92

Ventricular: —

## 8. AV DELAY

Intrinsic P Wave – Ventricular Pacer: —

Atrial Pacer – Ventricular Pacer: —

Atrial Pacer – Intrinsic QRS: 0.24 seconds

## 9. FUSION/PSEUDOFUSION BEATS

Present: No

## 10. UNEXPECTED PAUSES

Present: No

## 11. SENSING FUNCTION

Atrial: Indeterminable (no atrial sensing)

Ventricular: —

## 12. CAPTURE FUNCTION

Atrial: Normal

Ventricular: —

## 13. DATA ANALYSIS

An underlying intrinsic atrial mechanism is not present. Mechanical pacemaker spikes are immediately followed by a P wave, consistent with a mechanical atrial pacemaker (presumably atrial "demand" or AAI). The AV delay is constant but prolonged at 0.24 seconds. All QRS complexes result from intrinsic conduction of the descending supraventricular impulse. Atrial pacemaker capture function is normal. Sensing function cannot be assessed from this rhythm strip.

## 14. INTERPRETATION

Mechanical atrial pacemaker (presumably AAI) with first degree AV block

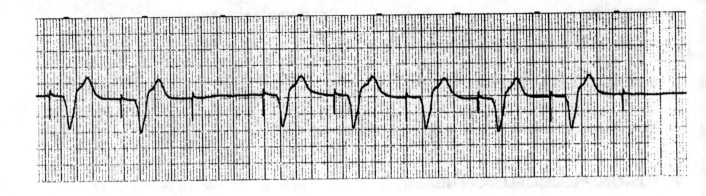

Figure 3-13A

# ECG PACEMAKER STRIP #13

## INTRINSIC

### I. RHYTHM

Atrial:

Ventricular:

### 2. RATE

Atrial:

Ventricular:

### 3. P WAVE

Present:

Configuration:

Consistency:

Relation to QRS:

### 4. P-R INTERVAL

Duration:

Consistency:

### 5. QRS COMPLEX

Present:

Configuration:

Consistency:

Duration:

## MECHANICAL PACEMAKER

### 6. MECHANICAL PACEMAKER SPIKES

Present:

Immediately Followed by P Wave:

Immediately Followed by QRS:

Consistently Preceded by P Wave:

### 7. MECHANICAL PACEMAKER RATE

Atrial:

Ventricular:

## 8. AV DELAY

Intrinsic P Wave – Ventricular Pacemaker:

Atrial Pacer – Ventricular Pacer:

Atrial Pacer – Intrinsic QRS:

## 9. FUSION/PSEUDOFUSION BEATS

Present:

## 10. UNEXPECTED PAUSES

Present:

## 11. SENSING FUNCTION

Atrial:

Ventricular:

## 12. CAPTURE FUNCTION

Atrial:

Ventricular:

## 13. DATA ANALYSIS

## 14. INTERPRETATION

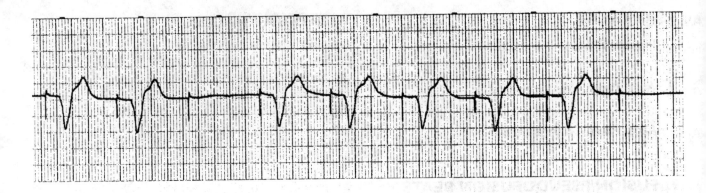

Figure 3-13B

# ECG PACEMAKER STRIP #13

## INTRINSIC

### 1. RHYTHM

Atrial: No intrinsic atrial rythm

Ventricular: Irregular (due to pauses)

### 2. RATE

Atrial: No intrinsic atrial rhythm

Ventricular: Overall less than 65

### 3. P WAVE: No intrinsic P waves

Present:

Configuration:

Consistency:

Relation to QRS:

### 4. P-R INTERVAL: No intrinsic P-R interval

Duration:

Consistency:

### 5. QRS COMPLEX

Present: Yes, except post pacer spikes #3 and #9

Configuration: Abnormal

Consistency: Yes, when present

Duration: 0.16 seconds

## MECHANICAL PACEMAKER

### 6. MECHANICAL PACEMAKER SPIKES

Present: Yes

Immediately Followed by P Wave: Yes

Immediately Followed by QRS: No

Consistently Preceded by P Wave: No

### 7. MECHANICAL PACEMAKER RATE

Atrial: 65

Ventricular: —

## AV DELAY

Intrinsic P Wave – Ventricular Pacer: —

Atrial Pacer – Ventricular Pacer: —

Atrial Pacer – Intrinsic QRS: 0.20 seconds

## FUSION/PSEUDOFUSION BEATS

Present: No

## UNEXPECTED PAUSES

Present: Yes

## SENSING FUNCTION

Atrial: Indeterminable (no atrial sensing)

Ventricular: —

## CAPTURE FUNCTION

Atrial: Probably Normal

Ventricular: —

## 13. DATA ANALYSIS

An underlying intrinsic atrial mechanism is not present. Mechanical pacemaker spikes are present at a rate of 65 per minute. There is slight deformity of the baseline immediately following the pacer spikes, suggestive of P waves and therefore implying the presence of a mechanical atrial pacemaker. Clinically the presence of postpacer spike P waves should be confirmed with a 12 lead ECG 0.20 seconds following pacer spikes #1, #2, #4, #5, #6, #7, and #8, wide QRS complexes, not immediately preceded by a pacer spike, occur. These complexes represent abnormal, intrinsic intraventricular depolarization consistent with underlying bundle branch block (probably LBBB). A 12 lead ECG is needed to confirm this. A QRS complex is "dropped" 0.20 seconds following atrial pacer spikes #3 and #9. Since the AV delay remains constant in the conducted impulses, the findings are consistent with Mobitz II second degree AV block. Atrial capture function appears normal. Atrial sensing function cannot be assessed from this rhythm strip.

## 14. INTERPRETATION

Mechanical atrial pacemaker (presumably AAI) with Mobitz II second degree AV block and underlying bundle branch block

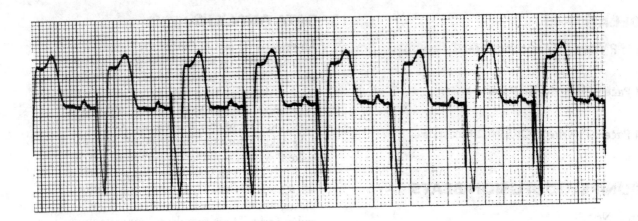

Figure 3-14A

# ECG PACEMAKER STRIP #14

## INTRINSIC

### 1. RHYTHM

Atrial:

Ventricular:

### 2. RATE

Atrial:

Ventricular:

### 3. P WAVE

Present:

Configuration:

Consistency:

Relation to QRS:

### 4. P-R INTERVAL

Duration:

Consistency:

### 5. QRS COMPLEX

Present:

Configuration:

Consistency:

Duration:

## MECHANICAL PACEMAKER

### 6. MECHANICAL PACEMAKER SPIKES

Present:

Immediately Followed by P Wave:

Immediately Followed by QRS:

Consistently Preceded by P Wave:

### 7. MECHANICAL PACEMAKER RATE

Atrial:

Ventricular:

## 8. AV DELAY

Intrinsic P Wave – Ventricular Pacemaker:

Atrial Pacer – Ventricular Pacer:

Atrial Pacer – Intrinsic QRS:

## 9. FUSION/PSEUDOFUSION BEATS

Present:

## 10. UNEXPECTED PAUSES

Present:

## 11. SENSING FUNCTION

Atrial:

Ventricular:

## 12. CAPTURE FUNCTION

Atrial:

Ventricular:

## 13. DATA ANALYSIS

## 14. INTERPRETATION

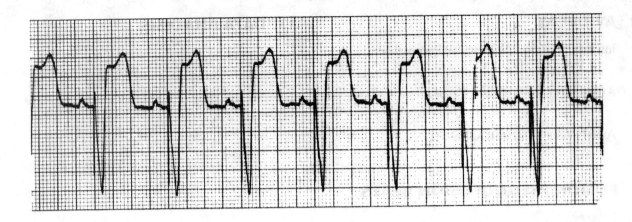

Figure 3-14B

# ECG PACEMAKER STRIP #14

## INTRINSIC

### 1. RHYTHM

Atrial: Regular

Ventricular: No intrinsic QRS complexes

### 2. RATE

Atrial: 75

Ventricular: No intrinsic rhythm

### 3. P WAVE

Present: Yes

Configuration: Normal

Consistency: Yes

Relation to QRS: 1:1

### 4. P-R INTERVAL: No intrinsic P-R interval

Duration:

Consistency:

### 5. QRS COMPLEX: No intrinsic QRS complexes

Present:

Configuration:

Consistency:

Duration:

## MECHANICAL PACEMAKER

### 6. MECHANICAL PACEMAKER SPIKES

Present: Yes

Immediately Followed by P Wave: No

Immediately Followed by QRS: Yes

Consistently Preceded by P Wave: Yes

### 7. MECHANICAL PACEMAKER RATE

Atrial: No atrial pacing

Ventricular: 75

## 8. AV DELAY

Intrinsic P Wave – Ventricular Pacemaker:
0.16 seconds

Atrial Pacer – Ventricular Pacer: —

Atrial Pacer – Intrinsic QRS: —

## 9. FUSION/PSEUDOFUSION BEATS

Present: No

## 10. UNEXPECTED PAUSES

Present: No

## 11. SENSING FUNCTION

Atrial: Normal

Ventricular: Indeterminable (no ventricular
sensing)

## 12. CAPTURE FUNCTION

Atrial: Indeterminable (no atrial pacing)

Ventricular: Normal

## 13. DATA ANALYSIS

The underlying atrial mechanism is sinus at 75
per minute. Pacemaker spikes are immediately
followed by QRS complexes, consistent with
mechanical ventricular pacing, and are consistently preceded by P waves with a constant AV
delay, consistent with atrial sensing and tracking.
The findings are consistent with a dual chamber
pacemaker. Atrial sensing and ventricular capture
function are normal. Atrial capture and ventricular sensing function cannot be assessed from this
rhythm strip.

## 14. INTERPRETATION

Sinus rhythm with dual chamber pacemaker
(presumably DDD) functioning in the atrial
synchronous mode (VAT)

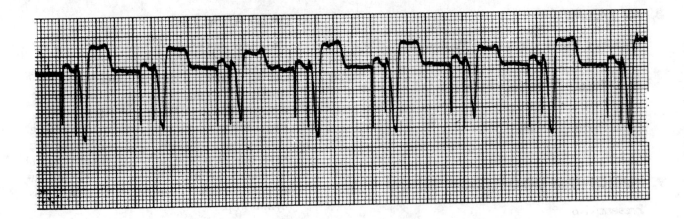

Figure 3-15A

## ECG PACEMAKER STRIP #15

### INTRINSIC

#### 1. RHYTHM

Atrial:

Ventricular:

#### 2. RATE

Atrial:

Ventricular:

#### 3. P WAVE

Present:

Configuration:

Consistency:

Relation to QRS:

#### 4. P-R INTERVAL

Duration:

Consistency:

#### 5. QRS COMPLEX

Present:

Configuration:

Consistency:

Duration:

### MECHANICAL PACEMAKER

#### 6. MECHANICAL PACEMAKER SPIKES

Present:

Immediately Followed by P Wave:

Immediately Followed by QRS:

Consistently Preceded by P Wave:

#### 7. MECHANICAL PACEMAKER RATE

Atrial:

Ventricular:

## 8. AV DELAY

Intrinsic P Wave – Ventricular Pacemaker:

Atrial Pacer – Ventricular Pacer:

Atrial Pacer – Intrinsic QRS:

## 9. FUSION/PSEUDOFUSION BEATS

Present:

## 10. UNEXPECTED PAUSES

Present:

## 11. SENSING FUNCTION

Atrial:

Ventricular:

## 12. CAPTURE FUNCTION

Atrial:

Ventricular:

## 13. DATA ANALYSIS

## 14. INTERPRETATION

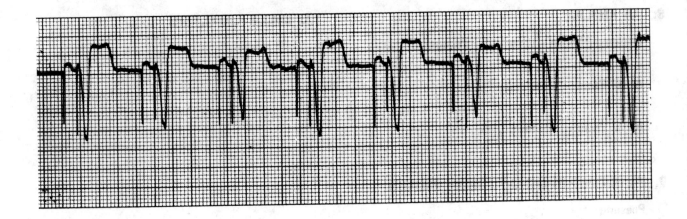

Figure 3-15B

## ECG PACEMAKER STRIP #15

### INTRINSIC

**1. RHYTHM:** No intrinsic rhythm

    Atrial:

    Ventricular:

**2. RATE:** No intrinsic rhythm

    Atrial:

    Ventricular:

**3. P WAVE:** No intrinsic P waves

    Present:

    Configuration:

    Consistency:

    Relation to QRS:

**4. P-R INTERVAL:** No intrinsic P-R intervals

    Duration:

    Consistency:

**5. QRS COMPLEX:** No intrinsic QRS complexes

    Present:

    Configuration:

    Consistency:

    Duration:

### MECHANICAL PACEMAKER

**6. MECHANICAL PACEMAKER SPIKES**

    Present: Yes

    Immediately Followed by P Wave: Yes

    Immediately Followed by QRS: Yes

    Consistently Preceded by P Wave: Yes

**7. MECHANICAL PACEMAKER RATE**

    Atrial: 70

    Ventricular: 70

## 8. AV DELAY

Intrinsic P Wave – Ventricular Pacemaker: —

Atrial Pacer – Ventricular Pacer: 0.14 seconds

Atrial Pacer – Intrinsic QRS: —

## 9. FUSION/PSEUDOFUSION BEATS

Present: No

## 10. UNEXPECTED PAUSES

Present: No

## 11. SENSING FUNCTION

Atrial: Indeterminable (no atrial sensing)

Ventricular: Indeterminable (no ventricular sensing)

## 12. CAPTURE FUNCTION

Atrial: Normal

Ventricular: Normal

## 13. DATA ANALYSIS

An underlying intrinsic atrial mechanism is not present. Two mechanical pacemaker spikes for each P-QRS complex are apparent. The 1st pacing spike is immediately followed by a P wave, the 2nd pacing spike is immediately followed by a wide QRS, and the AV delay is constant. The findings are consistent with a dual chamber pacemaker. Atrial and ventricular capture function are normal. Atrial and ventricular sensing function cannot be assessed from this rhythm strip.

## 14. INTERPRETATION

Dual chamber pacemaker (presumably DDD) functioning in the A-V sequential mode

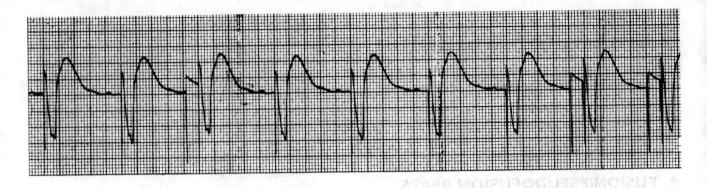

Figure 3-16A

## ECG PACEMAKER STRIP #16

### INTRINSIC

#### 1. RHYTHM

Atrial:

Ventricular:

#### 2. RATE

Atrial:

Ventricular:

#### 3. P WAVE

Present:

Configuration:

Consistency:

Relation to QRS:

#### 4. P-R INTERVAL

Duration:

Consistency:

#### 5. QRS COMPLEX

Present:

Configuration:

Consistency:

Duration:

### MECHANICAL PACEMAKER

#### 6. MECHANICAL PACEMAKER SPIKES

Present:

Immediately Followed by P Wave:

Immediately Followed by QRS:

Consistently Preceded by P Wave:

#### 7. MECHANICAL PACEMAKER RATE

Atrial:

Ventricular:

## 8. AV DELAY

Intrinsic P Wave – Ventricular Pacemaker:

Atrial Pacer – Ventricular Pacer:

Atrial Pacer – Intrinsic QRS:

## 9. FUSION/PSEUDOFUSION BEATS

Present:

## 10. UNEXPECTED PAUSES

Present:

## 11. SENSING FUNCTION

Atrial:

Ventricular:

## 12. CAPTURE FUNCTION

Atrial:

Ventricular:

## 13. DATA ANALYSIS

## 14. INTERPRETATION

423

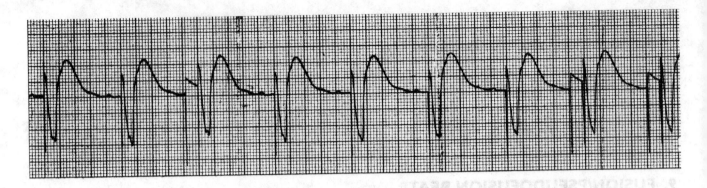

Figure 3-16B

# ECG PACEMAKER STRIP #16

## INTRINSIC

### I. RHYTHM

Atrial: "Irregular"

Ventricular: No intrinsic QRS complexes

### 2. RATE

Atrial: Overall less than 60

Ventricular: No intrinsic rhythm

### 3. P WAVE

Present: Yes (prior to QRS #1, #2, #4, #5, #6, #7)

Configuration: Normal

Consistency: Yes

Relation to QRS: 1:1 when present

### 4. P-R INTERVAL: No intrinsic P-R intervals

Duration:

Consistency:

### 5. QRS COMPLEX: No intrinsic QRS complexes

Present:

Configuration:

Consistency:

Duration:

## MECHANICAL PACEMAKER

### 6. MECHANICAL PACEMAKER SPIKES

Present: Yes

Immediately Followed by P Wave: Some

Immediately Followed by QRS: Yes (all)

Consistently Preceded by P Wave: Yes (all)

### 7. MECHANICAL PACEMAKER RATE

Atrial: 60

Ventricular: 60

## 8. AV DELAY

Intrinsic P Wave – Ventricular Pacemaker:
0.20 seconds

Atrial Pacer – Ventricular Pacer: 0.16 seconds

Atrial Pacer – Intrinsic QRS: —

## 9. FUSION/PSEUDOFUSION BEATS

Present: No

## 10. UNEXPECTED PAUSES

Present: No

## 11. SENSING FUNCTION

Atrial: Normal

Ventricular: Indeterminable (no ventricular sensing)

## 12. CAPTURE FUNCTION

Atrial: ? (see analysis below)

Ventricular: Normal

## 13. DATA ANALYSIS

The underlying atrial mechanism appears to be sinus. Following QRS complexes #2 and #7 a mechanical pacemaker spike occurs at the time the next sinus P wave is expected. This is an atrial pacemaker spike because a 2nd pacemaker spike occurs after an AV delay of 0.16 seconds, which captures the ventricles (as indicated by the occurrence of a QRS complex immediately following the 2nd spike). The findings are consistent with a dual chamber pacemaker. Most likely, sinus arrhythmia is present. With even slight slowing of the sinus rate the atrial pacing component discharges since both the sinus rate and pacing rate are 60 per minute. Atrial sensing function is normal since each sinus P wave is consistently followed by a ventricular pacing spike (atrial tracking). Although there is a deflection of the baseline following each atrial pacing spike (beats #3, #8, #9), the unequivocal occurrence of a P wave cannot be demonstrated from this rhythm strip. A 12 lead ECG is needed to further evaluate atrial capture function. Ventricular capture function is normal. Ventricular sensing function cannot be assessed from this rhythm strip.

## 14. INTERPRETATION

Probable sinus arrhythmia, dual chamber pacemaker (DDD) functioning in the atrial synchronous (VAT) and A-V sequential modes

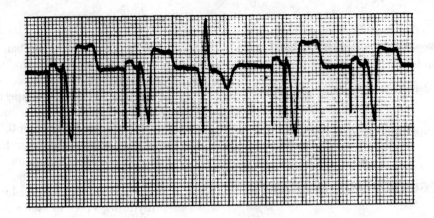

Figure 3-17A

# ECG PACEMAKER STRIP #17

## INTRINSIC

### 1. RHYTHM
Atrial:

Ventricular:

### 2. RATE
Atrial:

Ventricular:

### 3. P WAVE
Present:

Configuration:

Consistency:

Relation to QRS:

### 4. P-R INTERVAL
Duration:

Consistency:

### 5. QRS COMPLEX
Present:

Configuration:

Consistency:

Duration:

## MECHANICAL PACEMAKER

### 6. MECHANICAL PACEMAKER SPIKES
Present:

Immediately Followed by P Wave:

Immediately Followed by P Wave:

Consistently Preceded by P Wave:

### 7. MECHANICAL PACEMAKER RATE
Atrial:

Ventricular:

## 8. AV DELAY

Intrinsic P Wave – Ventricular Pacemaker:

Atrial Pacer – Ventricular Pacer:

Atrial Pacer – Intrinsic QRS:

## 9. FUSION/PSEUDOFUSION BEATS

Present:

## 10. UNEXPECTED PAUSES

Present:

## 11. SENSING FUNCTION

Atrial:

## 12. CAPTURE FUNCTION

Atrial:

Ventricular:

## 13. DATA ANALYSIS

## 14. INTERPRETATION

427

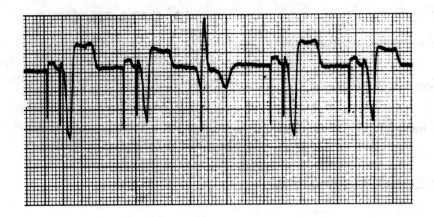

Figure 3-17B

## ECG PACEMAKER STRIP #17

---

### INTRINSIC

#### 1. RHYTHM

Atrial: No intrinsic atrial rhythm

Ventricular: One intrinsic QRS

#### 2. RATE

Atrial: No intrinsic atrial rhythm

Ventricular: One intrinsic QRS

#### 3. P WAVE: No intrinsic P waves

Present:

Configuration:

Consistency:

Relation to QRS:

#### 4. P-R INTERVAL: No intrinsic P-R interval

Duration:

Consistency:

#### 5. QRS COMPLEX

Present: One (beat #3)

Configuration: Abnormal

Consistency: —

Duration: 0.14 seconds

### MECHANICAL PACEMAKER

#### 6. MECHANICAL PACEMAKER SPIKES

Present: Yes

Immediately Followed by P Wave: Yes

Immediately Followed by QRS: Yes

Consistently Preceded by P Wave: Yes

#### 7. MECHANICAL PACEMAKER RATE

Atrial: 70

Ventricular: 70

## 8. AV DELAY

Intrinsic P Wave – Ventricular Pacer: —

Atrial Pacer – Ventricular Pacer: 0.14 seconds

Atrial Pacer – Intrinsic QRS: —

## 9. FUSION/PSEUDOFUSION BEATS

Present: Yes, QRS #3 (pseudofusion)

## 10. UNEXPECTED PAUSES

Present: No

## 11. SENSING FUNCTION

Atrial: Indeterminable (no atrial sensing)

Ventricular: Normal

## 12. CAPTURE FUNCTION

Atrial: Normal

Ventricular: Normal

## 13. DATA ANALYSIS

An underlying intrinsic atrial mechanism is not present. Except for QRS complex #3, two mechanical pacemaker spikes are associated with each P-QRS complex. The 1st pacing spike is immediately followed by a P wave, the 2nd pacing spike is immediately followed by a wide QRS, and the AV delay is constant. The findings are consistent with a dual chamber pacemaker. The 3rd QRS complex is wide, premature in the established QRS cycle, and not preceded by a P wave. This beat is a PVC. An atrial pacer spike appropriately occurs on time since no atrial activity occurs to inhibit atrial pacemaker discharge. The PVC is, however, appropriately sensed by the ventricular lead, hence a ventricular pacing spike does not follow the atrial pacing spike The occurrence of the atrial pacing spike "into" the PVC (QRS #3) gives the "appearance" of fusion (pseudofusion). Atrial and ventricular capture function and ventricular sensing function are normal. Atrial sensing function cannot be assessed from this rhythm strip.

## 14. INTERPRETATION

Dual chamber pacemaker (presumably DDD) functioning in A-V sequential mode (DVI) with PVC

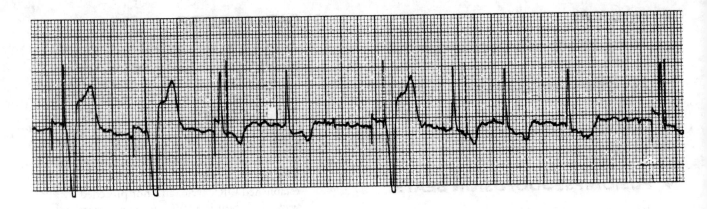

Figure 3-18A

# ECG PACEMAKER STRIP #18

## INTRINSIC

### 1. RHYTHM

Atrial:

Ventricular:

### 2. RATE

Atrial:

Ventricular:

### 3. P WAVE

Present:

Configuration:

Consistency:

Relation to QRS:

### 4. P-R INTERVAL

Duration:

Consistency:

### 5. QRS COMPLEX

Present:

Configuration:

Consistency:

Duration:

## MECHANICAL PACEMAKER

### 6. MECHANICAL PACEMAKER SPIKES

Present:

Immediately Followed by P Wave:

Immediately Followed by QRS:

Consistently Preceded by P Wave:

### 7. MECHANICAL PACEMAKER RATE

Atrial:

Ventricular:

## 8. AV DELAY

Intrinsic P Wave – Ventricular Pacemaker:

Atrial Pacer – Ventricular Pacer:

Atrial Pacer – Intrinsic QRS:

## 9. FUSION/PSEUDOFUSION BEATS

Present:

## 10. UNEXPECTED PAUSES

Present:

## 11. SENSING FUNCTION

Atrial:

Ventricular:

## 12. CAPTURE FUNCTION

Atrial:

Ventricular:

## 13. DATA ANALYSIS

## 14. INTERPRETATION

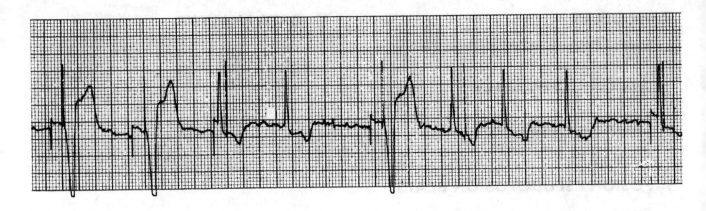

Figure 3-18B

## ECG PACEMAKER STRIP # 18

### INTRINSIC

### 1. RHYTHM

Atrial: Irregular

Ventricular: Irregular

### 2. RATE

Atrial: Indeterminable

Ventricular: 70

### 3. P WAVE: No (discrete P waves not present)

Present:

Configuration:

Consistency:

Relation to QRS:

### 4. P-R INTERVAL: No intrinsic P-R intervals

Duration:

Consistency:

### 5. QRS COMPLEX

Present: Yes

Configuration: Normal

Consistency: Yes

Duration: 0.08 seconds

### MECHANICAL PACEMAKER

### 6. MECHANICAL PACEMAKER SPIKES

Present: Yes

Immediately Followed by P Wave: Some

Immediately Followed by QRS: Some

Consistently Preceded by P Wave: No

### 7. MECHANICAL PACEMAKER RATE

Atrial: 60

Ventricular: 60

## 8. AV DELAY

Intrinsic P Wave – Ventricular Pacer: —

Atrial Pacer – Ventricular Pacer: 0.16 seconds

Atrial Pacer – Intrinsic QRS: —

## 9. FUSION/PSEUDOFUSION BEATS

**Present:** Yes , QRS #3, #9 (pseudofusion)

## 10. UNEXPECTED PAUSES

**Present:** Yes (but can be explained by hysteresis)

## 11. SENSING FUNCTION

**Atrial:** Indeterminable (in setting of atrial fibrillation)

**Ventricular:** Abnormal?

## 12. CAPTURE FUNCTION

**Atrial:** Indeterminable (in setting of atrial fibrillation)

**Ventricular:** Normal

## 13. DATA ANALYSIS

The underlying atrial mechanism is atrial fibrillation with an overall intrinsic ventricular rate of approximately 70 per minute. Two different mechanical pacemaker spikes are apparent. In complex #1 the 1st spike is predominantly negative in polarity, deflects the baseline upward stimulating a P wave, and is followed by a 2nd pacemaker spike after an AV delay 0.16 seconds. The 2nd pacemaker spike is predominantly positive in polarity and is immediately followed by a wide QRS complex. The findings are consistent with a dual chamber pacemaker. In the first two complexes the pacemaker is functioning in the A-V sequential mode at a rate of 60 per minute. Following QRS complexes #4 and #8 there are unexpected pauses that are terminated by discharge of the atrial and ventricular pacing components at a rate equivalent to 50 per minute. These findings can be best explained by the presence of a hysteresis feature in which atrial and ventricular pacing at a rate of 60 per minute does not occur until the intrinsic rate falls below 50 per minute. Mechanical pacing than continues at a rate of 60 per minute until the intrinsic rate increases above 60 per minute. Although there is upward deflection of the baseline (simulating P waves) following the atrial pacing spikes, atrial capture is not possible in the presence of atrial fibrillation so atrial capture function cannot be assessed. Due to the variable amplitude of the fibrillatory waves in atrial fibrillation, atrial sensing function cannot be assessed. Ventricular capture function appears normal. At first glance it appears ventricular sensing malfunction exists since QRS complexes #3, #6, and #9 "are not sensed." Careful inspection of QRS #6 reveals that an atrial pacer spike is present. Furthermore all three "unsensed" QRS complexes (#3, #6, #9) occur "between" an atrial pacer spike and a ventricular pacer spike. Some dual chamber pacemakers have specific features that can explain the occurrence of ventricular pacing discharge following atrial pacing discharge even though an intervening intrinsic QRS has occurred. In other words ventricular sensing malfunction may not be present on this rhythm strip. QRS complexes #3 and #9 may be called pseudofusion beats since these are distorted by the atrial pacer discharge.

## 14. INTERPRETATION

Atrial fibrillation with controlled ventricular response, dual chamber pacemaker (presumably DDD) with hysteresis, possible ventricular sensing malfunction and pseudofusion beats

# • Part IV •

## Continuing Education

# SELF-ASSESSMENT EXAMINATION

## Pure Practice for ECGs

## HOW TO OBTAIN CONTINUING EDUCATION CREDIT

Registered nurses may receive 14.5 contact hours by completing the rhythm strip analysis in Parts I, II, and III and successfully answering the post-test questions in Part IV.

## TAKING THE TEST

1. Read each test question and record your answer on the answer sheet provided. **Do not duplicate this answer sheet, a photocopy will be rejected by the scanner.**

2. Follow the instructions on the answer sheet exactly. Use only a **No. 2 pencil,** and do not make any stray marks on the answer sheet. It is important that you PRINT your name, address, and Social Security number correctly; failure to do so will result in rejection of your answer sheet by the computer.

**Payment:**
Check or money order in the amount of $50.00.
Payable to: Mosby

**Mail to:**
Mosby
Division of Continuing Education
11830 Westline Industrial Drive
St. Louis, MO 63146-3318

## CONTINUING EDUCATION

Mosby, Division of Continuing Education and Training (DCET) is accredited as a provider of continuing education in nursing by the American Nurses Credentialing Center Commission on Accreditation. This approval is reciprocal in all states and for all specialty organizations who recognize the ANCC approval process.

Mosby, DCET contact hours are applicable for recertification/relicensure requirements for all professional associations and in all states requiring mandatory continuing education that recognize the ANCC approval process.

## RECEIVING YOUR RESULTS

Your posttest will be graded, and you will be advised of your results by postcard within 90 days of receipt of your completed answer sheet. A score of 70% or higher is required.

PLEASE KEEP THE POSTCARD; IT IS YOUR CERTIFICATE OF CONTACT HOURS EARNED.

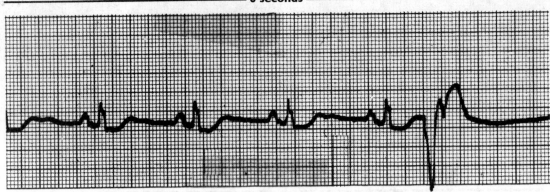

Lead II

6 seconds

Figure 4-1

Test strip #1

# ECG TEST RHYTHM STRIP #1

1. The atrial rate is:

    a.   40
    b.   50
    c.   56
    d.   60
    e.   65

2. The duration of the P-R interval is

    a.   0.12 seconds
    b.   0.16 seconds
    c.   0.20 seconds
    d.   0.24 seconds
    e.   0.28 seconds

3. The abnormal complex in the strip is

    a.   a premature ventricular beat
    b.   a junctional escape beat
    c.   a premature atrial beat
    d.   a premature junctional beat
    e.   none of the above

4. The wave immediately following the abnormal complex is

    a.   a biphasic T wave
    b.   a negative U wave preceding the T wave
    c.   a negative P wave preceding the T wave
    d.   a superimposed junctional beat
    e.   an artifact

5. The underlying rhythm is

    a.   sinus arrhythmia
    b.   atrial rhythm
    c.   sinus bradycardia
    d.   junctional rhythm
    e.   none of the above

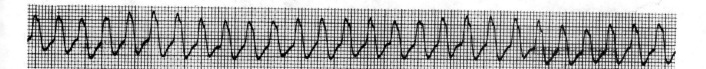

Figure 4-2

# ECG TEST RHYTHM STRIP #2

6. The atrial rate is

   a. 120
   b. 150
   c. 210
   d. 260
   e. indeterminable

7. The ventricular rate is

   a. 120
   b. 150
   c. 210
   d. 260
   e. indeterminable

8. The duration of the QRS complexes is

   a. indeterminable
   b. 0.08 seconds
   c. 0.10 seconds
   d. 0.12 seconds
   e. 0.14 seconds

9. The duration of the P-R interval is

   a. indeterminable
   b. 0.12 seconds
   c. 0.14 seconds
   d. 0.16 seconds
   e. 0.18 seconds

10. The dysrhythmia is

   a. junctional tachycardia
   b. ventricular tachycardia
   c. ventricular flutter
   d. artial flutter with 1:1 conduction
   e. supraventricular tachycardia

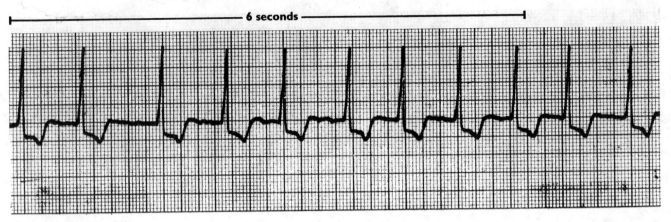

6 seconds

Figure 4-3

## ECG TEST RHYTHM STRIP #3

11. The atrial rate is

   a.   90
   b.   110
   c.   250
   d.   300
   e.   indeterminable

12. The ventricular rate is

   a.   80
   b.   90
   c.   100
   d.   110
   e.   indeterminable

13. The ventricular rhythm is

   a.   regular
   b.   regularly irregular
   c.   irregularly irregular
   d.   irregular with pattern of group beats
   e.   indeterminable

14. The QRS complex is

   a.   normal in appearance
   b.   abnormal in height
   c.   abnormal in width
   d.   inconsistent
   e.   0.12 seconds in duration

15. The dysrhythmia is

   a.   atrial flutter
   b.   wandering pacemaker
   c.   atrial fibrillation
   d.   sinus rhythm
   e.   junctional tachycardia

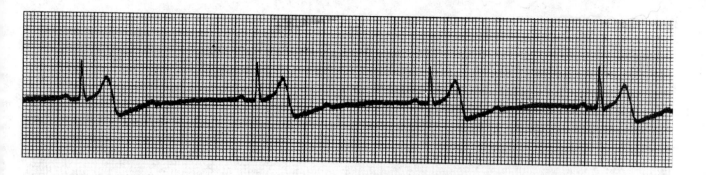

Figure 4-4

# ECG TEST RHYTHM STRIP #4

16. The atrial rate is

    a.   50
    b.   70
    c.   40
    d.   60
    e.   indeterminable

17. The ventricular rate is

    a.   30
    b.   40
    c.   50
    d.   60
    e.   indeterminable

18. The relationship of the P wave to the QRS complex is

    a.   1:1
    b.   2:1
    c.   1:2
    d.   indeterminable

19. The duration of the P-R interval is

    a.   0.10 seconds
    b.   0.14 seconds
    c.   0.18 seconds
    d.   0.22 seconds
    e.   0.26 seconds

20. The dysrhythmia is

    a.   sinus rhythm with second degree AV block
    b.   sinus rhythm with first degree AV block and second degree AV block
    c.   sinus rhythm with second degree AV block and third degree AV block
    d.   sinus rhythm with third degree AV block
    e.   sinus rhythm with first degree AV block and third degree AV block

6 seconds

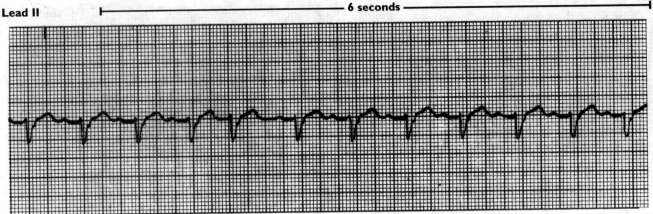

Figure 4-5

## ECG TEST RHYTHM STRIP #5

21. The atrial rate is

    a.   indeterminable
    b.   60
    c.   75
    d.   90
    e.   100

22. The abnormal values include

    a.   regularly irregular ventricular rhythm
    b.   a ventricular rate of 110
    c.   a variable relationship of P to QRS
    d.   a prolonged P-R interval of 0.22 seconds
    e.   an inconsistent QRS complex

23. The 5th beat in this strip is

    a.   a premature junctional beat
    b.   a premature atrial beat
    c.   a junctional escape beat
    d.   a sinus capture beat
    e.   none of the above

24. The wide, abnormal QRS complex complexes can be attributed to

    a.   a right bundle branch block
    b.   a left bundle branch block
    c.   ventricular ectopic beats
    d.   an intraventricular conduction delay
    e.   none of the above

25. The underlying rhythm is

    a.   sinus arrhythmia with first degree AV block
    b.   sinus rhythm with first degree AV block
    c.   atrial flutter with varying conduction ratios
    d.   accelerated idioventricular rhythm with AV dissociation
    e.   junctional tachycardia with aberrant ventricular conduction

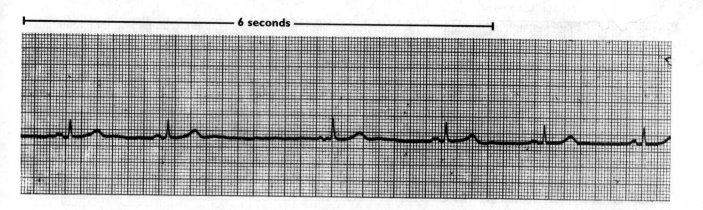

6 seconds

Figure 4-6

## ECG TEST RHYTHM STRIP #6

26. The atrial rate and ventricular rates are

    a.  30
    b.  40
    c.  50
    d.  different
    e.  indeterminable

27. The P wave is

    a.  smooth in configuration
    b.  notched in configuration
    c.  consistent in configuration
    d.  unrelated to the QRS complex
    e.  inconsistently related to QRS

28. The P-R interval is

    a.  indeterminable
    b.  inconsistent
    c.  0.12 seconds
    d.  0.16 seconds
    e.  0.20 seconds

29. The third beat in this strip is

    a.  a sinus beat
    b.  an atrial premature beat
    c.  an atrial escape beat
    d.  a junctional escape beat
    e.  none of the above

30. The cause of the slow rate is

    a.  sinus rhythm with SA exit block, type I (Wenckebach)
    b.  sinus arrhythmia with wandering pacemaker
    c.  sinus arrest with wandering pacemaker
    d.  sinus bradycardia with sinus arrhythmia
    e.  sinus bradycardia with sinus arrest

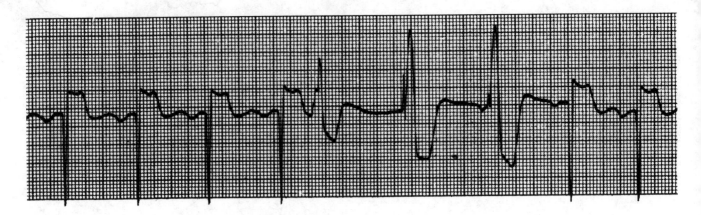

Figure 4-7                                                                 Test strip #7

## ECG TEST RHYTHM STRIP #7

31. The intrinsic atrial rate is

    a.   50
    b.   60
    c.   70
    d.   80
    e.   90

32. The intrinsic P-R interval is

    a.   0.12 seconds
    b.   0.16 seconds
    c.   0.21 seconds - 0.24 seconds
    d.   0.26 seconds - 0.28 seconds
    e.   0.30 seconds - 0.34 seconds

33. QRS complex #5 is

    a.   a PAC
    b.   a PVC
    c.   a fusion beat
    d.   a PAC with aberrancy
    e.   an artifact

34. QRS complexes #6 and #7 are

    a.   wide
    b.   immediately preceded by a pacemaker spike
    c.   are due to a mechanical ventricular pacemaker at a rate of 60 per minute
    d.   are not consistently preceded by P waves
    e.   all of the above

5. The correct interpretation of this strip is

    a.   junctional rhythm, PAC, ventricular demand (VVI) pacemaker
    b.   probable sinus rhythm, PVC, ventricular demand (VVI) pacemaker
    c.   probable sinus rhythm, I° AV block, PVC, ventricular demand (VVI) pacemaker
    d.   artrial flutter, PVC, ventricular demand (VVI) pacemaker
    e.   atrial fibrillation, PAC, ventricular demand (VVI) pacemaker